LITERACY AND DEAFNESS

Listening and Spoken Language

Second Edition

LITERACY AND DEAFNESS

Listening and Spoken Language

Second Edition

LYN ROBERTSON, PhD

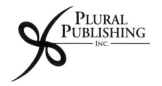

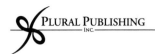

5521 Ruffin Road
San Diego, CA 92123

e-mail: info@pluralpublishing.com
Website: http://www.pluralpublishing.com

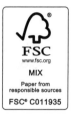

Typeset in 11/13 Garamond by Flanagan's Publishing Services, Inc.
Printed in the United States of America by McNaughton & Gunn, Inc.

Library of Congress Cataloging-in-Publication Data

Robertson, Lyn, author.
  Literacy and deafness : listening and spoken language / Lyn Robertson, author.
—Second edition.
      p. ; cm.
  Includes bibliographical references and index.
  ISBN-13: 978-1-59756-557-8 (alk. paper)
  ISBN-10: 1-59756-557-1 (alk. paper)
  I. Title.
  [DNLM: 1. Education of Hearing Disabled. 2. Adolescent. 3. Child.
4. Educational Status. 5. Hearing Aids. 6. Language. 7. Speech. HV 2430]
  HV2430
  371.91'246—dc23
                                        2013019939

CONTENTS

Preface   *xv*

Contributors   *xxi*

1 A History of Reading Achievement in People   1
with Hearing Loss

Before the development of technology that delivers
good, usable sound to people with hearing loss, literacy
achievement was reported to be at primary school
levels, but higher levels of achievement have been
reported in the last 40 years, particularly in children
with hearing loss who learn to listen. The progression
of studies in this area is presented and analyzed.

Introduction   1

A Review of Selected Studies   3

Higher Academic Achievement and Spoken Language   12

Conclusion   19

References   19

2 Literacy Theories   23

Literacy theories draw from theoretical work in
a variety of disciplines explained in this chapter:
behaviorism, linguistics, psycholinguistics, cognitive
psychology, sociolinguistics, literary criticism,
and critical theory. The ongoing debate between
approaching reading through phonics instruction
versus approaching reading through sight word
instruction is discussed by putting these word identifi-
cation processes together on one end of the spectrum of
approaches and meaning construction on the other.

Introduction   24

Theorizing About Reading   24

Definitions of Reading   25
Word Identification   27
Comprehension   29
An Interactive Theory   34
Many Disciplines Study Reading   35
Conclusion   40
References   40

3 Technology and Listening   43

Carol Flexer, PhD, LSLS CERT. AVT

The context for the use of amplification technology as a critical condition for literacy development for today's infants and children with hearing loss is detailed in this chapter. Topics discussed include the neurologic basis of listening and literacy; computer analogy for understanding technology; overview of amplification technologies; auditory feedback loop; distance hearing; and finally, a different way to look at the terms deaf and hard of hearing.

Introduction   43
Neurologic Basis of Listening and Literacy   44
Computer Analogy for Understanding Amplification   48
    Technology
Overview of Amplification Technologies—   49
    A New Context
Cochlear Implants   58
Auditory Feedback Loop   59
Distance Hearing and Incidental Learning   59
New Context for the Word "Deaf"   60
Conclusion   61
References   61

4 Spoken Language   67

Literacy theory links knowledge of the spoken language to be read with learning to read that language and explains why establishing listening and spoken language is a promising preparation for literacy.

Introduction   67
Learning the Sounds of a Spoken Language   68
Beyond the Sounds of Language   70
What About Bridging from American Sign Language?   71

Learning Spoken Language   73
Two Extended Studies of Children's Language   75
    Learning and Later Academic Achievement
"Advantaged" and "Disadvantaged" Parents   79
Conclusion   81
References   82

5 **Hearing, Listening, and Literacy**   **85**
Hearing is connected to listening, and listening
is connected to literacy. Reading and writing are
language acts and can be theorized as extensions of
listening and speaking.
Introduction   85
Phonological Awareness   87
Phonological Processing Capabilities   88
The Auditory-Verbal Approach   91
Principles of Listening and Spoken Language   93
    Specialist Auditory-Verbal Therapy
    (LSLS Cert. AVT)
Principles of Listening and Spoken Language   96
    Specialist Auditory-Verbal Education
    (LSLS Cert. AVEd)
Conclusion   98
References   99

6 **Issues in Child Development**   **101**
Gina Dow, PhD
Understanding the importance of early identification
and the developmental stages of childhood in children
with typical hearing is important for those who work
with and parent children with hearing loss and
provides needed background knowledge for thinking
about language and reading instruction.
Introduction   101
    Sensitivity in the Caregiving Relationship   104
Part I: Early Identification   106
    Attunement and Early Identification of   106
        Hearing Loss
    Early Identification and Intervention: How Early   106
        Is Early Enough?
    Early Identification in the United States   107

From Screening to Identification to Intervention   108
Concluding Remarks and Recommendations   112
Part II: Typical Development—Birth to Age Five   113
Cognitive Development and Play   113
Motor Development   114
Development of Self-Help Skills   115
Developmental Context   116
The Family Context as the Child's Immediate   116
    Environment
The Social and Economic Context   116
The Cultural Context   117
When Hearing Impairment Co-Occurs with   117
    Other Conditions
Useful Links on Developmental Milestones,   117
    Developmental Disabilities, and Hearing
    Impairment
References   119

7   Learning to Read   125

*Pedagogies employed in introducing children to
reading grow out of theories about hearing, listening,
and speaking.*

Introduction   126
Constructivism in Action   127
Shared Book Reading   129
Establishing a Rich Literacy Environment   136
Reading Comprehension and the Child   137
Practical Ideas for Helping Children Learn to Read   139
Conclusion   151
References   152

8   Reading Aloud With Children   155

*The interaction between the adult and child in
reading aloud is powerful in creating the foundation
for the child to learn to read. Reading aloud should
start early.*

Introduction   155
When Should Reading Aloud Begin?   156
How—and Why—Should Reading Aloud Begin?   157
Reading Aloud Is an *Indirect* Way of Teaching a   158
    Child How to Read

Reading Aloud Is Also a *Direct* Way of Teaching a Child How to Read — 158

How to Read Aloud with a Child with Hearing Loss — 161

An Extraordinary Example of Reading Aloud: The 1,000-Day Reading Streak — 166

Conclusion — 168

References — 168

9 Learning to Write — **171**

Pedagogies employed in introducing children to writing grow out of theories about hearing, listening, and speaking.

Introduction — 171

Writing and the Auditory-Verbal Approach — 173

A Word About Development — 178

Practical Ideas for Helping Children Learn to Write — 179

Conclusion — 185

References — 186

10 Creating and Using Language Experience Books — **189**

Language Experience Books are easy and satisfying to make. This chapter discusses creating books that fit each child.

Introduction — 189

Start and End with Listening — 190

A Spiral Progression through Using Language Experience Books — 190

Deciding on the Content for an LEB Entry — 193

An Example — 193

Conversations About Making and Using Language Experience Books — 193

General Comments from Teachers and Therapists About Using Language Experience Books — 196

Similarities and Differences Among Children With and Without Hearing Loss — 198

Using Background Knowledge — 201

Experiences of Teachers Who Have Been Trying Language Experience Books — 205

A Mother's Experience with Language Experience Books — 212

Conclusion   214
References   214

11 **Proceeding Through School**   **215**

*Much has been written about young children with
hearing loss and less about older students in upper
elementary, middle, high school, and college/
university. This chapter visits problems such students
experience, for example, the "fourth grade slump"
in which many students, with and without typical
hearing, plateau in reading. Other problems such
as access to spoken and written information, study
approaches, and school adjustment are discussed in
this chapter.*

Introduction   215
The "Fourth-Grade Slump"   216
Phonological Awareness, Vocabulary, and Reading   218
    Achievement
Academically Successful Young Adults with   227
    Hearing Loss
Conclusion   213
References   231

12 **Parents, Therapists, and Teachers Working**   **233**
Together

*The people in children's lives can come to under-
standings that facilitate learning for children in the
school environment.*

Introduction   233
Emotional Connectedness and a Team Approach   235
IDEA and IEPs   237
Using Mediation and Mediation Skills   238
Practical Ways for the Team to Communicate   244
Conclusion   246
References   246

13 **English Language Learners and Bilingualism**   **249**

*Many teachers and therapists are facing for the first
time the problems presented by children with hearing
loss whose families speak a language at home that*

is different from the language spoken at school.
Multilingual and multicultural theories and analyses
can be put to use in thinking about children who use
hearing technologies.

Introduction 249
Can Children with Hearing Loss Learn More Than 251
    One Spoken Language?
Learning to Read in the First Language First 254
Multilingual Mastery Is Possible 256
Hearing or Deaf, Language Learning Is Possible 258
Conclusion 259
References 259

14 **Music Learning and Spoken Language** **261**
Development
Listening to and making music are associated with
language and literacy development. Music lessons
enhance working memory, verbal memory, visio-
spatial processing, harmony, rhythm, melody, and
phonemic awareness.

Introduction 261
Issues Involved in Learning About Music 262
Music Learning in Children with Hearing Loss 264
Music Learning in Children with Typical Hearing 265
    and Its Association with Literacy
Music Lessons for Children with Hearing Loss 266
    Who Are Learning to Listen
The Work of Two Talented Therapists 268
The Suzuki Approach and Literacy 270
Conclusion 272
References 273

15 **Assessment Issues and Approaches** **275**
Theories of assessment are important in thinking
about children's progress in literacy.

Introduction 275
Norm-Referenced Standardized Tests 276
Criterion-Referenced Tests 278
The Relative Value of Norm-Referenced and 278
    Criterion-Referenced Tests

Practical Reading Assessments for Teachers to Use 279
Conclusion 286
References 286

16 Promising Literacy Practices 287

Emphasis on comprehension should be incorporated into a school's literacy practices for a child with hearing loss.

Introduction 287
Four General Suggestions 289
Before, During, and After Reading 294
Basic Elements of a Lesson Plan 294
Specific Steps for Meeting Literacy Goals 298
Reading and Writing as Thinking: The Basis of 302
    Good Programs in Reading
Conclusion 303
References 303

17 Educational Settings for Children with Hearing Loss 305

Ideally, the child with hearing loss should be placed in classes with children with typical hearing. Other placements can be suitable, as well.

Introduction 306
The Optimal Placement 306
What If the Optimum Is Not Possible? 308
Schooling Is Not the Only Source of Education 309
A Letter to a Mainstream Classroom Teacher 310
Conclusion 312

18 Parenting a Child with Hearing Loss 315

Parenting a child with hearing loss is a worthy challenge that can make your family strong and happy.

Introduction 315
Some Precepts to Consider 316
Conclusion 323
References 323

19 **Where Are They Now? Listening and Spoken**   **325**
Language Outcomes

*When working with and possibly worrying about
a child with hearing loss, it can be helpful to meet
or hear from a person who has mastered spoken
language and literacy. This chapter is comprised of the
stories of several young adults with hearing loss.*

Introduction   325
The Questions   326
The Respondents   327
Reference   335

20 **Thoughts From Two Founders of the**   **337**
Auditory-Verbal Approach

*Long before technology was developed that brought
clear sound to individuals with hearing loss, pioneers
such as Helen Beebe and Daniel Ling were developing
theory concerning the relationship between hearing,
listening, and spoken language and facilitating
listening and speaking in children with hearing loss,
even children with profound hearing losses.*

Introduction   337
Foreword, 1990, by Daniel Ling, PhD   338
An Auditory-Verbal Retrospective: A Personal   340
       Account of Individual Effort and
       International Organization, 1989, by
       Helen Hulick Beebe, CCC/SP
References   346

Appendix A. Knowledge Needed by Listening and Spoken   349
       Language Specialists
Appendix B. Listening and Spoken Language Specialist   357
       (LSLS) Domains Addressed in This Book
Appendix C. Description, Approaches, and Practice of   359
       Listening and Spoken Language Specialists

Index   363

PREFACE

I am pleased to have been asked to create a second edition of *Literacy and Deafness: Listening and Spoken Language*, and I am happy to report that prospects are multiplying rapidly for individuals with hearing loss. For those who choose a listening and spoken language approach, deafness in all its audiogrammatic forms can be treated in some way. Infants and toddlers discovered to be deaf or hard of hearing can be aided or implanted with state-of-the-art technology, and the people in these children's lives can learn to enrich and accentuate their access to sound and learn how to help them listen. These children can learn more than one spoken language and can learn to read, write, sing, and play musical instruments. Unless deafness is the desired outcome for a particular child, no child needs to remain in silence or even in partial sound. This book is about choosing listening and speaking as the most promising route to reading and writing, and I hope it serves to inform and persuade some to make the conscious choice of providing sound and spoken language to children with hearing loss. My intention is that this book be helpful to both parents and professionals.

Literacy and Deafness deals with the evidence of persistent low literacy levels in many individuals with hearing loss and with evidence of higher literacy levels in those with hearing loss who have learned to listen. I have attempted to pull together the dominant literacy research done in the "hearing world" and apply it to the situation of hearing loss. This rich research stretches back many years, and throughout this book I cite what have become classic works along with newer research.

Providing appropriate technology to a child with hearing loss and using it during every waking hour is an essential beginning on the way to literacy, but doing so is not sufficient to stimulate high levels of listening capacity. Education of the parent(s) and child is necessary, and much listening practice is required. The Alexander Graham Bell Academy for Listening and Spoken Language is working diligently to certify Listening and Spoken Language Specialists (LSLS) to work with parents and children in the clinic and in the classroom. The LSLS Cert. AVT (Auditory Verbal Therapist) "works one-on-one with children and families in all intervention sessions," and the LSLS Cert. AVEd (Auditory Verbal Educator) "involves the family and works directly with children in individual, group or classroom settings." A complete description of these certification categories can be found at The Alexander Graham Bell Listening and Spoken Language Knowledge Center (http://www.agbell.org/AcademyDocument.aspx?id=541).

The LSLS Cert. AVT and the LSLS Cert. AVEd must master the same foundational knowledge, complete the Certification Route, and pass the qualifying examination; the certifications differ according to the setting in which the LSLS will practice. In particular, I hope that this book will help individuals in their preparation for Domain 9, Emerging Reading, of the qualifying examination for LSLS certification.

The Plan of the Book

Before the development of technology that delivers good, usable sound to people with hearing loss, literacy achievement was routinely reported to be at primary school levels, but higher levels of achievement have been reported in the last 40 years, particularly in children with hearing loss who learn to listen. Chapter 1 presents and comments upon the progression of studies in this area. Chapter 2 describes literacy theories and how they draw from theoretical work in behaviorism, linguistics, psycholinguistics, cognitive psychology, sociolinguistics, literary criticism, and critical theory. It discusses the debate between approaching reading through phonics instruction versus approaching reading through sight word instruction by putting these word identification processes together on one end of the spectrum of approaches and meaning construction on the other end. Chapter 3, written by audiologist Carol Flexer, addresses the necessity of hearing technology that delivers sound to the brain and puts into context the use of amplification technology as a critical condition for literacy development for today's infants and children with hearing loss. Dr. Flexer discusses the neurologic basis of listening and literacy, a computer analogy for understanding technology, amplification technologies, the auditory feedback loop, distance hearing, and a different way to look at the terms "deaf" and "hard of hearing." Chapter 4 explores how literacy theory links knowledge of the spoken language to be read with learning to read that language and explains why establishing sign language as the first language and then beginning spoken language instruction through the introduction of print is a less promising approach than establishing a spoken language as preparation for literacy. Chapter 5 discusses how hearing connects to listening and listening to literacy. It explains reading and writing as language acts that can be theorized as extensions of listening and speaking. Chapter 6 is contributed by Dr. Gina Dow, a researcher in child development. Having an understanding of early identification of hearing loss and the developmental stages of childhood in children with typical hearing is important for parents and for those who work with parents of children with hearing loss, and this chapter provides background knowledge needed for thinking about the introduction of language and reading. Chapters 7, 8, 9, and 10explore pedagogies employed in introducing children to reading and writing that grow out of theories about hearing, listening, and speaking. Chapter 8 is new and explains why reading aloud with children is foundational to language learning and literacy development. Chapter 10 is new, as well, and provides practical direction for creating Language Experience Books and experiences with such books related by practicing therapists and teachers.

Much has been written about young children with hearing loss and less about older students in upper elementary, middle, high school, and college/university. Chapter 11 visits the problems such students experience, for example, the "fourth grade slump" in which many students, with and without typical hearing, plateau in reading achievement. Other problems such as access to spoken and written information, study approaches, and school adjustment are also discussed in this chapter. Chapter 12 demonstrates how the people in children's lives can come to understandings that facilitate learning for children in the school environment.

Many teachers and therapists are facing for the first time the problems presented by children with hearing loss whose families speak a language at home that is different from the language spoken at school, and Chapter 13 deals with the application of multilingual and multicultural theories and analyses with children who use hearing technologies. Chapter 14 is another new chapter; it expands upon a brief section in the first edition of *Literacy and Deafness* and makes the argument that if learning music helps children with typical hearing learn to read and write, the same can happen with children who are learning to listen. Chapter 15 describes theories of assessment and their importance in thinking about children's progress in literacy. Chapter 16 answers the question of what to look for in a reading program in terms of promising literacy practices for children with hearing and argues for putting emphasis on reading comprehension. Chapter 17 takes the position that, ideally, the child with hearing loss should be placed in classes with children with typical hearing, noting that other placements can be suitable, depending upon the situation. Chapters 18 and 19 are new; in Chapter 18, I express some of my thoughts about parenting a child with hearing loss, and Chapter 19 is comprised of reflections by young successful professionals on their lives and hearing loss. Long before technology was developed that brought clear sound to individuals with hearing loss, pioneers such as Helen Beebe and Daniel Ling were developing theory concerning the relationship between hearing, listening, and spoken language and facilitating listening and speaking in children with hearing loss, even children with profound hearing losses. Chapter 20 ends the book with two pieces by Daniel Ling and Helen Beebe written nearly 30 years ago that remain vitally relevant to us today.

A Few Words About Language

In thinking about a new world of accessibility to sound and hearing, we must think about the labels we use. Is a person "deaf" who cannot hear without the cochlear implant in place, but who can hear well with it on? Is a person "hard of hearing" who hears little inside the speech range without a hearing aid, but hears nearly all of it with the hearing aid functioning well? These questions may be a matter of semantics, but I think they also signal the possibility of some categorical changes in the way we think about the phenomenon of hearing loss. Where we used to resign ourselves to a generally diminished use of spoken language and concomitant lesser academic achievement among people with hearing loss, we can now expect language, literacy, and learning achievement commensurate with that of their hearing peers. And so, our language must change. A person can be physical "deaf," but function as a hearing person with the support of technology.

Throughout this book, I refer to the person or people I am writing about first, realizing that at times doing so results in a kind of wordiness that takes up more space than I might like. Instead of referring to a child as a "deaf child," I refer to the child as a "child with hearing loss," or a "child who is deaf or hard of hearing." This distinction on paper may seem slight, but the distinction in thinking about the child first as a person and second as an individual who has something different about his or her hearing is a tribute to personhood. The same goes for language that includes both male and female. Instead of allowing pronouns such as "he" and "him" to stand for all people, I endeavor to use language throughout that is inclusive of boys and girls, men and women.

When I refer to parents, I also mean siblings, grandparents, aunts, uncles, neighbors, and caregivers, as all the people in a child's life need to contribute to helping the child learn to listen. All who *interact* with the child using spoken language contribute to the child's learning of that language, and everyone in the child's life can collaborate about this.

In this book, I make the argument that helping a child learn to listen provides the best possibility that he or she will learn to read and write. I come at this from both a research-based and a personal point of view, as I am an academic as well as the parent of a now adult daughter in whom a severe-to-profound hearing loss was diagnosed at age 15 months.

With all this in mind, it is my hope that you will find this book to be a celebration of literacy, deafness, and personhood!

Lyn Robertson
Department of Education
Denison University
Granville, Ohio

CONTRIBUTORS

Gina Annunziato Dow, PhD
Associate Professor
Department of Psychology
Denison University
Granville, Ohio
Chapter 6

Carol Flexer, PhD, CCC-A, LSLS Cert. AVT
Distinguished Professor Emerita
The University of Akron and
Northeast Ohio Au.D. Consortium (NOAC)
Akron, Ohio
Chapter 3

Chapter 1

A HISTORY OF READING ACHIEVEMENT IN PEOPLE WITH HEARING LOSS

There is no frigate like a book
To take us lands away,
Nor any coursers like a page
Of prancing poetry.

This traverse may the poorest take
Without oppress of toll; How frugal is the chariot
That bears a human soul!

Emily Dickinson (American poet, 1830–1886)

Introduction

The desirability of knowing how to read is taken for granted by most people. We can look back in history and find cogent references to the hope and faith that people attach to this ability. Thomas

1

Jefferson, for example, put great stock in education for all, reasoning that an educated, literate citizenry would be the preservation of democracy: "Where the press is free and every man able to read, all is safe" (Jefferson, as cited in Lee, 1961, p. 81). In his view, " . . . were it left to me to decide whether we should have a government without newspapers, or newspapers without a government, I should not hesitate a moment to prefer the latter. But I should mean that every man should receive those papers and be capable of reading them" (Jefferson, as cited in Lee, 1961, p. 102).

Reading opens worlds to us that are not available first hand, keeps knowledge and experience safely recorded for perusal at any time, and allows us to communicate with each other over time and space. Literacy enriches us personally by putting us in contact with wisdom and with beauty. On a practical level, literacy equips us to take on responsible jobs and to support ourselves and others. Indeed, adults who read at low levels are likely to live in poverty and suffer frequent unemployment. A study commissioned by Congress and published by the National Institute for Literacy (1998) presents the sobering estimate that 21 to 23%, or 40 to 44 million Americans over 16 read at the lowest level, Level 1. Some readers at Level 1 are able to do some tasks involving simple reading, but all have difficulty with reading tasks needed in daily living, such as finding more than one item of information in an article or table and filling out applications (p. 4). A report from the National Assessment of Adult Literacy (2003) finds 14%, or 30 million Americans at the below-basic level in prose reading, and 29%, or 63 million Americans at the basic level in prose reading. The NAAL reports for 1992 and 2003 differ from each other only slightly. The below-basic level represents employing no more than the most simple and concrete literacy skills; at the basic level, a person can perform only simple and everyday literacy activities. It is difficult to define and measure a population's literacy levels, so such reports yield only broad descriptions of our national situation. The attainment of literacy brings with it all manner of opportunities and pleasures, whereas the neglect of it leaves people in dependence on others for their communication needs. The illiterate or merely functional reader is closed out of much that life offers in our present complex society, and low literacy levels are associated with unemployment and poverty.

In the past, as you will read in this chapter, people who were deaf or hard of hearing did not learn to read as well as people with typical hearing, and this resulted in their not being expected to learn to read. Lower reading achievement followed low expectations and even produced judgments of diminished intelligence. Fortunately, intelligence is now defined differently by psychologists than in the past, but, despite that progress in our thinking, low expectations for literacy development in people with hearing loss continue in many settings today; they just are not linked as closely to conclusions about an individual's intelligence.

In the thinking of psychologists, researchers, and teachers who deal mainly with learners with typical hearing, it is abundantly clear that knowledge of the spoken language to be read is a major prerequisite of learning to read that language (see, for example, such classic work as Adams, 1994; Ruddell & Ruddell, 1994; Scarborough, 2002; and Snow, Burns, & Griffin, 1998). Many people who are deaf or hard of hearing do not learn a spoken language, and, consequently, learning to read presents a real challenge for them. For this reason, reading and learning to read are bound up in the controversy over signing versus speaking. Researchers on both sides of this divide seek just the right approach to teaching reading (see, for example, Robertson, 2000; and Stewart & Clarke, 2002), each subscribing to different underlying theory. One side says "learn to speak and use that language to learn to read," and the other says, "learn to read and use that skill to learn the spoken language." My understanding is that the spoken language route to literacy is the one best supported by the body of research we have available.

In the following section, I describe studies of learning and literacy achievement in children with hearing loss with publication dates as early as 1916. Some of these deal with language learning, but, as you will see, connecting literacy to the learning of spoken language has been a more recent development. This series of studies is as exhaustive as my sources have allowed, and I acknowledge there may be other pertinent studies I have not discovered. As you read, you will find the studies are not cohesive, yet they are interesting in light of some common threads of thought they display.

A Review of Selected Studies

One of the earliest studies of the academic ability of children who were deaf was conducted by Pintner and Paterson (1916). Their focus was not reading, but Digit-Symbol and Symbol-Digit testing, which they regarded as a measure of learning ability. In their study, these tests were administered without the use of spoken language or written instruction, and Pintner and Paterson assumed that knowledge of language was not involved in responding to the test items. How to do the test was demonstrated repeatedly for the children until the researchers were satisfied that most of the children understood what to do. Although Pintner and Paterson did not describe the tests they used in great detail, they may have been similar to the WAIS-III Digit Symbol-Coding subtest, whose scores are associated mainly with speed of processing, but also with memory (Joy, Kaplan, & Fein, 2004). In all, the study involved 1624 students, ages 8 to 26, in three large schools for the deaf. Pintner and Paterson considered their work to be investigating "native ability," and concluded that "the deaf child is about three years behind the hearing child in learning ability, as tested by the rapidity and accuracy of forming associations between numbers and forms" (p. 22). They found that children who lost their hearing post-lingually did slightly better on the tests than children who were born deaf, but the number of such children in their study was very small, and the authors did not make much of this finding; in fact, in their conclusion, they reported "the congenitally deaf and the adventitiously deaf are equal in learning ability" (p. 22). Pintner and Paterson's work is pertinent to us today for at least two reasons. First, this study posited the value of learning a spoken language: "It is the learning of language that forms the greatest obstacle in the education of the deaf child" (Pinter & Paterson, 1916, p. 1). Second, and, unfortunately, they gave scientific credibility to holding low expectations for the academic achievement of children who are deaf or hard of hearing, for they were working during a time when great faith was being placed in the new, but now discredited, idea that intelligence could be measured and children's education should be fitted to their "native ability." The desire to label children innately "bright," "normal," "backward," and "dull" (Pinter & Paterson, 1916, p. 12), and then to tailor their education accordingly, although not confined to the authors of this study, has done a disservice to both children with hearing loss and those with typical hearing. (You may wish to consult Gould 1981 for a comprehensive discussion of how the concept of intelligence and intelligence testing itself came to be misused in education in the United States.)

Pintner and Paterson must have been busy, for they published another study in 1916. In this one, they wrote, "*As is natural* [author's italics], the comparison with hearing children shows a retardation in every class" (p. 421), underlining indelibly the low expectations held for children with deafness. As in their previous article, these researchers reported data from digit-symbol and symbol-digit tests and a number of other non-language tests, and termed this category "intelligence," assuming that no language was involved in performing the digit/symbol tests. In this study, they also looked at language ability, using tests of following directions and a commonly employed language scale. These authors understood intelligence to be separate from language and, this time, wrote generously, "The uneducated deaf child may have no language, but still possess considerable general intelligence" (p. 428). On a test involving printed directions, the scores of children with deafness showed wide disparity compared to children with typical hearing, whereas the scores of children who were hard of hearing were much higher, sometimes as high or almost as high as those of children with typical hearing. On the Trabue Language Scale, a sentence completion task, none of the children with deafness scored above 4th grade level.

Pintner (1918) used the Trabue Scales again, this time with 1,098 children in four schools for the deaf, and found, "Third-grade hearing children are able to accomplish as much on these language tests as the highest grades in these schools for the deaf" (p. 757). He concluded that language acquisition was "strikingly" more difficult for children with deafness than for children with hearing (p. 763). Pintner's work is found throughout the mid-to-late teens and the 1920s and seems to have set the scene for low expectations for literacy achievement among children with deafness.

A report by Grover Farquhar (1928) details the responses of 41 boys and girls with hearing loss whose average age was 16 to a test involving paragraphs, sentences, and words. As in the studies discussed above, the results are difficult to describe as they are expressed in raw data. Farquhar concluded that students with deafness displayed three "faults": "carelessness in following directions," "a deficient vocabulary range," and "inability to perceive accurately the antecedents of personal and relative pronouns" (pp. 271–272). He resolved, "There must be constant practice and eternal vigilance in detecting opportunities for error, of which in every way our

English language abounds" (p. 272) and asserted "it should be our aim to achieve for the deaf an approximation to the attainments of the normal child" (p. 264), although he did not offer explicit guidance for doing so.

In a speech to the 26th Meeting of the Convention of American Instructors of the Deaf in 1929, Percival Hall, president of Gallaudet College, described the results of testing of the college's most recent freshman and preparatory classes. This involved 62 students whose average hearing was expressed as "18% to 19%," which seems to have meant a severe-to-profound hearing loss. These students were given the New Stanford Achievement Tests designed for "common school hearing boys and girls, particularly those in grades 4 to 9" (p. 390). The lowest scores for both groups were in paragraph meaning, and they were "far down the scale in public school grade" (p. 393). Hall concluded that schools for the deaf should work harder to prepare their students for college.

Skipping the 1930s, as no studies of reading achievement during that time emerged in my search, we move to the 1940s where we find another study of reading achievement termed, instead, "intelligence" (Morrison, 1940). It is important to reiterate that we now distinguish between achievement and potential for achievement, but in these studies, achievement was equated with intelligence. Using the Ontario School Ability Examination, which is not described in the report, Morrison concluded, " . . . the percentage of deaf children belonging to the normal or superior groups is lower than it is for hearing children. It follows from this that the percentage of children in the dull, borderline, and feeble-minded groups is large" (p. 188).

In 1941, a short piece in the *American Annals of the Deaf* applauded the increasing use of standardized testing with individuals with hearing loss: "It is a great satisfaction to know that research activity in the education of the deaf is gaining momentum" (Elliott, 1941, p. 242). In this piece, Elliott listed chronologically 82 studies published from 1912 to 1941, about seven of which appear to use standard tests of reading. It can be surmised that not much was expected in terms of reading achievement for children with deafness, as this lengthy list of tests spanning a 30-year period includes many tests of nonverbal intelligence, language ability, personal interest, personality, social maturity and adjustment, and artistic ability, but only these seven attempted to deal with reading achievement.

One of the studies listed by Elliott is a study published in 1941 by Richard Brill. As did Pintner and Paterson, Brill began with the premise that learning spoken language is "the most important function of a school devoted to teaching the deaf" (p. 227). Brill's purpose was to discover a way of predicting which children would learn to read and which would not. This study correlates scores on the Keys and Pedersen Visual Language Test with scores taken five years later on the same students, using the reading batteries of the Stanford Achievement Test. Brill concluded that the instruments test the same processes, thus establishing a link between a test formulated for children with hearing loss and a test developed for children with typical hearing. Brill's analysis of the correlations led him to assert that children with hearing loss of around "40%" before the age of six fare no better in language learning and reading than children whose hearing loss is greater. Ultimately, Brill set scores of 80 and below on the Visual Language Test as indicating that the child had "practically no chance of successfully learning language or reading in the next five years" (p. 238). Of importance in this study is the connecting of learning the spoken language to learning to read, yet Brill also fell into the trap of concluding that innate intelligence may be more important than the degree of hearing in learning language, particularly when instruction involves more advanced stages of language acquisition (p. 239).

Jean Walter (1955) conducted a study of the sentence construction of children ages 6 to 10 with profound deafness, using pictures that could be described using only 41 words, not wanting vocabulary limitations to overshadow children's ability to express themselves in sentences (pp. 238–239). Of particular interest to Walter was the children's ability to use parts of speech appropriately, and she catalogued the children's achievement according to five stages that emerged in the children's written responses to pictorial prompts. The progression of stages reported extends from the absence of verbs to the use of simple sentences to the use of compound sentences. Her report of 102 cases cites 6 children using "at least one correct compound sentence with a conjunction," 26 "attempting to use compound sentences with conjunctions and using at least one correct simple sentence," 33 "either attempting to use compound sentences with conjunctions or using at least one correct simple sentence, 25 "neither attempting to use compound sentences with conjunctions nor using correct sentences," 7 " not attempting to use sentences with verbs," and 5 displaying "no written language" (p. 243). Approximately 63% of the children tested wrote at least one correct simple sentence using a small corpus of words; the remaining 37% did not write a simple sentence, did not use verbs, or did not produce written language. The contribution of the study was the establishment of a predictable set of stages through which the writing of a child with profound deafness would be expected to progress.

Wrightstone, Aronow, and Moskowitz (1963) conducted a study designed to formulate norms for use in comparing children with hearing loss with each other, rather than with children with typical hearing. They used the scores of 5,307 children in 73 schools for the deaf in the United States and Canada on a reading subtest of the Metropolitan Achievement Tests, Elementary Level. In a very straightforward response to this study, Furth argued that the achievement of children with deafness should be compared to the achievement of children with typical hearing and presented data that showed that of 5,224 students with deafness, aged 10.5 to 16.5 years, the highest mean grade equivalent was 3.5, with only 12% of the oldest students scoring at 4.9 grade level or better (1966, p. 461). Furth observed that tests below grade 4 "sample only fragmentary aspects of language and present a purposely simplified language which is not used in natural life" (pp. 461–462) and surmised that guessing could have contributed to the scores obtained. He reasoned forcefully that such low scores could not be associated with lack of intelligence, as so many students were tested, and the researchers had been careful to eliminate children who were thought to be less intelligent. He asserted, "The low reading level of the deaf does not constitute a reading deficiency but linguistic incompetence," and concluded refreshingly, "The better this fact is realized the sooner we shall be able to face the problem and its full implications" (p. 462).

In a study that involved only children with hearing loss, Vernon and Koh (1970) compared the achievement of 79 children in a manual group with 190 in an oral group. The manual group was comprised of children with hearing loss whose parents were deaf and with whom signing and finger spelling had been used from the time they were infants. The oral group's parents had typical hearing, and these parents did not use sign language. On two subtests of the Stanford Achievement Test (paragraph meaning and word meaning), and on reading average and general average, the students in the manual group scored higher than the children in the oral group, although neither group came close to the norms for children with typical hearing. The education levels of the parents were included in the study. The oral parents with typical hearing had far more education than the manual parents who were deaf: 30% of the oral group's parents had attended college, 33% had attended high school and 38% had completed 8th grade or below. In the manual group, 88% of the parents had only 8th grade or below. On the basis of the performance of the manual group, the researchers concluded:

> Thus, although the hearing parents of the oral group had much more to give their children educationally, their oral communication limitations apparently prevented their doing it. By contrast, the deaf parents who had far less to offer educationally had a communication method that enabled them to exchange information with their children. Consequently their children obtained much more, especially in the development of basic language competence. (p. 532)

This study is commonly cited by those who argue for the use of signing with children with hearing loss by adults who know the particular sign language in its mature form, but without pointing out that both the signing group and the oral group in this study fell far short of the academic achievement of children with typical hearing.

Conrad (1979) reported on 468 students, ages 15 to 16, as they left school in England and Wales. Only five were reading at levels appropriate for their ages; the group achieved an average appropriate for a nine-year-old (as interpreted in Power & Leigh, 2000), which translates approximately to a fourth grade reading level.

In a chapter in *Deaf Children in America*, Allen (1986) reported on two large norming projects, answering questions regarding average reading achievement levels of 36,868 children (ages 8–18) with hearing loss (92.8% prelingual), achievement trends from 1974 to 1983, and how to account for the measured achievement levels. Using scaled scores on the Reading Comprehension portion of the Stanford Achievement Test (6th and 7th editions), Allen reported slightly better achievement for the 1983 norming group compared to the 1974 group, with both "'leveling off' in their reading comprehension achievement at about the third grade level" (p. 164) by age 18. Scores for children in local schools where they were getting special services were better than for children in special schools (p. 197), and scores were better for children with more hearing than those with severe and profound losses (p. 201). Allen's discussion ends with the caveat that the norming samples represent children who persist in special education, so those children with hearing loss who achieved higher scores may have moved out of special education and thus not been included in this sample. Allen concludes in a hopeful manner: " . . . it should not be concluded of any young hearing impaired student that he or she will never achieve beyond a certain level" (p. 205).

Holt (1993) reported on the norming sample scores for "various groups of deaf and hard of hearing students" on the 8th Edition of the Stanford Achievement Test Reading Comprehension subtest (p. 172). The sample was composed of students ages 8 to 20 reported as not having "mental retardation" who were in special education programs across the United States. The 17-year-olds in the group had the highest average score, 619, which was judged to equal a grade equivalent of 4.5. The highest scores were achieved by students integrated into local schools. Students in special schools and students in local schools with no integration with children with typical hearing scored significantly lower. Establishing a familiar and predictable hierarchy, students with less-than-severe hearing losses generally scored higher than students with severe losses, and those with severe losses in general scored better than those with profound losses. Students with "additional educationally relevant handicaps" scored less well than those without them (p. 175).

In 2000, Traxler discussed results of the Gallaudet Research Institute's norming of the 9th edition of the Stanford Achievement Test, again using a national sample of students with deafness and hardness-of-hearing:

> The median Reading Comprehension scores, by age, for the entire group of deaf and hard-of-hearing students in the norming sample fall largely in the Level 4: Below Basic area. Many of these students are indeed placed below grade level in school, when compared to hearing students of the same age. The 80th percentile line, which lies just below the border between Level 1 and Level 2, shows that many of the top fifth

of the deaf and hard-of-hearing students in the national norming sample (whose scores lie above the 80th percentile) were
likely functioning at about the Level 2: Basic level or higher.
(pp. 342–343)

In 2008, the Gallaudet Research Institute continued to have on its
website a report of this norming sample: "For the 17-year-olds and
the 18-year-olds in the deaf and hard of hearing student norming
sample, the median Reading Comprehension subtest score corresponds to about a 4.0 grade level for hearing students" (Gallaudet Research Institute, 2008), but this information has now been
removed due to concerns about the accuracy of the data reported
(Gallaudet Research Institute, 2011).

Pausing to Think About These Studies

Throughout these studies, the degree of hearing loss has been used
as a variable, with recognition given to the fact that children with
more hearing usually achieve higher levels of reading than children
with more severe hearing losses. Learning the spoken language
to be read has also been given some attention in these studies,
but the underlying assumption was, and has continued for some
to be, that most of the children would naturally use little spoken
language. Curiously, this state of affairs has been remarked upon
and accepted, abandoning children with hearing loss to the low
expectations thus created in their parents and teachers, as well as
in society at large.

And yet, in thinking about these studies that began nearly
100 years ago, it is apparent that progress in reading has been
made. The children in the earliest studies seem to have had little
language of any sort, visual or audible (signing or spoken), and,
consequently and unfairly, they were regarded as having very low
intelligence. In the intervening years, increased use and popularity
of sign language(s) have contributed to bringing average reading
achievement scores to about the fourth grade level. Still, two important questions arise:

1. Why does development plateau at that point for so many
   individuals?

2. Is a fourth grade reading level enough to equip children for all the challenges, adventures, and satisfactions of life as adults in the 21st century?

Higher Academic Achievement and Spoken Language

In the 1970s, articles dealing with children with hearing loss who were developing spoken language began to appear. A 1974 article by Lane and Baker reports higher reading achievement scores among children with hearing loss. They announced, "Better reading achievement for deaf children is possible" (p. 489). Their study, conducted at the Central Institute for the Deaf, begins with a catalogue of the low literacy achievement expectations held for children with hearing loss. Subjects in this study were 132 students, ages 10 to 16 years, 92 of whom had graduated from CID at eighth grade. The length of time spent at CID averaged 10.1 years for the group overall and 10.4 years for the graduates of CID in the group. Ninety percent of the subjects had profound deafness, and the hearing losses of the remaining 10% were in the severe range. Five consecutive years of grade-level scores for each subject on the Sentence and Word Meaning and Paragraph Meaning subtests of the American School Achievement Series were studied, yielding a comparison between the students with deafness and students with typical hearing. Over a four-year period, the average scores of the group as a whole increased 2.5 grade levels to 5th grade, 8 months, and the average scores of the 92 graduates increased 2.7 grade levels to 6th grade, 2 months. Although the rate of growth was slower than that expected statistically for children with typical hearing, this study demonstrated the possibility of a sustained rate of growth compared to the Wrightstone, Aronow, and Moskowitz (1963) study that reported very little growth between the ages of 10 years, 6 months and 16 years, 6 months. More significantly, children with deafness had been found who were reading at 5th and 6th grade levels. These children were "taught language through oral-aural channels and learned to communicate verbally" (pp. 497–498). The authors recommended putting children into classes with children with typical hearing when they are able to communicate well using spoken language.

Reich, Hambleton, and Houldin (1977) did a study of 195 children with hearing loss across three types of educational placement: fully integrated, itinerant help, and hard of hearing classes, in the case of the elementary students, and fully integrated, itinerant help, and partial integration, in the case of the secondary students. They found that students in fully integrated classes, both in elementary and secondary school, were scoring very near their peers with typical hearing on the Language Usage and Structure and the Reading Comprehension portions of the California Achievement Tests. At the elementary level, the 63 students had an average reading level about half a year ahead of their peers with typical hearing and an average language level a few months ahead. The secondary students scored close to grade level, with an average of one month below their peers with typical hearing. This study cautioned that children with hearing loss needed much special assistance at school and a good deal of support from parents in order to be successful in an integrated setting (p. 542).

Doehring, Bonnycastle, and Ling (1978) studied the relationship between rapid reading skills and language and naming skills in children in Montreal, ages 6 to 13 years, 11 with severe hearing loss and 10 with profound loss, who were integrated into regular classrooms where English was spoken. The children were given the Slosson Oral Reading Test; tests of oral reading, comprehension, spelling, and visual scanning; the receptive and expressive portions of the Northwestern Syntax Screening Test; and the Peabody Picture Vocabulary Test. Doehring, Bonnycastle, and Ling reported:

> The profoundly hearing-impaired children were at or above normal grade level as a group on all of the 11 reading-related tests, except oral syllable reading and sentence comprehension. Their oral word reading on the standardized Slosson Test was excellent, being more than one year above normal. Their oral words and sentence reading was also above normal, and oral letter reading was normal. The group median was one year below normal in oral syllable reading and sentence comprehension, the four oldest children being particularly deficient in this regard. (p. 404)

The children with severe losses did not perform as well as those with profound losses, and the researchers attributed that outcome to their not having been identified as early and not having had training using auditory-oral methods before age three (p. 405).

Moog and Geers (1985) reported on an experimental oral program, EPIC (Experimental Project in Instructional Concentration), spanning three years and involving 15 students with prelingual hearing loss, hearing loss greater than 85 dB, average to above-average nonverbal intelligence, expressive language at or above the 45th percentile, reading skills no more than one year behind children with typical hearing, and ages between 6;1 to 8;11 at the project's beginning. The children received instruction in language, speech production and perception, reading, and math, with science and social studies added for the older students. Eighteen children from two other programs were in a control group. At the beginning, the experimental and control groups differed on only 2 of 13 measures. The intent of the project was to create the most favorable learning conditions possible for the experimental group, and so the following were employed: homogenous grouping according to subject matter achievement, flexible groupings ranging from six or seven children to one-to-one arrangements, mastery learning, and allocation of time according to students' needs. By the third year, the experimental group outperformed the control group on 10 of 13 measures, with the children who were then ages 9 to 11 scoring in paragraph meaning at an average 4th grade level (p. 267) and gaining with consistency 0.73 grade levels each year.

A few years later, Geers and Moog (1989) reported academic achievement scores of 100 students, ages 16 and 17, from 26 states and 3 Canadian provinces who were orally educated. Their pure tone audiograms ranged in better-ear averages from 85 to 128 dB. The students were brought in smaller groups to four Reading Research Camps at Central Institute for the Deaf (CID) in St. Louis, Missouri, where they were given 14 different reading, writing, and speaking tests. On the California Achievement Test, using norms for students with typical hearing, the average grade level for vocabulary was 7.6, with a range of 3.0 to 12.9, the maximum score. On the Stanford Achievement Test, the average comprehension score was 8th grade, with a range from 2.3 to 12.9, again the maximum score. Thirty percent achieved grade level scores (10th grade), and 50% scored at or above 7th grade level. Using norms for students with hearing impairment, 98% of the scores were above the 50th percentile, and 56% were above the 90th percentile (pp. 75–76). The authors concluded that children with hearing impairment who have "at least average nonverbal intellectual ability, early oral education management and auditory stimulation, and middle-class family environment with strong family support" have potential for greater literacy achievement than had up until then been reported for children with hearing loss, and they end their article with:

> The primary factors associated with the development of literacy in this orally educated sample are good use of residual hearing, early amplification and educational management, and —above all—oral English language ability, including vocabulary, syntax, and discourse skills. (p. 84)

About the same time, Carol Flexer and I were doing an exploratory study of parents' responses to a survey concerning their children's literacy development (Robertson & Flexer, 1993). In this work, the target population was children with whom the auditory-verbal approach had been used, and we found good achievement in these children with hearing loss in comparison to children with typical hearing. Families were contacted through their auditory-verbal therapists, and the study describes the contents of 54 usable surveys returned from all regions of the United States and Toronto, Canada, and 29 from Germany and Switzerland. Eighty-one percent of the children described had a severe-to-profound or profound hearing loss; the children were between the ages of 6 and 19; half were male and half female. Parents were queried about their children's hearing loss and history, school(s), extracurricular activity, the quality of contact they had with children with typical hearing, whether they read to their children, and whether their children liked to read. Eighty-one percent (44) of the children were mainstreamed totally in their school placements. Ninety-four percent (51) of the parents reported having read daily to their children as infants and preschoolers, 93% (50) described their children as reading beyond schoolwork every week, and 86% (46) reported their children read as well or better than the average hearing child. All but one child was described as being involved in extracurricular activities with hearing peers and having regular contact with hearing peers, and 76% (41) were described as liking to read. Parents were also asked to submit scores of standardized reading tests their children had been administered at school, and 37 of the United States and Canadian parents did so; none of the German and Swiss parents could send test scores, as standardized tests were not in wide use in their countries, and their children had not been tested in this way. Thirty of the 37 children for whom test results were received had scored at the 50th percentile or higher on reading tests normed on children with typical hearing, for example, the Gates-McGinitie, the Stanford Achievement Test, and the Iowa Tests. We did not claim to generalize from these children to a larger population, but did think we were contributing to an understanding of the relationship between learning spoken language and learning to read, simply by finding some children with hearing loss who were comparable in their achievement to children with typical hearing.

Also in 1993, Goldberg and Flexer reported on a survey in which they had attempted to locate as many graduates of auditory-verbal programs as possible. Criteria for participation included being age 18 or older and having been in an auditory-verbal program for at least three years. Of the 366 surveys sent out through auditory-verbal therapists to distribute to their graduates, 157 that could be used were returned, yielding a 42.9% response rate. Among the 157, 93% described their hearing losses as being in the severe-to-profound range, and over 95% reported their losses as prelingual, defined as occurring at age three or younger. Most had been mainstreamed in school (78.5% in elementary, 86.7% in middle, and 86.2% in high school), and 152 had graduated from high school. More than 95% (139) had continued with postsecondary education, with 124 of those in colleges or universities whose students mainly have typical hearing. Fifteen (12.1%) were students at National Technical Institute for the Deaf or Gallaudet University (Goldberg, & Flexer, 1993). Although this study did not deal directly with literacy, higher literacy levels are implied by the graduates' academic attainment by participating in higher education at mainstream institutions alongside students with typical hearing.

In the same year, Daniel Ling (1993) reflected on his auditory-verbal work in the 1950s with 6- to 12-year-old children in Reading, England, and reported his finding that academic progress was entirely possible. In his words:

> Standardized tests of reading, math, and spelling confirmed that most of the children were rapidly closing the educational gap between themselves and their normally hearing peers. After a few years, most, with continuing support from a visiting specialist teacher, successfully followed academic subjects alongside hearing children of the same age. Friendships with such children, formed in the classes they shared and during

play breaks, led to extensive social relationships and confor-
mity with behaviors observed among children at large. The
children's speech and language skills increased rapidly to meet
the standards of communication required to function effectively at home and in school. (p. 190)

Roberts and Rickard (1994) also reported a survey study, this
one done in Australia. Theirs involved 100 7- to 17-year-olds who
had completed an auditory/oral preschool program. Seventy-one of
the children had severe or profound hearing loss. Fifty-five attended
school in integrated (mainstreamed) settings, 37 attended in unit
(pull-out) settings, and 8 attended in segregated settings. Eighty-
three percent of the children "perceived their overall academic
progress to be 'average' or 'above average' as compared to their
class peers" (p. 207), a self-perception that the authors conceded
could have been better than it was in reality (p. 219). Nearly two-
thirds reported their peer group was composed of children with
typical hearing, construed by the authors to mean the children were
comfortable in their oral communication skills (p. 221).

Wray, Flexer, and Vaccaro (1997) studied 19 children who had
completed an auditory-verbal intervention program whose main
goal was to ready children for mainstream education. At the time
of the study, the children were age 5 years, 5 months to 15 years,
2 months; 14 of the children had severe or severe-to-profound
hearing loss, and 5 had moderate and moderately severe loss. All
had attended preschool with children with typical hearing and then
continued full time in the mainstream, receiving support services as
necessary. The teachers of these students were surveyed on a variety of educational matters. Findings included evidence that communication improved over time, as the older children were judged
stronger in this area than the younger. Of the 19 children, 16 (84%)
read "at or above the level of their normally hearing peers" (p. 116),
and 7 of these 16 read at above-average levels. Three of the 19 read
below grade level, but they were still "within acceptable ranges for
their classes" (p. 116). Four of the students with severe or profound
hearing losses were in gifted or honors classes.

In a follow-up of the study I did with Carol Flexer, I located 38
children, from preschool to university age, with prelingual severe or
profound hearing loss and no other problems such as visual impairment, learning disability, or developmental delay; all were enrolled
in school settings with peers with typical hearing (Robertson,

2000). These children had been diagnosed with hearing loss by the age of three, had begun wearing hearing aids between 2 and 20 months, and began receiving auditory-verbal therapy between 5 and 48 months. They lived in Denver, Toronto, and Easton, Pennsylvania. Each child completed the appropriate grade-level form of the Gates-McGinitie Reading Test for his or her grade placement in school, and each child in fourth grade and beyond (n = 23) produced a writing sample in response to the prompt, "write about something that interests you." Of the 38 children, 11 were one year older than their hearing peers with whom they attended school; their parents had chosen to "hold them back" by having them begin kindergarten or first grade one year later than usual. The children's mean score on the vocabulary portion of the test was the 55th percentile; on the reading comprehension test, the mean score was the 57th percentile. The spread of scores was from the 1st to the 99th percentile. The writing samples were evaluated by in-service teachers practiced at holistic scoring of hearing students' writing in comparison to an established grade-level performance scale. Only 3 of the 23 writing samples were judged not to be at the grade level of their writers.

In a presentation at the 2002 Alexander Graham Bell Association for the Deaf and Hard of Hearing Conference, Rattigan discussed a study of 43 children in Australia who used cochlear implants (Rattigan, Reed, & Lee, 2002). The reading achievement of more than half of the children was age-appropriate, and 5 of the children read above age-level. These authors concluded that "word reading efficiency was related to the children's phonological awareness, rapid naming, phonological memory skills and receptive vocabulary," and they found a connection between receptive vocabulary and phonological awareness skills.

Jean Moog (2002), in writing about outcomes among 17 children between 5 and 11 years in age who had received cochlear implants, stated, "The progress of children with implants in the areas of speech perception, speech production, language, and reading has far exceeded the expectations of even the most optimistic" (p. 138). She used the Gates-MacGinitie Reading Test (3rd edition) for children younger than 8 years and the Stanford Achievement Tests (9th edition) for children 8 and older and reported that, "more than 70% of the students scored within the average range for their age" (p. 142).

Conclusion

It should be clear from an examination of these studies that literacy achievement as measured by standardized tests has improved for children with hearing loss since 1916. For a very long time, expectations have been low for children with varying degrees of deafness, and most children have scored at far lower levels than their peers with typical hearing, with the gap growing as the children progressed through the grades. Some heroic instances of children progressing faster and further began to be reported in the 1970s, and these involved children in whom spoken language was being cultivated. It has taken advances in technology in the form of smaller, more effective hearing aids and cochlear implants, and the concomitant discovery of some children reading at levels commensurate with children with typical hearing to spur the understanding of a link between listening and spoken language and literacy. Simultaneously, researchers studying children with typical hearing have come to an agreement that knowledge of the syntax and semantics of the language to be read and the ability to manipulate the sounds of the language comprise the necessary foundation for reading achievement to progress beyond the beginning stages. Researchers at Gallaudet University are coming to a similar conclusion about the necessity of knowing important components of the language to be read: "Regardless of the primary language of the child, a strong knowledge of the vocabulary and the syntax and grammar of the language of print are both (independently) critical for reading success" (Morere, 2011). We proceed to these matters in the next chapters.

References

Adams, M. (1994). *Beginning to read*. Cambridge, MA: MIT Press.

Allen, T. E. (1986). Patterns of academic achievement among hearing impaired students: 1974 and 1983. In A. N. Schildroth & M. A. Karchmer (Eds.), *Deaf children in America* (pp. 161–206). San Diego, CA: College-Hill Press.

Brill, R. (1941). The prognosis of reading achievement of the deaf. *American Annals of the Deaf, 86*, 227–241.

Conrad, R. (1979). *The deaf school child*. London, UK: Harper Row.

Dickinson, E. (1993). *The collected poems of Emily Dickinson* (introduction by M. Bianchi). New York, NY: Barnes and Noble.

Doehring, D., Bonnycastle, D., & Ling, D. (1978) Rapid reading skills of integrated hearing-impaired children. *Volta Review, 80*(6), 399–409.

Elliott, A. (1941). Standardized tests used with the deaf. *American Annals of the Deaf, 86*, 242–249.

Farquhar, G. (1928). A study of a reading test. American *Annals of the Deaf, 73*, 264–272.

Furth, H. (1966). A comparison of reading test norms of deaf and hearing children. *American Annals of the Deaf, 111*, 461–462.

Gallaudet Research Institute. *Literacy and deaf students*. Retrieved February 8, 2008, from http://gri.gallaudet.edu/Literacy/#reading

Gallaudet Research Institute (2011). Retrieved from http://research.gallaudet.edu/Archive/

Geers, A. S., & Moog, J. S. (1989). Factors predictive of the development of literacy in profoundly hearing-impaired adolescents. *Volta Review, 91*, 69–86.

Goldberg, D., & Flexer, C. (1993). Outcome survey of auditory-verbal graduates: Study of clinical efficacy. *Journal of the American Academy of Audiology, 4*, 189–200.

Gould, S. (1981). *The mismeasure of man*. New York, NY: W. W. Norton.

Hall, P. (1929). Results of recent tests at Gallaudet College. *American Annals of the Deaf, 74*, 389–395.

Holt, J. (1993). Stanford Achievement Test, 8th edition: Reading comprehension subgroup results. *American Annals of the Deaf, 138*(2), 172–175.

Joy, S., Kaplan, E., & Fein, D. (2004). Speed and memory in the WAIS-III Digit Symbol-Coding subtest across the adult lifespan. *Archives of Clinical Neuropsychology, 19*, 759–767.

Lane, H., & Baker, D. (1974). Reading achievement of the deaf: Another look. *Volta Review, 76*, 488–499.

Lee, G. (Ed.). (1961). *Crusade against ignorance: Thomas Jefferson on education*. New York, NY: Teachers College.

Ling, D. (1993). Auditory-verbal options for children with hearing impairment: Helping to pioneer an applied science. *Volta Review, 95*, 187–196.

Moog, J. (2002). Changing expectations for children with cochlear implants. *Annals of Otology, Rhinology, and Laryngology, 111*, 138–142.

Moog, J. S., & Geers, A. S. (1985). EPIC: A Program to accelerate academic progress in profoundly hearing-impaired children. *Volta Review, 87*, 259–277.

Morere, D. (2011). *National Science Foundation Science of Learning Center on Visual Language and Visual Learning, Research Brief Number 4:*

Reading Research and Deaf Children. Retrieved from http://vl2.gallaudet .edu/assets/section7/document141.pdf

Morrison, W. (1940). The Ontario school ability examination. *American Annals of the Deaf, 85,* 184–189.

National Assessment of Adult Literacy. Retrieved from http://nces.ed.gov/ naal/kf_demographics.asp#3

National Institute for Literacy. (1998). *The state of literacy in America: Estimates at the local, state, and national levels.* Washington, DC: Author.

Pintner, R. (1918). The measurement of language ability and language progress of deaf children. *Volta Review, 20,* 755–764.

Pintner, R., & Paterson, D. (1916). Learning tests with deaf children. *Psychology Monographs, 20.*

Pintner, R., & Paterson, D. (1916). The survey of a day-school for the deaf. *American Annals of the Deaf, 61,* 417–433.

Power, D., & Leigh, G. (2000). Principles and practices of literacy development for deaf learners: A historical overview. *Journal of Deaf Studies and Deaf Education, 5*(1), 3–8.

Rattigan, K., Reed, V., & Lee, K. (2002). *An investigation into the phonological processing and literacy skills of children using a cochlear implant in an oral educational setting.* Paper presented at the meeting of the Alexander Graham Bell Association for the Deaf and Hard of Hearing, St. Louis, MO.

Reich, C., Hambleton, D., & Houldin, B. (1977). The integration of hearing-impaired children in regular classrooms. *American Annals of the Deaf, 122,* 534–543.

Roberts, S., & Rickards, F. (1994). A survey of graduates of an Australian integrated auditory/oral preschool, part II: Academic achievement, utilization of support services, and friendship patterns. *Volta Review, 96,* 207–236.

Robertson, L. (2000). *Literacy learning for children who are deaf or hard of hearing.* Washington, DC: Alexander Graham Bell Association for the Deaf and Hard of Hearing.

Robertson, L., & Flexer, C. (1993). Reading development: A survey of children with hearing loss who developed speech and language through the auditory-verbal method. *Volta Review, 95,* 253–261.

Ruddell, R., & Ruddell, M. (1994). Language acquisition and literacy processes. In R. Ruddell, M. Ruddell, & H. Singer (Eds.), *Theoretical models and processes of reading* (4th ed., pp. 83–101). Newark, DE: International Reading Association.

Scarborough, H. (2002). Connecting early language and literacy to later reading (dis)abilities: Evidence, theory, and practice. In S. Neuman & D. Dickinson (Eds.), *Handbook of early literacy research* (pp. 97–110). New York, NY: Guilford Press.

Snow, C., Burns, M., & Griffin, P. (Eds.). (1998). *Preventing reading difficulties in young children*. Washington, DC: National Academy Press.

Stewart, D., & Clarke, B. (2003). *Literacy and your deaf child: What every parent should know*. Washington, DC: Gallaudet University Press.

Traxler, C. (2000). The Stanford Achievement Test, 9th edition: National norming and performance standards for deaf and hard-of-hearing students. *Journal of Deaf Studies and Deaf Education, 5*(4), 337–348.

Walter, J. (1955). A study of the written sentence construction of a group of profoundly deaf children. *American Annals of the Deaf, 100*, 235–252.

Wray, D., Flexer, C., & Vaccaro, V. (1997). Classroom performance of children who are deaf or hard of hearing and who learned spoken communication through the auditory-verbal approach: An evaluation of treatment efficacy. *Volta Review, 99*(2), 107–119.

Wrightstone, J., Aranow, M., & Muskowitz, S. (1963). Developing reading test norms for deaf children. *American Annals of the Deaf, 108*, 311–316.

Vernon, M., & Koh, S. (1970). Early manual communication and deaf children's achievements. *American Annals of the Deaf, 115*, 527–537.

Chapter 2

LITERACY THEORIES

Reading is the complex act of constructing meaning from print. We read in order to better understand ourselves, others, and the world around us; we use the knowledge we gain from reading to change the world in which we live.

Becoming a reader is a gradual process that begins with our first interactions with print. As children, there is no fixed point at which we suddenly become readers. Instead, all of us bring our understanding of spoken language, our knowledge of the world, and our experiences in it to make sense of what we read. We grow in our ability to comprehend and interpret a wide range of reading materials by making appropriate choices from among the extensive repertoire of skills and strategies that develop over time. These strategies include predicting, comprehension monitoring, phonemic awareness, critical thinking, decoding, using context, and making connections to what we already know.

National Council of Teachers of English

. . . there is not a single process involved in reading, but instead several operating interactively. Reading research cannot simply track a single process but must study its interaction with other processes over time, as skill unfolds.

Padden & Hanson, 2000, p. 444

Introduction

People who know how to read carry with them ideas about how the process works, and when they think about teaching reading, they usually think about doing so in terms of their own personal understandings. Such informal theorizing works best in the context of knowledge of studies done by researchers and theorists who have published their ideas for intellectual scrutiny, so as you read, keep in mind what you already think you know about reading and writing, and see where you can either fit in more ideas or alter some thoughts you have had. This chapter sets aside deafness for the moment in order to lay out theories of literacy as they have been developed for children and adults with typical hearing, and then Chapter 4 begins making connections essential to understanding the relationship between literacy, deafness, and listening.

Theorizing About Reading

Reading has been studied from many perspectives, including behaviorism, linguistics, psycholinguistics, cognitive psychology, sociolinguistics, literary criticism, and critical theory, and all have something to contribute to our understanding of literacy in the context of deafness. Theories in all of these areas include assumptions about the necessity of development in the reader of the language to be read. By age five, six, or seven, the child with typical hearing who has not been deprived of language in some way has caught on to all of the spoken structures voiced in his or her presence (Fry, 1966, p. 187). By age seven or eight, the child can understand and construct sentences using conventional word order and use the parts of speech in the same ways adults do (Ling, 1989, p. 4). Throughout life, through direct experience and educational experiences, the individual adds conceptual knowledge to this linguistic knowledge in the form of an ever-expanding network of vocabulary. When this child with typical hearing goes to school at age five or six, he or she may be presented with one approach to reading or to a combination of approaches, but all approaches depend on the learner knowing the spoken language to be read and seek to remediate language gaps and delays where they are discovered.

In the United States, the matter of teaching children to read has been and remains controversial, which makes it very interesting. Some of the controversy appears to be at root a power struggle in the political realm, and other aspects of it involve differing definitions of reading and the fact that research done from different points of view produces different results. This chapter begins with definitions of reading and then focuses on word identification and comprehension, which are involved in the two major "camps" in the discussion. Then it discusses the contributions of numerous academic disciplines that study reading. I hope you will see there are many, many ways to think about reading and that you will come to appreciate how they can fit together.

Definitions of Reading

At first glance, it seems easy to define reading. It is the getting of meaning from print. Or, it's the pronouncing of words as they are seen on the page. Or, it's connecting what one sees in print to what one already knows. But could it be an act of interpretation? Could the reader be *bringing* meaning to the print instead of getting meaning from it? The more one thinks about it, the more complex and interesting it gets. How one thinks about reading underlies how one studies it and how one formulates ways of teaching it to children and adults. In this section, we look at various ways some influential researchers have defined reading. These definitions are standing up over time because they deal well with questions that arise about reading as a process and the needs of learners as they acquire reading ability.

During the process of reading, "a mental representation is constructed of the discourse in memory, using both external and internal types of information, with the goal of interpreting (understanding) the discourse" (van Dijk & Kintsch, 1983, p. 6, as cited in Hacker, 2004). This is a goal-oriented definition involving combining information found both within and beyond the reader.

Marie Clay, who developed Reading Recovery, writes about reading:

> . . . as a message-getting, problem-solving activity which
> increases in power and flexibility the more it is practiced. My

> definition states that within the directional constraints of the printer's code, language and visual perception responses are purposefully directed by the reader in some integrated way to the problem of extracting meaning from cues in a text, in sequence, so that the reader brings a maximum of understanding to the author's message. (Clay, 1991, p. 6)

Clay goes on to observe that mature reading may be the result in different readers of their having learned its components in different orders and in different ways (p. 16). Therefore, she does not insist on only one approach to teaching reading.

Smith (2004), author of six editions of *Understanding Reading*, maintains that reading is a natural process of "interpreting experience," and that people do this interpreting continuously from infancy in all facets of their lives, not only in dealing with print (p. 2). The reader recognizes something and fits it into his or her knowledge so that, "All reading of print is interpretation, making sense of print" (p. 3). Smith sees reading as a set of active processes employed as needed in different contexts with readers finding what they seek on the page:

> Readers find letters in print when they ask one kind of question and select relevant visual information; they find words in print when they ask another kind of question and use the same visual information in a different way; and they find meaning in print, in the same visual information, when they ask a different kind of question again. (p. 181)

From Smith's point of view, fluent reading is related to being able to answer the questions one is asking while reading (p. 182).

In the often cited text, *Beginning to Read,* Adams (1990) writes:

> In the course of proficient reading, the processes supporting orthographic, phonological, and semantic identification of words occur interactively and interdependently; without the complete and proper operation of all three, the reader is left with neither capacity nor support for comprehension. (p. 8)

Stanovich sees these definitions of reading as different levels of processing, with one involving perception and the other involving reasoning (1994, p. 261). At the same time that he writes of the importance of word recognition, he terms reading, "a special type of constrained reasoning" (1994, p. 264).

These views come from different directions, and in some respects they seem truly at odds with each other. I find taking them together to be useful in not getting caught up in arguing about different reading approaches, particularly because accounts of how reading proceeds may or may not be related directly to how reading might be taught. For example, although it may be apparent that the typical reader looks at the letters in the words being read, this understanding may not require teaching reading in a letter-by-letter fashion. It is clear that children with typical hearing learn to read by engaging in many different reading programs (Clay, 1991, p. 3). An ever-present difficulty is that they do not all learn to read at high levels, regardless of the approach or materials used. Given this reality, there is room for definitions that feature word identification and for definitions whose focus is comprehension, *as both are necessary*. It is useful to understand the thinking underlying both.

Word Identification

Word identification is often called "bottom-up" reading; the metaphor proceeds from the text up to the reader, suggesting that letters and words are driving the process. The reader is seen as taking in every letter (Adams, 2002, p. 69) and applying rules that result in constructing the word-by-word speech message of the writer. It is as though the reader "hears" the writer's voice, or as though the reader is identifying words as whole units and then "hears" the results. Pointing to research done beginning with LaBerge and Samuels (1974), Schwanenflugel et al. (2006) argue that fluency in word identification is the underpinning for comprehension, and that practice in decoding leads to fluency (p. 499). In this view, the goal is reading without thinking about identifying the words. This goal is accomplished by moving, over time and with practice, from identifying words at the letter-to-letter level to identifying them as sets of letters in predictable units. Those who work from this point of view rely on studies that show that readers who can identify words automatically are better at comprehension, and they judge that automaticity in word identification leaves more cognitive processing time for understanding the message of the text (Schwanenflugel et al., 2006; Stanovich, 1980). Stanovich's report that better readers identify words with much less difficulty, "either by direct visual recognition or phonological recoding," thus giving them more time to decide on meaning (1980, p. 64) serves as reason for some that reading instruction should begin with direct and systematic phonics instruction.

At issue when the subject is word identification is how the reader comes to an understanding of the rules for identifying words by matching letters to sounds. Some argue for direct phonics instruction (Adams, 1990, for example), and others argue for a whole language approach that incorporates phonics along with other aspects and experiences of reading (Weaver, 2002, for example). In any case, it is the alphabetic principle that needs to be developed, the concept that letters stand for the sounds heard in words. Coming to this understanding on the basis of a few letters usually allows children to understand this principle and apply it to the rest of the sound-symbol relationships (Byrne, cited in Adams, 2002, p. 76).

Coming to know all of the relationships is a very large task, and the way some letters "sound" is dependent on their places among other letters as well as certain features of the language being represented in print. The word "frigate" in Emily Dickinson's poem that begins Chapter 1 looks as though it ought to rhyme with "fry" and "gate," rather than as "fri-git" with two "short" i sounds and a "hard" g. The "ea" in "bears" sounds different from the "ea" in "search." These pronunciations depend on the other letters in the word, as well as on speech conventions that have developed over the years. Clymer (1963) identified 121 generalizations in English being taught in basal reading programs and investigated 45 of them to determine their utility, which he then expressed in percentage terms. (A basal reading program is a program produced by a publisher for the purpose of developing reading in elementary children. Programs are based on presenting children with texts, workbooks, and other materials of increasing difficulty, and teachers are guided in instructing their students by teachers' manuals.) Clymer found many of the rules presented in basal series hold true a small percentage of the time, so the task in pronouncing "frigate," or "bears," for example, is one of working with approximations in comparison to the instances when the generalizations work.

In the case of learning words by sight, the explanation is that of paired-associate memorization of whole words. In both cases, many judge that a great deal of practice with isolated letters and words is necessary.

Comprehension

Comprehension is the point of reading, the end goal of any reading event. Otherwise, the reader is simply pronouncing words. Returning to the "frigate" example, even if the reader pronounces the word conventionally, he or she needs to have at least two kinds of knowledge in order to grasp that in this poem Dickinson sees reading as a vehicle for traveling around in the world in a "virtual" way: (1) that a frigate is a ship, and (2) that we can use a comparison of unlike entities to get an idea across.

It is possible for a person to know the basic rules of pronunciation in a language other than his or her own and to be capable of doing an oral reading that makes use of the rules, but without any understanding of what is being read. Children who do not have a well-developed grasp of the language they are reading may be able to sound somewhat convincing in reading aloud, but comprehension may not be taking place. Even in fluent readers, it is also possible in reading aloud to be devoting so much cognitive effort to the performance that little is processed in a meaningful way. Think back to the last time you read something aloud that you had not read silently beforehand, or to the last time you were at the podium reading something to a large crowd. Quite possibly, you sounded fluent, but understood less than would be the case ordinarily for you. Clearly, just pronouncing words is not enough.

Comprehension is often associated with "top-down" processing. Here, the metaphor calls up an image of memory structures in the reader driving meaning *making*, as opposed to meaning *identificiation*. Comprehension is a constructivist process, and regarding it in this way is useful in the instruction of comprehension (Stanovich, 1994, p. 260). Constructivism is an idea developed by Jean Piaget, who posited that children learn by assimilation and by accommodation. Both involve building on existing memory structures. When an idea is assimilated, it is brought into a person's background knowledge in much the way it is encountered, as long as it fits with other background knowledge. When an idea is accommodated, it is because it does not fit neatly with background knowledge currently held by the person. Either existing knowledge or the new knowledge itself is changed in some way until the person feels that it "makes sense." Of course, a child or an older person could make a similar or a different meaning compared to someone else, and one could discover the reasons for that understanding through conversation. Comprehension evolves in one's thinking, with the person being an active creator of successive iterations of a given idea. In reading the Emily Dickinson poem we have been examining, the reader who does not know what a frigate is could guess and come to some idea about a book taking one far away from one's normal life, and that would suffice. But, there is much more to think about in Dickinson's words. The reader who realizes that several comparisons are being made, but who doesn't know the words because they are not used frequently today, may seek help from a dictionary or from an older person. Finding out that a frigate was a ship, in fact, a powerful warship that escorted other ships, punches up the comparison to a book. So does the word "courser," a word for a fast horse. Then, there is the matter of the traverse (travel) the poorest can take without paying a toll (in other words, for free). In Dickinson's view, a book is available to everyone and is as powerful as warships, fast horses, and chariots in taking the human soul to places unknown. This is a lovely statement about the power of reading. The more the reader works with the language of this poem, the more layers of meaning can be developed. So, we can see how learning the conventions of one's social and cultural setting is an important task for children so they can communicate easily with others. Once everyone knows conventionally what frigates, coursers, tolls, and chariots are, and what it means to traverse, then everyone can share common ideas about those meanings.

Another way of thinking about this is in terms of "schema theory," a cognitive psychological construct that provides a robust account of how people use their existing knowledge in order to add to it. Schemata (the plural of schema) are overlapping and interconnecting structures of memory developed by each person on the basis of life experiences. Put more simply, schemata constitute a person's background knowledge. If one does not know "frigate," "coursers," "traverse," "toll," and "chariot," the poem is harder to read. But once these are added to the person's network of knowledge, the poem is much more accessible. The reverse happens, as well; experience in constructing increasingly sophisticated ideas about the poem can establish those previously unknown words in the person's set of schemata. Another sort of schema relevant in this case is that of understanding how one word or concept can be compared to another in order to make a larger point. This is a procedural schema; for this poem, it has to do with figuring out the simile that compares books to powerful entities in order to comment on how much a book can change a person.

Schemata can be semantic (the meaning a person constructs, often, but not always, in a conventional sense), then, and they also can be procedural (how to do something, for example, how to hold a book right-side up). They help us recognize conventional and nonconventional knowledge and behaviors. An often cited schema involves behavior in a restaurant (Anderson, 2004). Depending on whether the establishment is a fast food outlet or a place for fine dining, the conventions for eating there are different, but each is predictable within its own environment: one goes to the counter in a fast food place, and one waits for the waiter to present the menu in a nice restaurant. Naturally, people have different experiences, and so they carry around different schemata with which to interpret whatever they encounter. Therefore, because different people have developed different schemata, they can have differing interpretations of the same reading. Many fascinating studies have been done to illustrate this point (see, for example, Anderson, 2004). Subjects have been given passages to read in which all the words are identifiable and all the sentences conventional and complete, but without some relevant piece of information they are incomprehensible, demonstrating that word identification is not enough. For example:

> The procedure is actually quite simple. First you arrange things into different groups. Of course, one pile may be sufficient depending on how much there is to do. If you have to go somewhere else due to lack of facilities that is the next step, otherwise you are pretty well set. It is important not to overdo things. That is, it is better to do too few things at once than too many. In the short run this may not seem important but complications can easily arise. A mistake can be expensive as well. At first the whole procedure will seem complicated.

Soon, however, it will become just another facet of life. It is difficult to foresee any end to the necessity for this task in the immediate future, but then one never can tell. After the procedure is complete one arranges the materials into different groups again. Then they can be put into their appropriate places. Eventually they will be used once more and the whole cycle will then have to be repeated. However, that is part of life. (Bransford & Johnson, 1972, p. 722)

If you have not seen this passage before, you are probably wondering what it is about, and you may have decided that it is just badly written. Subjects who were supplied the topic ("Washing Clothes"), though, were able to comprehend and then remember it better than subjects who did not receive the title before reading the passage. If you have had experience doing laundry, you probably had a moment of recognition on seeing the title. If you have not, you are still in the dark! If you go back and reread with the title in mind, you will probably find that every idea in the passage is now accounted for—and it makes sense to you, as long as you have done laundry. Chances are that you can even remember it now well enough to retell it to someone else, because the title enables you to fit the steps together.

Schemata are thought to have numerous properties (Anderson, 2004, pp. 598–599). First, they provide slots that foster assimilation. In the fine-dining schema, there is a place for the entrée, and so one expects a main dish. New information that fits easily into an existing slot such as this will be easily learned and remembered. One is not surprised to see conventional categories such as meat, poultry, and seafood on the menu and can use that knowledge to scan the menu instead of reading everything on it. Second, a schema helps one know what is most important and where to put one's attention. It could tell the reader that knowing what was eaten for dinner is not important to the story at hand and so not to dwell on those details. Third, a schema helps one make inferences. For example, the kind of dinner a character consumes might be a clue to the person's personality or social status. Fourth, a schema helps one do a memory search in order to reconstruct the events in the text. The character got into his car, waited for everyone else to get in, pulled out his car key, started the car, drove to the restaurant, and so on. If a step is left out, the story works less well. Fifth, a schema helps a reader decide what to keep and what to leave out in retelling the story. The crux of the story may be that a mother and father took their family out to dinner to celebrate their child's birthday. And, sixth, a schema allows for figuring out what must have happened. In this hypothetical story, there was probably a special birthday cake involved.

Another important aspect of reading involves metacognition, which is thinking about the meaning one is making while reading. Such thinking about one's thinking can also be called comprehension monitoring or self-regulated comprehension (Hacker, 2004).

Does the reading make sense (do the parts fit together logically)? Can one construct an image or a list of reasons for a character's actions or an experiment's outcome? If not, then the reader needs to figure out what is happening. Usually, the reader depends on the text to be sensible, or "considerate." In other words, one ordinarily doesn't think a text has been written in order to try to trick the reader. So, in comprehension monitoring, the reader asks questions of the text: What does "tear" mean in this context (is it moisture from one's eyes or a rip in some fabric?) Do I know enough about the topic? (What happens in making and flying a kite?) What could I ask someone or look up in a dictionary or on the Internet using Google so that I can understand this? Did I understand what it said about arranging things into piles? Where should I go back and read again? After exhausting such questions, a reader who has not found satisfaction may determine that the text actually does not make sense, which, of course, may or may not be the case for other readers with different background knowledge and different metacognitive capabilities. The reader uses knowledge of the world (content schemata) and knowledge of procedures (process schemata) while reading by figuratively stepping back and examining the meaning he or she has made and then proceeding from there. Increasing skill in doing this allows a reader to question the sense he or she is making of a text over increasingly larger stretches of text, and, over time, the reader expands a personal set of strategies to use in self-regulated comprehension. Verbal representations (words, phrases, sentences, and paragraphs) are translated into text propositions that are stored in memory as a representation of the text. World knowledge is brought to bear on the propositions, and a gist of the text is constructed. This gist serves to modify subsequent meaning making with the text, and readers begin to set standards for themselves for what constitutes comprehension (Hacker, 2004, pp. 760–761).

It should be obvious that different readers will construct different meanings based on their differing knowledge of the topic at hand, their differing ways of reasoning, differing understanding of word meanings, and their differing purposes for reading. When readers' constructions overlap, and they do surprisingly often, they find they agree with each other about the meaning of the text (Hacker, 2004, pp. 765–766).

An Interactive Theory

In 1977, Rumelhart proposed an interactive theory, and Stanovich followed up in 1980. These models posit a simultaneous synthesis of information from many sources:

> A pattern is synthesized based on information provided *simultaneously* from several knowledge sources (e.g., feature extraction, orthographic knowledge, lexical knowledge, syntactic knowledge, semantic knowledge). (Stanovich, 1980, p. 35)

In this explanation, reading involves an interaction of bottom-up and top-down processes, a view that should end the debate concerning whether reading is predominantly word identification or predominantly comprehension and all the processes attendant to it. It is not a matter of one being more important than the other; *they are both necessary, and they interact.*

Related to this position, but with a slightly different explanation, Adams (2002) cites research on parallel distributed processing as demonstrating that all "levels of processing are assumed to be active and interactive at once, working in mutual coordination with each other" (p. 69). This would include responding to orthographic, phonological, and semantic information simultaneously during any instance of reading. Using the example of identifying the word "cat," Adams posits a context processor (interpretation) that interacts with a semantic processor (meaning). The semantic processor, an orthographic processor (that deals with written language), and a phonological processor (that deals with spoken language) all interact with one another. Seeing the word *cat* sets off all the reader's prior knowledge of cats, but if the reader is already expecting the word *cat* from the context, the meaning is already in process, and the spoken word will be drawn from memory. *All parts of the memory system will affect all the others.* "Moreover, as soon as any given set of memories reaches a critical level of activation dominance, it shuts off all competitors in winner-take-all fashion" (p. 71). The winner of the interactive race to meaning is the most efficient process on that particular reading occasion; sometimes a direct semantic route wins, and other times written or spoken forms are more successful. Goodman (1994, 1996), Smith, (2004), and Weaver (2002) use this reasoning to say that reading is mainly meaning-driven, and that the reader constantly hypothesizes about what is coming next, using background knowledge, including language knowledge to do so. In this explanation, the reader knows symbol-sound relationships, but dips into the symbols on the page only as necessary to confirm predictions. They argue that knowledge of the conventional sound-symbol relationships is learned in a variety of ways, including experience over time with them and direct instruction as needed. Even those focusing on fluency of word identification do not rule out meaningful reading experiences during instruction of beginners. Schwanenflugel et al. (2006) conclude, " . . . our findings support the importance of carrying out fluency-oriented instruction *alongside* comprehension instruction" (p. 519). As you may be aware, however, this interactive view has not ended the so-called "reading wars" concerning how to teach children how to read.

Many Disciplines Study Reading

Reading has been studied since the beginning of the 20th century as the field of psychology was beginning to develop. Over the years, numerous other disciplines have extended their work to include the study of reading and they, too, began attempting to explain this process and develop approaches for teaching it to children. For this reason, there is no single explanation or set of explanations for reading processes, and your task is to pull from each as you think about the children with whom you live and work. I have consulted three histories of reading research in formulating the following discussion and suggest reading them in their entirety if this is an interest of yours (Alexander & Fox, 2004; Allington & McGill-Franzen, 2004; Pearson & Stephens, 1994).

Behaviorist Psychology

B. F. Skinner's behaviorism was the prevailing view in the 1960s, and thinking about reading was fairly well settled at that time. A behaviorist sees reading as a matter of responding to letters on the page (written code) in order to turn them into a spoken code. Then, the reader listens to the result, just as he or she would listen to spoken language. Behaviorists don't venture into speculating about what is going on in thought processes, as behaviorism limits itself to observing and experimenting with external behaviors in people. Therefore, language processes in the reader are not a part of the investigation, and reading is seen as a stimulus-response perceptual activity: the reader sees, and the reader responds, pairing sight with sound in a linear fashion through a text. In this view, the reader needs to practice making appropriate (conventional) responses until accuracy is achieved with increasingly difficult texts. Behaviorists, therefore, are concerned with word *identification*, which translates as phonics instruction for identifying words pronounced conventionally and whole word instruction for those that are not (Pearson & Stephens, 1994).

Linguistics and Psycholinguistics

Beginning in the late 1950s and into the 1960s, linguists began challenging behaviorist ideas about language. As might be expected, linguists start with spoken language, not with reading, and so they see language as the necessary underpinning of reading. They point out that language acquisition is too complex and too natural to be accounted for by perception of repeated pairings of stimuli and responses. In 1965, Noam Chomsky proposed that children come into the world "hard-wired," or innately equipped to learn language and then to learn to read that language, also in natural ways, just by being exposed to it (Alexander & Fox, 2004; Pearson & Stephens, 1994). Infants begin life capable of discriminating among sounds found in all the world's languages. They learn quickly to differentiate among the specific sounds of their native language(s), and by 10 to 12 months of age, they lose the ability to discriminate among the sounds specific to other languages (Werker & Tees, 2005).

Psycholinguistics grew from these efforts, and investigations began of children's language acquisition. Psycholinguists observe that children don't just copy other people's utterances, but they also experiment with producing utterances of their own, testing their way into learning the language through using it meaningfully, and that, in the absence of problems such as deafness, they learn the language well by the age of five, without any special sort of intervention from the people around them. The next psycholinguistic step is to infer that reading is an extension of spoken language that can be developed by children through interacting with meaningful texts. Far different from the behaviorists, psycholinguists think about and try to get an understanding of what a person is doing with language, whether spoken or written. Kenneth Goodman developed "miscue analysis" as a way of understanding an individual's language and semantic processing while reading aloud. Rather than thinking of a misread word as a mistake, Goodman terms it a "miscue" and uses the semantic, graphophonemic, and syntactic information surrounding it to derive an understanding of whether and how the reader is making sense of the text. If, for example, the text says, "Jennifer was excited to ride the big white horse," and the child utters, "Jennifer was excited to ride the big white *pony*," that is deemed a more acceptable and meaningful miscue than, "Jennifer was excited to ride the big white *house*," as a pony can actually be ridden, but a house cannot. In this sense, reading is not just about "sounding out" the words, but about making meaning. Reading "house" for "horse" and remaining satisfied with it may signify something about identifying letters, but it certainly implies that the reader is not expecting to make logical sense of the sentence in relation to the conventions of the world.

Another psycholinguist, Frank Smith, writes of readers learning to read by reading in the presence of mature readers, just as they have learned to talk by talking with mature users of spoken language. In his view, readers make use of interactive cueing systems (the orthographic, syntactic, semantic, and visual), in order to make predictions, verify or reject them, and construct meaning. He famously asserted that reading is "only incidentally visual," which flies in the face of word identification conducted in a linear fashion and suggests that the reader continuously uses prior knowledge along with the cuing systems to make predictions and then checks with the visual text itself in order to confirm or disconfirm decisions about meaning (Alexander & Fox, 2004; Pearson & Stephens, 1994).

Sociolinguistics

In the 1970s, sociolinguistics began to develop, as researchers began to investigate the differences in language that children bring to school. They look at the contextual setting of reading and focus particularly on children who come to school having spoken a dialect or language different from the school's language from an early age. The insight of the sociolinguist is that children are often making huge leaps in translating the language on the page into the language of their own dialects. The child who reads "wif" for "with," for example, is not misidentifying the letters "th" as "sounding like "f," but is identifying meaning that he or she understands prior to reading and pronounces as "wif." The sociolinguist sees this as a difference, not a deficit, and suggests that children not be made to feel their language is unacceptable at school, while at the same time the children need to be introduced to standard language so that they can switch back and forth using both home and school language: home language at home where it is used and understood, and school language at school where it is used and understood. Shirley Brice Heath contributes the understanding that children live and attend school in social environments, and these environments interact with the social understandings they bring with them. The reaction of the school to the child can make a real difference in whether and how the child learns reading and content (Alexander & Fox, 2004; Pearson & Stephens, 1994).

Cognitive Psychology

Also in the 1970s, cognitive psychology began to develop ways of looking into the workings of the mind: "perception, attention, comprehension, learning, memory, and executive control of all cognitive processes" (Pearson & Stephens, p. 30). In studying reading, cognitive psychologists began to investigate the underlying structures of narrative and expository texts and how people make sense of them. Most important, they asked questions about what the reader brings to a text in the way of prior knowledge, and this resulted in the development of schema theory (Pearson & Stephens, 1994) that I explored earlier in this chapter.

Literary Criticism

Literary criticism in the form of Louise Rosenblatt's work (Rosenblatt, 1978) takes on the question of where meaning resides, which, of course, is connected to comprehension. Is meaning constructed in the mind of the reader or does it stay in one form on the page in the book? How can differences in comprehension be understood? Rosenblatt suggests that meaning results from a transaction between the reader and the text, resulting in the "poem," her figurative language for meaning. Every reading event, even when the same reader reads the same text, is a transaction, always resulting in a different meaning. The reader responds a bit differently on each occasion, constructing at least slightly different meanings each time. Although reading may feel like identifying an author's thoughts on the page, it is all about interpretation. As the interpreter changes—by mood, by age, by experience—so does the transaction between him or her and the text. Your interpretation of the Emily Dickinson poem about frigates and books may be quite different from mine. This happens not only with more complex text, but also with texts read by beginning readers.

Critical Theory and Pedagogy

Critical theory and pedagogy advanced by Paulo Freire (1981) and bel hooks [sic] (1994) causes us to think about the political aspects of reading. These thinkers ask questions about who has access to literacy, to texts of all sorts, and to the Internet—in short, to information and literature—and who does not. They see literacy as empowerment and have come to the conclusion that the oppressed of the world are systematically, and often subtly, kept from literacy.

Their argument is for equal and equitable educational opportunity for all, regardless of their status in society or condition of potential disability. Although they do not write about deafness as a category, they remind those of us who are concerned about deafness to think carefully about how access to language and literacy either helps or hinders people in being full participant citizens in society at large.

Conclusion

I hope I have made it clear that there are many fascinating ways to think about reading. Arguing over which one or ones are correct is not the point, and doing so is not very useful. Each comes out of a particular set of assumptions and contributes a different sort of understanding, and I do not find them to be mutually exclusive. The most important aspect of each theory for our purposes is this: *all of these theories rely on knowledge of the spoken language being read* built over time from experience with the language. There is no more critical understanding to cultivate than that, particularly when we are thinking about children with hearing loss and their prospects for learning how to read, write, and get along in a world where literacy confers power and control over one's life, and illiteracy is synonymous with powerlessness.

References

Adams, M. (1990). *Beginning to read.* Cambridge, MA: MIT Press.

Adams, M. (2002). Alphabetic anxiety and explicit, systematic phonics instruction: A cognitive science perspective. In S. Neuman & D. Dickinson (Eds.), *Handbook of early literacy research* (pp. 66–80). New York, NY: Guilford Press.

Alexander, P., & Fox, E. (2004). A historical perspective on reading research and practice. In R. Ruddell & N. Unrau (Eds.), *Theoretical models and processes of reading* (5th ed., pp. 33–68). Newark, DE: International Reading Association.

Allington, R., & McGill-Franzen, A. (2004). Looking back, looking forward: A conversation about teaching reading in the 21st century. In R. Ruddell

& N. Unrau (Eds.), *Theoretical models and processes of reading* (5th ed., pp. 5–32). Newark, DE: International Reading Association.

Anderson, R. (2004). Role of the reader's schema in comprehension, learning, and memory. In R. Ruddell & N. Unrau (Eds.), *Theoretical models and processes of reading* (5th ed., pp. 594–606). Newark, DE: International Reading Association.

Bransford, J., & Johnson, M. (1972). Contextual prerequisites for understanding: Some investigations of comprehension and recall. *Journal of Verbal Learning and Verbal Behavior, 11*(6), 717–726.

Clay, M. (1991). *Becoming literate: The construction of inner control.* Portsmouth, NH: Heinemann.

Clymer, T. (1963). The utility of phonic generalizations in the primary grades. *Reading Teacher, 16,* 252–258.

Freire, P. (1981). *Pedagogy of the oppressed.* New York, NY: Continuum.

Fry, D. (1966). The development of the phonological system in the normal and the deaf child. In F. Smith & G. Miller (Eds.), *The genesis of language: A psycholinguistic approach* (pp. 187–206). Cambridge, MA: MIT Press.

Goodman, K. (1994). Reading, writing, and written texts: A transactional sociopsycholinguistic view. In R. Ruddell, M. Ruddell, & H. Singer (Eds.), *Theoretical models and processes of reading* (4th ed., pp. 1093–1130). Newark, DE: International Reading Association.

Hacker, D. (2004). Self-regulated comprehension during normal reading. In R. Ruddell & N. Unrau (Eds.), *Theoretical models and processes of reading* (5th ed., pp. 755–779*)*. Newark, DE: International Reading Association.

Hooks, B. (1994). *Teaching to transgress: Education as the practice of freedom.* New York, NY: Routledge.

LaBerge, D., & Samuels, S. (1974). Toward a theory of automatic information processing in reading. *Cognitive Psychology, 6,* 293–323.

Ling, D. (1989). *Foundations of spoken language for hearing-impaired children.* Washington, DC: Alexander Graham Bell Association for the Deaf.

National Council of Teachers of English. Retrieved from http://www.ncte .org/positions/statements/positiononreading

Padden, C., & Hanson, V. (2000). Search for the missing link: The development of skilled reading in deaf children. In K. Emmorey & H. Lane (Eds.), *The signs of language revisited: An anthology to honor Ursula Bellugi and Edward Klima* (pp. 435–447). Mahwah, NJ: Lawrence Erlbaum.

Pearson, P., & Stephens, D. (1994). Learning about literacy: A 30-year journey. In R. Ruddell, M. Ruddell, & H. Singer (Eds.), *Theoretical models and processes of reading* (pp. 22–42). Newark, DE: International Reading Association.

Rosenblatt, L. (1978). *The reader, the text, the poem: The transactional theory of the literary work.* Carbondale, IL: Southern Illinois University Press.

Rumelhart, D. (1977). Toward an interactive model of reading. In S. Dornic (Ed.), *Attention and performance VI.* Hillsdale, NJ: Erlbaum Associates.

Schwanenflugel, P., Meisinger, E., Wisenbaker, J., Kuhn, M., Strauss, G., & Morris, R. (2006). Becoming a fluent and automatic reader in the early elementary school years. *Reading Research Quarterly, 41*(4), 496–522.

Smith, F. (2004). *Understanding reading* (6th ed.). Mahwah, NJ: Lawrence Erlbaum Associates.

Stanovich, K. (1980). Toward an interactive-compensatory model of individual differences in the development of reading fluency. *Reading Research Quarterly, 1*, 32–71.

Stanovich, K. (1994). Constructivism in reading education. *Journal of Special Education, 28*(3), 259–274.

Weaver, C. (2002). *Reading process and practice* (3rd ed.). Portsmouth, NH: Heinemann.

Werker, J., & Tees, R. (2005). Speech perception as a window for understanding plasticity and commitment in language systems of the brain. *Developmental Psychobiology, 46*, 233–251.

Chapter 3

TECHNOLOGY AND LISTENING

Carol Flexer, PhD, LSLS CERT. AVT

Hearing loss is not about the ears; it's about the brain.

Cole & Flexer, 2011, p. 6

Introduction

We hear with the brain; the ears are just a way in. A primary problem is that hearing loss keeps sound from reaching the brain. If amplification technologies can be used during early childhood to access, stimulate and grow auditory centers, then the secondary negative effects of hearing loss such as language, reading, and academic difficulties can be ameliorated (Joint Committee on Infant Hearing, 2007).

The purpose of this chapter is to create a context for the use of amplification technology as a critical condition for literacy development for today's infants and children with hearing loss. To that end, the following topics will be discussed: the neurological basis of listening and literacy; a computer analogy for understanding technology; an overview of amplification technologies; the auditory feedback loop; distance hearing; and finally, a different way to look at the concept and context of deafness in this day and age.

Neurological Basis of Listening and Literacy

Hearing is powerful! There is substantial evidence that "hearing" (auditory brain development) is the most effective modality for the teaching of spoken language (speech), literacy and other cognitive skills. Child development is positively influenced if "hearing" is emphasized and negatively affected if hearing is minimized.

Studies in brain development show that sensory stimulation of the auditory centers of the brain is critically important, and indeed, influences the actual organization of auditory brain pathways (Berlin & Weyand, 2003; Boothroyd, 1997; Chermak, Bellis, & Musiek, 2007). The fact is, the brain can organize itself only around the stimuli that it receives. If complete acoustic events are received, then that is how the brain will be organized. Conversely, if hearing loss filters some or all speech sounds from reaching auditory centers of the brain, then the brain will be organized differently. "When we want to remember (or learn) something we have heard, we must hear it clearly because memory can be only as clear as its original signal . . . muddy in, muddy out." (Doidge, 2007, p. 68). Signal enhancement, such as that provided by amplification technology, is really about brain stimulation with subsequent development of auditory–neural pathways.

Neural imaging has shown that the same brain areas—the primary and secondary auditory areas—are most active when a child listens and when a child reads. That is, phonological or phonemic awareness, which is the explicit awareness of the speech sound units of language structure, forms an important basis for the development of literacy skills (Pugh, 2005; Strickland & Shanahan, 2004; Tallal, 2004).

It is important to recognize that children are not small adults; they are not able to listen like adults listen. Indeed, children bring different listening capabilities to a communicative and learning situation than do adults in two main ways. First, human auditory brain structure is not fully mature until about age 15 years; thus a child does not bring a complete neurological system to a listening situation (Bhatnagar, 2002; Boothroyd, 1997). Second, children do not have the years of language and life experience that enable adults to fill in the gaps of missed or inferred information. (Such filling in of gaps is called auditory/cognitive closure.) Leibold and Neff (2011) found that children require years of listening experience to learn to focus on the most informative aspects of complex speech sounds in the presence of interfering noise. Therefore, because children require more complete, detailed auditory information than adults, all children need a quieter room and a louder signal (Anderson, 2004). The goal is to *develop* the brains of children, unlike adults where sound enters a *developed* brain.

Janet Werker, a developmental, cognitive neuroscientist summarizes the following points from numerous scientific studies that investigate the development of infant speech perception, early word learning, and cognitive development (Bernhardt, Kemp, & Werker, 2007; Vouloumanos, & Werker, 2007; Werker, 2006; Werker & Byers-Heinlein, 2008). I comment on some of Werker's points below:

- Infants acquire native languages by listening, and are neurologically "hardwired" to talk.
- Because the inner ear is fully developed by the 20th week of gestation, a typical infant is born with about 20 weeks of listening experience. That is, the infant's brain has been stimulated with sound in utero for 20 weeks. As a result, at birth, infants prefer their mother's speech, and songs and stories heard before birth. *An infant whose hearing loss occurred embryologically and whose inner ear did not fully develop, is already 20 weeks behind in auditory exposure at birth. Therefore, amplification needs to be provided as soon as possible, followed by an enriched and embellished auditory learning environment designed to stimulate and grow auditory neural pathways.*
- During the first 6 months of life, babies are universal language learners. That is, they can distinguish all speech sounds. However, by the end of the first year, the brain undergoes a functional reorganization to discriminate language-specific phonemes; infants become language-specific listeners between 6 and 12 months of age. This neural reorganization improves and tunes the phonetic

categories required for their language, and attenuates those distinctions not required. *Therefore, if multiple spoken languages are desired by the family (e.g., if the home language is different from the language to be used in school) we need to begin enriching both languages at birth.*

■ Fetuses hear mostly the low frequency acoustic features of their mother's speech in utero—so the acoustic spotlight is on rhythmic elements. *Therefore, even if initial amplification can access only low frequency sounds, from a developmental perspective, there is substantial value to using that signal.*

■ At birth, infants listen at multiple levels at the same time. They learn to distinguish rhythm, phonemes, and phonologic elements all at once. *Therefore, we should speak to the infant in complete sentences/phrases with a great deal of melody.*

■ Infants' speech perception acuity predicts their vocabulary. The more precisely an infant can hear phonemic elements, the better chance he or she has of learning new words.

■ Infants use their phonetic categories to bootstrap learning new words.

■ Phonetic distinctions guide new word learning at 17 months.

■ The model is: phonetic categories > phonological processes > lexical-semantic use > reading and higher order language use. *Therefore, listening experience in infancy forms the basis for literacy development.*

To summarize, listening experience in infancy is critical for adequate language and literacy development. Anything we can do to access and "program" those critical and powerful auditory centers of the brain with acoustic detail will expand the infant/child's opportunities to acquire language and develop literacy skills. Amplification technology must be used to access the auditory centers of the brain of a child with hearing loss; there is no other way to reach those centers.

Practice, Practice, Practice

Skills mastered by the child as close as possible to the time of intended biological preprogramming results in developmental synchrony (Robbins et al., 2004). That is, children are organically receptive to developing specific skills during certain times of development. If those skills can be accessed and supported at the intended point in time, a developmental rather than a remedial paradigm of intervention will be in effect because we are working harmoniously with the child's structure. Furthermore, mastery of any developmental skill depends on *cumulative practice;* each practice opportunity builds on the last one. Therefore, the more delayed the age of acquisition of a skill, the farther behind children are in the amount of cumulative practice they have had to perfect that skill. The same concept holds true for cumulative auditory practice. Delayed auditory development leads to delayed language skills, and both deficits will necessitate using a remedial rather than a developmental paradigm of intervention.

The brain demands many practice opportunities to develop neural connections. Becoming expert in a skill means that the brain has developed specialized connections through repeated practice (Pugh, 2005, 2006). The amount of practice required to continually wire and rewire the brain for higher-order language skills and the acquisition of knowledge is enormous. Gladwell (2008), Levitin (2006), and others report 10,000 hours of practice are needed to become an expert in a particular skill. Hart and Risley (1999, 2003) report that, by the age of 4 years, children need to have heard 46 million words to be ready for school. Dehaene (2009) reports that 20,000 hours of listening are necessary in infancy and early childhood as a basis for reading.

Neuroplasticity, the ability of the brain to develop neural connections with repeated stimulation, is greatest during the first 3½ years of life; the younger the infant, the greater the neuroplasticity (Sharma et al., 2005). Because the infant brain develops its patterns of activity rapidly, prompt intervention in the case of hearing loss is required. Typically, this includes amplification and a program to promote auditory skill development. In the absence of sound, the brain organizes itself differently so as to receive input from other senses, primarily vision. This process, called "crossmodal reorganization," reduces auditory neural capacity. Early amplification or implantation stimulates a brain that has not yet been reorganized, allowing it to be more receptive to auditory input, resulting in greater auditory capacity. Importantly, early auditory access allows for the many auditory and language practice sessions the brain requires for the neural growth that serves as the foundation for literacy.

This chapter offers evidence that "hearing" is the most effective modality for the teaching of spoken language (speech), literacy, and other cognitive skills. Furthermore, with today's amplification technologies, cochlear implants, and early identification and intervention, auditory brain access, stimulation, and development are available for the vast majority of babies with even the most profound deafness.

Computer Analogy for Understanding Amplification Technology

One way to create a context for understanding the negative effects of any type and degree of hearing loss on a child's language and literacy development and to clarify the character of amplification technology is to use a computer analogy. The primary concept is: data input precedes data processing.

An infant or toddler must have information or data fed to the brain in order to learn. A primary avenue for information entering into the brain is through the ears, via hearing. So, the ears can be thought of as analogous to a computer keyboard, and the brain can be compared to the computer "hard drive." As human beings, we are wired neurologically to code sound and hence to develop spoken language and certain reading skills through the auditory centers of the brain, the "hard drive." Because auditory data input is critical, it is worth making detailed auditory information available as soon as possible to a child with any degree of hearing loss. If data are entered inaccurately, incompletely, or inconsistently—analogous to using a malfunctioning computer keyboard or to having one's fingers on the wrong keys of the computer keyboard—the child's brain/hard drive will have incorrect or incomplete information to process. Amplification technology such as hearing aids, personal FM systems, or sound field systems (now called classroom audio distribution systems—CADS) and biomedical devices such as cochlear implants can all be thought of as keyboards, as means of entering acoustic information to the child's hard drive. Technology can be viewed as a more efficient keyboard, although not a perfect one. Technology is only as effective as the use to which it is put, and only as efficient as the people who use it. Conversely, without the technology and quality acoustic data input, auditory brain access is not possible for persons who are deaf or hard of hearing.

Overview of Amplification Technologies— A New Context

The purpose of hearing aids is to make the speech spectrum as audible as possible within the constraints of the child's residual hearing. If hearing aids cannot permit soft speech to be clearly audible at distances, then a cochlear implant should be considered —if the family's desired outcome is listening and talking. Stated another way, the first step in attainable and sustainable listening, spoken language and literacy outcomes is acoustic accessibility to the brain via amplification technology. Everything we do regarding intervention and teaching a child with hearing loss is predicated on the fact that speech (as clear and intact as possible) is sent to the brain. Therefore, we must be mindful about the technology that makes brain access possible.

Poor auditory brain access due to less than optimum technology is probably the weakest link in intervention for today's children.

For Literacy Development, First Things First: Optimize Detection of the Complete Speech Spectrum by Using Technology and Environmental Management

Sounds arrive at the brain by passing through the environment, the auditory system, and ultimately through any technology worn by the child. An acoustically poor environment and/or unmanaged hearing loss of any degree prevent some or all sounds from reaching the brain, thereby interfering with the development of language, literacy, and academic competencies (ASHA, 2005).

Speech intelligibility is based on the science of signal-to-noise ratio (S/N ratio) . . . the relationship of the desired signal to all background/competing noise; children need the desired signal to be 10 times, or approximately 15 to 20 dB, louder than background noise in order to clearly discriminate words (ANSI 2010). Due to noise, reverberation, and variations in teacher position, the S/N ratio in a typical classroom is unstable and averages out to only about +4 dB and may be 0 dB, often less than ideal even for adults with normal hearing (Nelson & Blaeser, 2010; Smaldino, 2011).

To make possible the reception of intact spoken language and environmental sounds, the following must occur: control and management of the listening environment by reducing noise; favorable positioning of the speaker—whether parent, teacher or clinician—so he or she is always within earshot of the baby or child; and consistent use of the appropriate amplification—hearing aids, cochlear implants and/or FM systems (Boothroyd, 2004). The child's technology must be optimally fit and managed, or auditory brain access will be faulty.

Hearing Aids/Instruments

Hearing aids, also called hearing instruments, are typically the initial technology used to access sound for a baby or child who experiences a hearing loss. Hearing aids do not actually correct the hearing loss. Rather, they function to amplify and shape the incoming sounds to make them audible to the child. The hearing aid fit needs to be evaluated functionally (speech perception) as well as electroacoustically (real-ear measurements).

There are many excellent resources for detailed descriptions and discussions of hearing aids, cochlear implants and FM technologies. For more information, the reader is referred to Madell and Flexer (2008, 2011), Dillon (2012), and to the *Pediatric Amplification Guideline* (2004).

New Context for Hearing Instruments

There is a new context for hearing instruments in today's world. In the "olden days," hearing aids may have had a negative context, a visible declaration that something was wrong. The small size feature of the hearing instrument was emphasized with the subtext that the hearing loss should be concealed. Now, "earwear" or "ear gear" is very common, popular, and highly visible everywhere.

Children and adults often are observed with cords, buttons, flashing blue devices, cell phones, iPods, and so forth. dangling from their ears. Hearing aids and cochlear implants attached to ears and heads are no longer a unique proclamation that "something is wrong." This is the electronic and technological age where gadgets and devices are the rule rather than the exception. In fact, technology is typically viewed as connection and information access, especially by the younger generation that has been raised with electronic entrée to the world. Therefore, using electronic technology (such as hearing aids, FM systems, and cochlear implants) for information access makes a positive statement to today's world. The child is "handicapped" without the use of technology, not with it. Technology is not the problem; amplification technology is the solution.

Hearing Instrument Fitting Issues

Appropriate hearing aid fitting and validation is a complex and ongoing process that must be accomplished by a pediatric audiologist who has expertise in evaluating and managing infants. The *Pediatric Amplification Protocol* and the *Pediatric Amplification Guideline (2004)* address the many relevant issues of candidacy, preselection issues and procedures, hearing aid circuitry and signal processing, electroacoustic verification and functional validation of the hearing aid fitting, hearing instrument orientation and training, and follow-up and referral. For continual updating of pediatric fitting and validation protocols, you should refer to the American Academy of Audiology's website (http://www.audiology.org) and to Application of The University of Western Ontario Pediatric Audiological Monitoring Protocol 2011 (UWO PedAMP) (http://www.audiologist.org/_resources/documents/publications/audiology_practices_exerpts/Bagatto_AP_Quarter4_2011.pdf).

How successful amplification might be for a given child depends on several interactive factors: the child's residual or remaining hearing; the length of auditory deprivation experienced by the child; the quality of the hearing aid fit; the baby's age at amplification; the quality and quantity of auditory-based therapy; the ability of family, therapists, and teachers to create an "auditory world" of enrichment and embellishment for the child; and the use of necessary additional technologies such as an FM system with a remote microphone to facilitate incidental hearing and distance learning (Dillon, 2012).

Digital Hearing Instruments: Description and Terminology

There is much discussion about digital equipment for children. The advantage of digital instruments is their flexibility and more precise fit. Digital hearing instruments have a computer controlled sound processor inside the hearing aid. Traditional analog hearing instruments, that are mostly unavailable in this day and age, have a limited number of control options or else the options are pre-set and unavailable for manipulation.

The following terms often are used when discussing digital hearing aids. First is *advanced signal processing*. Advanced signal processing automatically adjusts the amount of amplification (gain) provided by the hearing aid according to the loudness of the sound reaching its microphone. So, softer sounds are amplified more than louder sounds and the *compression component* constantly adjusts the amount of gain available so that softer sounds can be more easily heard, while avoiding discomfort from louder sounds. Different signal processing configurations can vary the amount of compression, as well as the loudness level at which compression is activated, providing some benefit in noisy situations. Wide dynamic range compression may help children hear conversations at different listening distances.

The amount of gain (amplification) a hearing instrument provides at each frequency is called its *frequency response*. Digital hearing instruments divide the frequency response into two or more channels of control called *multichannel capability*. Each channel can be adjusted independently so that different advanced signal processing schemes can be applied to each frequency region.

Many digital hearing instruments have memory, allowing them to store more than one frequency response or program, called *multimemory capability*. Multiple memories allow the child, parent, teacher, or therapist to choose from different frequency responses and signal processing options with a remote control, or by pressing a button on the hearing instrument—or the hearing aid may have the ability to switch programs automatically. Multiple memories can be useful for children who communicate in many different listening situations or have fluctuating hearing losses. For example, for a child who often has otitis media (fluid in the middle ear), one program in the hearing aid might have added gain to allow the child better access to sound when her hearing loss has been made worse by the addition of middle ear fluid.

Some digital hearing instruments have separate microphone settings (*multimicrophone capability*) that allow the child to pick up sound either from a broad area (omnidirectional) or from a narrower listening range (directional microphone), analogous to a camera having both a wide angle and a zoom lens. In noisy listening situations, the directional microphone can somewhat suppress sounds that come from behind (usually competing noise), and that suppression may improve the child's ability to hear speech that comes from the front. The assumption is that the most desirable speech comes from the front and is close but such is not always the case for children. Some instruments will automatically switch between microphone modes depending on the listening environment.

Some digital instruments are designed to identify noise and automatically reduce the amplification in the frequency regions where it is detected. This *noise reduction capability* may provide the child with some improved ease of listening in background noise—but the remote microphone of an FM system is still necessary.

Frequency compression is a term that describes the electronic shift of higher frequencies to lower ones while also compressing them in a frequency domain that leaves the lower frequencies untouched. Frequency compression is designed to restore audibility of previously unheard high frequencies by shifting them to the lower frequency range where the child's residual hearing allows better access to sound. Some children with severe to profound high frequency hearing losses benefit from this fitting protocol.

Wireless connectivity to the environment and to electronic devices is an exciting advancement for hearing aid wearers (Schum, 2010). Bluetooth (BT) technologies are having a significant impact on developments of wireless assistive devices (Levitt, 2004). Bluetooth is a proprietary open wireless technology standard for exchanging data using short wavelength radio transmissions in the 2.4 GHz frequency range to link computers and other digital devices together; it offers flexibility and increased access to multiple technologies (Beck & Fabry, 2011). Even though BT is the primary wireless technology used in cell phones and other electronics, BT wireless transmission poses a problem for hearing aids because the size of the transmitters and receivers is large compared to the components of hearing aids. In addition, BT transmission has high power requirements that exceed the capabilities of hearing-aid-size batteries, and limited bandwidth relative to dedicated FM systems. The current solution is to use a body-worn gateway device that accepts signals from various formats such as BT, direct audio input and FM, converts the input signal to a digital magnetic signal and then sends the signal to a digital magnetic receiver that is integrated in the electronics of the hearing aid (Nyffeler & Dechant, 2010).

To overcome some of the BT limitations, the hearing aid industry has developed new *dedicated wireless digital signal processing devices* that allow hearing aids to communicate directly with a programming device, companion microphone, television, cell phones or a second hearing aid worn on the opposite ear (Beck & Fabry, 2011). These technologies offer improved ease of use, more attractive cosmetics, and better performance but still cause the hearing aid to have a shorter battery life and increased expense. Nevertheless, the vision is to provide a universal standard for connectivity that is low cost, easy to use, and effective (Jespersen, 2012).

An additional feature to consider for hearing aids is their compatibility with FM devices. All hearing instruments that are fitted on children ought to be *"bootable."* Bootable means they have direct audio input capability for attachment of FM receivers directly to the hearing aid.

Hearing Aid Styles

Hearing aid styles include *behind the ear* (BTE) also called *ear level,* the most suitable for children; in the ear (ITE), in the canal (ITC), and completely in the canal (CIC). The last three are not usually appropriate for children due in part, to the inability of these styles to connect to personal FM systems (they are not "bootable"), and also to continual ear canal growth. A fourth style is body-worn, once the rule for children, but now rarely used due to today's small and powerful BTE hearing aids. However, sometimes for infants, a body-style hearing aid can best accommodate the usual infant behaviors of lying down and drooling, as well as their small and soft ears and small ear canals.

To summarize, hearing aids/instruments for infants and children should be capable of being flexibly programmed for frequency response and power requirements. Initial fittings typically need to be adjusted as the child becomes a more reliable hearing test-taker and listener. Of particular import is that a child's hearing loss could change over time, and/or the child can experience fluctuating hearing losses. These situations demand adjustable hearing aids.

Functional Measures of a Child's Speech Perception Capabilities With and Without Wearing Hearing Instruments

Functional speech perception measures should be obtained regularly to verify the effectiveness of hearing instruments (hearing aids and cochlear implants) with and without FM attachment in order to (Johnson & Seaton, 2012):

a. demonstrate the child's response to speech for parent education purposes
b. monitor the child's auditory progress
c. assess speech perception at soft (e.g., 35 dB HL) and at average conversational levels (e.g., 50 dB HL) in quiet and in the presence of noise to evaluate the effectiveness of amplification technology. Each hearing aid should be evaluated separately and then both tested together.

Because the purpose of technology is to enhance speech perception, speech perception and other auditory performance validation measures should be made every time hearing aids, cochlear implants, or FM technologies are evaluated and reprogrammed (Bagatto, 2011; Madell & Flexer, 2008, 2011). In addition, assessment of speech audibility should be performed using the Ling 6 Sound Test at varying distances (e.g., 2 feet through 40 feet). Distance hearing capability is critical for overhearing conversations and should be monitored because incidental learning is vital for social and emotional as well as linguistic growth.

Personal-Worn FM Technology

A personal-worn FM unit is a wireless personal listening device that includes a remote microphone placed near the desired sound source (usually the speaker's mouth, but it could also be a DVD player or TV) and a receiver for the listener who can be situated anywhere within approximately 50 feet of the person talking. No wires are required to connect the talker and listener because the unit is really a small FM radio that transmits and receives on a single frequency. Because the talker wears the remote microphone within 6 inches of his or her mouth, the personal FM unit creates a listening situation that is comparable to a parent or teacher being within 6 inches of the child's ear at all times, thereby allowing a positive and constant S/N ratio (Nguyen & Bentler, 2011).

Personal FM units are essential for a child with any type and degree of hearing loss, from minimal to profound, who is in any classroom or group learning situation (Anderson et al, 2005; ASHA, 2000; Flynn, Flynn, & Gregory, 2005). The most common styles currently used include one in which the FM receiver is built into the ear-level hearing-aid case and another in which a small FM receiver boot is attached directly to the bottom of the ear-level hearing aid, or to a cochlear implant speech processor.

FM Use at Home

In the past, personal FM systems have been used for school-aged children in classroom settings; however, accumulating evidence suggests that children, including infants and toddlers, also can benefit from personal FM systems used at home. Moeller, Donaghy, Beauchaine, and Lewis (1996) compared two groups of children, one group that was encouraged to use an FM system at home, and another group that used hearing aids alone. The families that wore the FM systems at home were provided with training regarding how to operate the units. Subjective reports from parents suggested appropriate use of the FM at home facilitated effective communication in a variety of listening situations. Another reported advantage was that two of the children felt an increased sense of security when they could hear their parents from a distance.

Classroom Audio Distribution Systems — CADS (Sound-Field Technology)

Sound-field technology, now often called Classroom Audio Distribution Systems (CADS) is an effective educational tool that allows control of the acoustic environment in a classroom, thereby facilitating acoustic accessibility of teacher instruction for all children in the room (Smaldino & Flexer, 2012). A CADS looks like a wireless public address system, but it is designed specifically to ensure that the entire speech signal, including the weak high frequency consonants, reaches every child in the room. Through the use of this technology, an entire classroom can be amplified by one, two, three, or four wall- or ceiling-mounted loudspeakers.

CADS facilitates the reception of consistently more intact signals than those received in an unamplified classroom, but signals are not as complete as those provided by using a personal FM unit (Smaldino & Flexer, 2012). In addition, the equipment, must be installed appropriately, especially the loudspeakers, and teachers must be given in-service training about the rationale and effective use of the technology.

A primary value of CADS is that it can focus the children and facilitate attention to relevant information. To that end, the effective use of the sound system's microphone can be a powerful teaching tool. Teachers need to be shown how to use the microphone to create a listening attitude in the room; the purpose of the microphone is to quiet and focus the room, not to excite or distract the students.

In many instances, the best listening and learning environment can be created by using both a CADS infrared (IR) and a personal-worn FM system at the same time. The CADS IR unit, appropriately installed and used in a mainstreamed classroom, improves acoustic access for all pupils and creates a "listening" environment in the room. The individual personal-worn FM system allows the particular child with hearing loss to have the most favorable S/N ratio within that environment. So, the CADS focuses and quiets the environment, and the personal FM provides the best S/N ratio directly to the ear of the child. Care must be taken to appropriately integrate the technologies so they do not interfere with each other.

Hearing Assistance Technology (HAT) Guidelines (American Academy of Audiology, 2008)

The American Academy of Audiology's *Clinical Practice Guidelines for Remote Microphone Hearing Assistance Technologies for Children and Youth Birth–21 Years* (2008) provides a rationale and comprehensive protocol for devices that use remote micro-phones such as personal-worn FMs, CADS and Loop Systems. The protocol contains a core statement that addresses the complex process of HAT selection, fitting, and management plus supplements that outline procedures for fitting and verification of ear level FM (Supplement A) and classroom audio distribution systems (CADS) (Supplement B). A third supplement for personal neck loops is under development.

The guidelines discuss regulatory considerations and qualifications of personnel as well as candidacy, fitting and verification protocols. Monitoring and managing equipment is discussed in detail including procedures for checking systems to be sure they are working. Strategies for implementing guidelines in the schools are offered.

For access to the full document, please refer to: http://www.audiology.org/resources/documentlibrary/Documents/HATGuideline.pdf

Cochlear Implants

The cochlear implant is very different from a hearing aid; hearing aids amplify sound, but cochlear implants compensate for damaged or nonworking parts of the inner ear (Niparko, 2004; Wolfe & Schafer, 2010).

A cochlear implant is a surgically inserted biomedical device designed to provide sound information to children and adults who experience severe to profound hearing loss (ASHA 2004; Wilson & Dorman, 2012). The cochlear implant bypasses some of the damaged parts (typically the hair cells) of the inner ear; coded electrical signals stimulate different hearing nerve fibers that then send information to the brain. Hearing through an implant might sound different from typical hearing, but a properly inserted and programmed cochlear implant can allow many children to develop complete spoken communication skills if they receive appropriate early intervention (Segal & Kishon-Rabin, 2011).

Like the hearing aid and hearing assistance technologies (HAT) discussed previously, a cochlear implant is only a tool, analogous to a computer keyboard that improves "data entry" to the brain. The ultimate effectiveness of the tool, however, is determined largely by the type and degree of listening and spoken language therapy and education that follow implantation (Cole & Flexer, 2011; Moog & Geers, 2003; Wolfe & Shafer, 2010; Zwolan et al, 2004). Is the child placed in an environment that emphasizes spoken communication? Are listening skills systematically developed and practiced? What are the expectations for the child's ultimate use of the cochlear implant? Nicholas and Geers (2006) found that a key variable is the age of the baby or child at implantation. Those children who were implanted at the youngest ages when the brain has the most neuroplasticity developed the highest skills if they received appropriate auditory-based intervention. In addition, the benefits of bilateral implantation have been receiving increasing attention (Litovsky, 2008; Zheng et al, 2011).

Auditory Feedback Loop

The auditory feedback loop is the process of self-monitoring (input) and correcting one's own speech (output). Auditory feedback is crucial for the attainment of auditory goals and fluent speech (Perkell, 2008). That is, a child must be able to hear his or her own speech clearly in order to produce clear speech sounds. Improving the S/N ratio of the child's own speech can boost the salience of the speech signal.

To facilitate development of the child's auditory feedback loop, place the microphone of the FM system within 6 inches of the child's mouth when she is speaking or reading aloud. Because speaking and reading are interrelated, speaking into the FM microphone will highlight the child's speech and allow her to monitor and control her speaking and reading fluency.

Distance Hearing and Incidental Learning

Incidental learning through "overhearing" refers to times when the child listens to speech that is not directly addressed to him or her, and learns from it. Very young children learn a great deal of information unintentionally if they have access to overhearing conversations that occur at distances. Akhtar, Jipson and Callanan (2001) found that children as young as two years of age with typical hearing can acquire new words from overheard speech, showing the active role played by children in learning language. Further, Knightly et al. (2003) found that childhood overhearing helped improve speech perception and phonologic production of all languages heard.

Unfortunately, without appropriate technology, children with hearing losses, even minimal ones, have reduced overhearing potential because they cannot receive intelligible speech well over distances. This reduction in distance hearing, also called "earshot," can pose substantial problems for life and classroom performance because distance hearing is necessary for the passive/casual/incidental acquisition and use of spoken language. Therefore, a child's distance hearing needs to be extended as much as possible through the use of technology (Cole & Flexer, 2011; Ling, 2002).

New Context for the Word "Deaf"

In this day and age, hearing aids and/or cochlear implants and FM technology can allow infants and children with even the most profound hearing losses to have access to the entire speech spectrum. Indeed, there is no degree of hearing loss that prohibits access to sound if cochlear implants are available. Degree of hearing loss as a limiting factor in auditory acuity is now an "old" acoustic conversation. That is, when one uses the word "deaf," the implication is that one has no access to sound, period. The word "deaf" in 1970 occurred in a very different context than the word "deaf" used today. Today's child who is "deaf" without using technology may function like a child with a mild to moderate hearing loss when he or she is using hearing aids or a cochlear implant because critical neural connections have been developed through meaningful auditory stimulation. Therefore, the words used to express hearing loss may need to be reconsidered.

For this new generation of children with hearing loss, the degree of hearing loss ought not determine their functional outcome. These are the new hearing children.

Conclusion

The purpose of this chapter has been to create a context for the blending of technology and listening. Because of newborn hearing screening programs, infants are now receiving amplification at a very young age, often before one month of age. Consequently, we can access, stimulate, and grow the auditory neural system in ways that were not possible a few years ago. Auditory language enrichment can be provided during critical periods of maximum brain neural plasticity—the first few years of life. Therefore, this new generation of babies and young children who are born deaf have incredible possibilities for achieving higher levels of spoken language, reading skills, and academic competencies than were available to most children in previous generations.

The stimulation of "hearing" literally means the stimulation and growth of neural connections throughout the brain. The earlier we channel meaningful sounds to the brain and provide numerous listening and spoken language practice opportunities, the more dramatic will be brain growth due to neural plasticity. Thus, early identification followed by early fitting of technology and auditory management all are essential ingredients.

To conclude, current research confirms several facts for families who desire a spoken language outcome for today's infant or toddler who experiences profound deafness. Families need to know that very early use of hearing aids or the insertion of a cochlear implant for severe to profound degrees of hearing loss to access, stimulate, and grow auditory centers of the brain during times of critical neuroplasticity, followed by thoughtful, intense, and ongoing auditory skill development activities to take advantage of developmental synchrony and cumulative practice, offer a high probability of reaching their desired outcome of age-appropriate spoken language and literacy skills.

References

Akhtar, N., Jipson, J., & Callanan, M. A. (2001). Learning words through overhearing. *Child Development, 72*(2), 416–430.

American National Standards Institute. (S12.60-2010). *Acoustical Performance Criteria, Design Requirements, and Guidelines for Schools*. New York, NY: American National Standards Institute (ANSI S12.60).

American Speech-Language-Hearing Association. (2000). *Guidelines for fitting and monitoring FM systems*. Retrieved from http://www.asha.org/members/deskref-journals/deskref/default

American Speech-Language-Hearing Association. (2004). *Cochlear implants*. Retrieved from http://www.asha.org/members/deskref-journals/deskref/default

American Speech-Language-Hearing Association. (2005). *Guidelines for addressing acoustics in educational settings*. Retrieved from http://www.asha.org/members/deskref-journals/deskref/default

Anderson, K. (2004). The problem of classroom acoustics: The typical classroom soundscape is a barrier to learning. *Seminars in Hearing, 25*(2), 117–129.

Anderson, K. L., Goldstein, H., Colodzin, L., & Inglehart, F. (2005). Benefit of S/N enhancing devices to speech perception of children listening in a typical classroom with hearing aids or a cochlear implant. *Journal of Educational Audiology, 12*, 14–28.

Bagatto, M. P. (2011). Application of The University of Western Ontario Pediatric Audiological Monitoring Protocol (UWO PedAMP). *Audiology Practices, 3*(4), 40–46. Retrieved from http://www.audiologist.org/_resources/documents/publications/audiology_practices_exerpts/Bagatto_AP_Quarter4_2011.pdf

Bhatnagar, S. C. (2002). *Neuroscience for the study of communicative disorders, Second Edition*. Philadelphia, PA: Lippincott Williams & Wilkins.

Beck, D. L., & Fabry, D. (2011). Access America: It's about connectivity. *Audiology Today, 23*(1), 24–28.

Berlin, C. I., & Weyand, T. G. (2003). *The brain and sensory plasticity: Language acquisition and hearing*. Clifton Park, NY: Thompson Delmar Learning.

Bernhardt, B. M., Kemp, N., & Werker, J. F. (2007). Early word–object associations and later language development. *First Language, 27*(4), 315–328

Boothroyd, A. (1997). Auditory development of the hearing child. *Scandinavia Audiology, 26*(Suppl.46), 9–16.

Boothroyd, A. (2004). Room acoustics and speech perception. *Seminars in Hearing, 25*(2), 155–166.

Chermak, G. D., Bellis, J. B., & Musiek, F. E. (2007). Neurobiology, cognitive science, and intervention. In G. D. Chermak & F. E. Musiek (Eds.), *Handbook of central auditory processing disorder: Comprehensive intervention, Volume II* (pp. 3–28). San Diego, CA: Plural.

Cole, E. & Flexer, C. (2011). *Children with hearing loss: Developing listening and talking, birth to six* (2nd ed.). San Diego, CA: Plural.

Dehaene, S. (2009). *Reading in the brain: The science and evolution of a human invention.* New York, NY: Penguin Group.

Dillon. H. (2012). *Hearing aids* (2nd ed.). New York, NY: Thieme Medical.

Doidge, N. (2007). *The BRAIN that changes itself.* London, UK: Penguin Books.

Flynn, T. S., Flynn, M. C., & Gregory, M. (2005). The FM advantage in the real classroom. *Journal of Educational Audiology, 12,* 35–42.

Gladwell, M. (2008). *Outliers: The story of success.* New York, NY: Little, Brown and Company.

Hart, B., & Risley, T. R. (1999). *The social world of children learning to talk.* Baltimore, MD: Brookes.

Hart, B., & Risley, T. R. (2003). *The early catastrophe: The 30 million word gap by age four.* Retrieved from http://www.aft.org/newspubs/period icals/ae/spring2003/hart.cfm

Jespersen, C. T. (2012). A review of wireless hearing aid advantages. *Hearing Review, 19*(2), 48–54.

Johnson, C. D. & Seaton. J. (2012). *Educational audiology handbook* (2nd ed.). Park, NY: Delmar-Cengage Learning.

Joint Committee on Infant Hearing. (2007). Year 2007 position statement: Principles and guidelines for early hearing detection and intervention programs. *Pediatrics, 102*(4), 893–921.

Knightly, L. M., Jun, S. A., Oh, J. S., & Au, T. K. (2003). Production benefits of childhood overhearing. *Journal of the Acoustical Society of America, 114*(1), 465–474.

Leavitt, H. (2004). Assistive listening technology: What does the future hold? *Volta Voices, 11*(1), 18–21.

Leibold, L. J., & Neff, D. (2011). Masking by remote-frequency noise band in children and adults. *Ear and Hearing, 32*(5), 663–666.

Levitin, D. J. (2006). *This is your brain on music: The science of a human obsession* (p. 233). New York, NY: Plume.

Ling, D. (2002). *Speech and the hearing impaired child* (2nd ed.). Washington, DC: Alexander Graham Bell Association of the Deaf and Hard of Hearing.

Litovsky, R.Y. (2008). *Benefits of bilateral hearing in children with cochlear implants.* Paper presented at the 2008 Research Symposium of the Alexander Graham Bell Association International Convention, Milwaukee, Wisconsin, June 29, 2008.

Madell, J. R., & Flexer, C. (2008). *Pediatric audiology: Diagnosis, technology, and management.* New York, NY: Thieme Medical.

Madell, J. R., & Flexer, C. (2011). *Pediatric audiology casebook.* New York, NY: Thieme Medical.

Moeller, M. P., Donaghy, K. F., Beauchaine, K. L., Lewis, D. E., & Stelmachowicz, P.G. (1996). Longitudinal study of FM system use in nonacademic settings: Effects on language development. *Ear and Hearing, 17*(1), 28–41.

Moog, J. S., & Geers, A. E. (2003). Epilogue: Major findings, conclusions and implications for deaf education. *Ear and Hearing, 24*(1S), 121S–125S.

Nelson, P. B., & Blaeser, S. B. (2010). Classroom acoustics: What possibly could be new? *ASHA Leader, 15*(11), 16–19.

Nguyen, H, & Bentler, R. (2011). Optimizing FM systems. *ASHA Leader, 16*(12), 5–6.

Nicholas, J. G., & Geers, A. E. (2006). Effects of early auditory experience on the spoken language of deaf children at three years of age. *Ear and Hearing, 27*(3), 286–298.

Niparko, J. K. (2004). Cochlear implants: Clinical application. In F. G. Zeng, A. Popper, & R. Fay (Eds.), *Cochlear implants: Auditory prosthesis and electric hearing* (pp. 53–100). New York, NY: Springer-Verlag.

Nyffeler, M., & Dechant, S. (2010). The impact of new technology on mobile phone use. *Hearing Review, 17*(3), 42–49.

Pediatric Amplification Guideline: Position Statement of the American Academy of Audiology. (2004*). Audiology Today, 16*(2), 46–53.

Perkell, J. S. (2008). *Auditory feedback and speech production in cochlear implant users and speakers with typical hearing.* Paper presented at the 2008 Research Symposium of the Alexander Graham Bell Association International Convention, Milwaukee, Wisconsin, June 29, 2008.

Pugh, K. (2005). *Neuroimaging studies of reading and reading disability: Establishing brain–behavior relations.* Paper presented at the Literacy and Language Conference at the Speech, Language and Learning Center, Beth Israel Medical Center, New York, NY, November 30, 2005.

Pugh, K. R., Sandak, R., Frost, S. J., Moore, D., & Mencl, W. E. (2006). Neurobiological investigations of skilled and impaired reading. In D. K. Dickinson & S. B. Neuman (Eds.), *Handbook of early literacy research* (Vol. II). New York, NY: Guilford.

Robbins, A. M., Koch, D. B., Osberger, M. J., Zimmerman-Philips, S., & Kishon-Rabin, L. (2004). Effect of age at cochlear implantation on auditory skill development in infants and toddlers. *Archives of Otolaryngology-Head and Neck Surgery, 130*(5), 570–574.

Schum, D. J. (2010). Wireless connectivity for hearing aids. *Advance for Audiologists, 12*(2), 24–26.

Segal, O., & Kishon-Rabin, L. (2011). Listening preference for child-directed speech versus nonspeech stimuli in normal-hearing and hearing-impaired infants after cochlear implantation. *Ear and Hearing, 32*(3), 358–372.

Sharma, A., Martin, K., Roland, P., Bauer, P., Sweeney, M. H., Gilley, P., & Dorman, M. (2005). P1 latency as a biomarker for central auditory development in children with hearing impairment. *Journal of the American Academy of Audiology, 16*, 564–573.

Shaywitz, S. E., & Shaywitz, B. A. (2004). Disability and the brain. *Educational Leadership, 61*(6), 7–11.

Smaldino, J. (2011). New developments in classroom acoustics and amplification. *Audiology Today, 23*(1), 30–36.

Smaldino, J., & Flexer, C. (2012). *Handbook of acoustic accessibility: Best practices for listening, learning, and literacy in the classroom.* New York, NY: Thieme Medical.

Strickland, D. S., & Shanahan, T. (2004). Laying the groundwork for literacy. *Educational Leadership, 61*(6), 74–77.

Tallal, P. (2004). Improving language and literacy is a matter of time. *Nature Reviews Neuroscience, 5,* 721–728.

Vouloumanos, A. & Werker, J. F. (2007). Listening to language at birth: Evidence for a bias for speech in neonates. *Developmental Science, 10*(2), 159–164.

Waltzman, S. (2005). Expanding patient criteria for cochlear implantation. *Audiology Today, 17*(5), 20–21.

Werker, J. (2006). *Infant speech perception and early language acquisition.* Paper presented at the 4th Widex Congress of Paediatric Audiology, Ottawa, Canada, May 19–21, 2006.

Werker, J. F., & Byers-Heinlein, K. (2008). Bilingualism in infancy: First steps in perception and comprehension. *Trends in Cognitive Sciences, 12*(4), 144–151.

Wilson, B., & Dorman, M. (2012). *Better hearing with cochlear implants: Studies at the Research Triangle Institute.* San Diego, CA: Plural.

Wolfe, J., & Schafer, E. (2010). *Programming cochlear implants.* San Diego, CA: Plural.

Zheng, Y., Koehnke, J., Besing, J., & Spitzer, J. (2011). Effects of noise and reverberation on virtual sound localization for listeners with bilateral cochlear implants. *Ear and Hearing, 32*(5), 569–572.

Zwolan, T. A., Ashbaugh, C. M., Alarfaj, A., Kileny, P. R., Arts, H. A., El-Kashlan, H. K., & Telian, S. A. (2004). Pediatric cochlear implant patient performance as a function of age at implantation. *Otology and Neurotology, 25*(2), 112–120.

Chapter 4

SPOKEN LANGUAGE

The links between the child's development of spoken language and the child's subsequent development of literacy are becoming increasingly well understood . . . the child's phonological development—the progression in representing in the brain the speech units that make up different words—is now recognized to play a causal role in the acquisition of literacy.

Goswami, 2002, p. 111

Introduction

The development of spoken language is of primary importance, as one cannot comprehend language whose underlying structures are not in memory waiting for retrieval. Greater oral language knowledge is associated with more semantic knowledge and is represented in vocabulary and syntactic knowledge. Children with limited memory structures (schemata) read less well than children with much spoken language and experience in their backgrounds (Whitehurst & Lonigan, 2002, p. 19). As reading progresses, children begin to be able to add to their oral language by reading, but a sufficient knowledge of oral language is necessary for the process to begin. How much is sufficient? The average five- or six-year-old with typical hearing knows the structures of his or her spoken language, and then spends a lifetime filling in hundreds of thousands of the words possible in the language. About this time, the average child with typical hearing comprehends 14,000 words (Dollaghan, C. as cited in Goswami, 2002, p. 113). Unless deprived in some way, children with typical hearing are thought to be ready to learn to read at about age six, having established this enormous base of spoken language. At this point, they can converse in complete sentences; comprehend, remember, and formulate stories they have heard using their own words; interact with some words in print; pretend to read and write; and use some invented spellings that they remember and assign meaning to (Ruddell & Ruddell, 1994, p. 83).

Learning the Sounds of a Spoken Language

Adams concludes that much of the aforementioned language use is done unconsciously: "For purposes of listening to language, therefore, it is fortunate that the processing of subunits—phonemes, syllables, and words—is automatic" (1990, p. 294), and "Deep down in the machinery of our brains and long before we get to school, each of us has established a thorough familiarity with the phonemes of our language" (1990, p. 65). But Adams is writing about children with typical hearing who have learned language without much deliberate work on the part of the adults in their lives. For the child with hearing loss, sufficient intentional interactions with people using well-formed spoken language must be taking place so that such listening and speaking processing is on its way to becoming automatic. Listening must develop to the extent that the child is aware of the syllables within words when they are spoken to him or her; speaking obviously involves producing the sounds and syllables in conventional order. Learning to do this happens over time. Most of us probably know a child with typical hearing who refers to "spaghetti" as "basghetti." The refinement that comes with experience enables the child to sort out the order of the sounds and then produce them in conventional adult ways.

Interestingly, being able to count syllables in spoken words is a strong predictor of whether a child will learn to read. Doing so probably represents the conscious ability to distinguish sounds from meaning, which allows for developing the alphabetic principle that sounds and symbols connect with one another. As listening and speaking progress, a working knowledge of the language system develops (Adams, 1990, pp. 300–301, 412). This working knowledge must be examined consciously in the process of learning to read. Well-developed oral language is also associated with phonological knowledge: the more words that are known, the greater the necessity of remembering them according to their parts, as the same word parts are found in flexible arrangements and rearrangements across the spoken language (Whitehurst & Lonigan, 2002, p. 19). Lexical restructuring theory (Metsala, 1999, Metsala & Walley, 1998) is proposed as a way of describing the process of learning to segment and specify what one hears. As the number of words in the child's vocabulary increases, the ways they are stored in memory must become increasingly efficient and compartmentalized so that the child can tell them apart when listening to them. According to Goswami (2002):

> There is considerable developmental pressure to represent these words in the brain in a way that will distinguish them from other words and allow the child to recognize them accurately and quickly during speech comprehension. For example, a 2-year-old probably knows the words "cot," "cat" and "cut," "hot," "not," and "lot," and "cough." All these words differ from "cot" by a single phoneme. To distinguish between these similar-sounding words both quickly and accurately, child linguists argue that children must begin to represent the sequences of sounds that constitute each known word in their brains. They must represent the "segmental phonology" of the words they know. (p. 113)

This "segmental phonology" represents knowledge of syllables in terms of their sounds. Without the discovery of such knowledge, a child's reading is stalled at a place of memorizing whole words as a word identification strategy (Snow, Burns, & Griffin, 1998, p. 54).

The flip side of this is in speech production, that is, in using the memory of the sounds to produce them in speech. None of this happens easily without knowing many words (Snow, Tabors, & Dickinson, 2001, p. 3). A growing vocabulary demands the recognition and segmentation of word parts in order to make the words distinguishable from one another. This segmentation is thought to underlie the phonological awareness that is linked to learning to read (Goswami, 2002, p. 114). At least one study reports that children can be taught to be aware of phonemes, the smallest sounds that distinguish one word from another, and to connect these sounds with alphabetic letters. The children in this study showed improved early reading and spelling skills compared to a control group (Ball & Blackman, 1991). The need for building these memory processes is the basis of a very strong argument for presenting the child who has hearing loss with spoken language, spoken language analysis, and constant opportunities to converse in a particular spoken language.

Beyond the Sounds of Language

Language is more than sounds, of course, and the content of the language used with children is very important. A study reported by Beals, De Temple, and Dickinson (1994) distinguishes between "immediate" and "nonimmediate" talk offered by mothers in low-income families reading to their children. "Immediate" talk focuses only on the book itself, and "nonimmediate" talk involves explaining characters' behavior, the meanings of words, making inferences and predictions, and making connections between the content of the book and the individual child's world (pp. 23–24). The greater the amount and proportion of "non-immediate" talk during book reading at age three, the better the children scored later on the Concepts About Print test (p. 35). The amount of "non-immediate" talk at age four also correlated positively with story comprehension and Peabody Picture Vocabulary Test scores at age five (p. 36). The study also investigated talk at mealtimes between children and their parents, and utterances were coded as "explanation" when they made connections between different kinds of information and "narrative" when they referred to a past or future event. The authors found that more explanatory and narrative talk provided to the four-year-olds resulted in larger receptive vocabularies at age five, and those who experienced more "narrative" talk achieved higher listening comprehension scores (p. 35). It is clear that talk that stretches children's thinking beyond the here and now provides them with cognitive challenges that help them increase their facility with all facets of language and word knowledge.

These findings demonstrate why a child with hearing loss should be able to hold meaningful spoken conversations with an adult and with peers before being instructed in reading. The work of establishing spoken language should be done first so as to provide the thinking and comprehension using language that one does when reading. Generally, a child can first understand what someone else says and then begin to produce similar utterances on his or her own, learning the language system through trial and error by using it for authentic communication. Language and reading acquisition spiral up through successively difficult structures of language until the control over vocabulary, syntax, and phonology that signal mature use of language in both spoken and written forms is achieved. At the beginning, children should not be presented with written words and their isolated sounds that have no meaning for them. Instead, they should be learning to read what they are able to listen to and speak with understanding. This makes it possible for them to make meaningful predictions based on vocabulary, word order, word sounds, and personal experience.

What About Bridging from American Sign Language?

American Sign Language (ASL) and other modes of signing are fine languages through which people can communicate beautifully and effectively. These languages follow established grammatical rules, they are passed down from parent to child, and they function very well culturally in establishing an individual's identity and in drawing together members of the Deaf community.

Proponents of teaching children American Sign Language as a first language argue that a spoken language can be learned through learning to read it, building their assertion from the general precept that establishing language is the essential criterion for the development of reading (Mayer & Wells, 1996, p. 93). This argument does not differentiate between audible and visual language. As can be seen in Chapter 13, it is well established that a secure and well-developed knowledge of a spoken first language provides a bridge to a spoken second language, yet it remains to be seen whether this can happen easily in producing a high level of achievement when the bridging is from a visual language to a spoken language. People have been using this theory in working with children for at least several decades, and average and median reading levels in these students have still not risen above fourth grade. Something is preventing acquisition of advanced levels of reading in this population, and I have come to understand the problem as stemming from an incomplete knowledge of the spoken language that will be read; one must know the spoken language, and know it very well, in order to learn to read it at high levels.

Imagine trying to learn to read Spanish at the same time you are learning Spanish. If you already know how to listen to English, you have an advantage, but if you do not know any spoken language, you are at a distinct disadvantage, as you must learn the mode as well as the system simultaneously.

Next is the matter of syntax. ASL does not use the same word or concept order as English or other spoken languages, so learning to read the spoken language is not a simple case of learning that a particular sign stands for a particular set of letters. Words in spoken languages are not interchangeable, either; translations from one spoken language to another are not one-to-one substitutions, and they often just provide a gist of the original intent. Words are ordered differently in different languages. "La Tour Eiffel" in French is "the Eiffel Tower" in English. "She's hungry" translates to the French, "Elle a faim," which literally is "She has hunger." A French person who wants to say, "I suspected it," says, "Je m'en doutais," whose literal translation is "I to myself about it doubted." "They miss their parents" is "Leurs parents leur manquent," or "Their parents to them are lacking" (O'Keefe, C., personal communication).

Yet another difficulty is the "window of opportunity" for learning language. If we wait to teach a child the spoken language until the age of five, six, or seven when reading is presented ordinarily to children, we are by then working with a closing "window" for acquiring spoken language. Children who have begun learning multiple languages by this age are more likely to become truly bilingual or multilingual than are individuals who attempt to learn a second language beginning in middle or high school. You might reflect on the ease of learning, or lack thereof, that you experienced if you first spoke English and then began studying Spanish, French, German, or any other spoken language after the age of 12.

The concept of shifting a child from a visual language to a spoken language is a difficult matter, involving more than study of what the brain can do in terms of language, as it is also a matter of identity and sociocultural values.

Despite all I have written here, I hope that people interested in helping children use ASL as a bridge to a spoken language will do more work and research toward the efficacy of this approach. Even though I am a proponent of spoken language, I have no objection if this way can be made to work in behalf of literacy.

Learning Spoken Language

Spoken language is learned in extended interaction with those who speak the language, usually from parents and other family members, and many sources document the need for the richest language environments possible from the earliest moments possible. (See, for example, International Reading Association and National Association for the Education of Young Children, 1998; Hart & Risely, 1995; Snow, Burns, & Griffin, 1998.) Children learn to attend to the utterances addressed to them as early as people start speaking to them. From the moment someone picks up an infant and starts cooing with him or her, the baby begins to learn about language. Usually, eye contact is established, and the baby responds with several kinds of baby sounds. The adult coos back, and the baby begins to learn how conversations work. This is the social interaction facilitative of language described by Vygotsky (D'Arcangelo, 2000). As time goes on, the adult involved begins using words and referencing objects and actions in the environment, all of which the infant is taking in and responding to. Gradually, the baby develops control over the musculature of speaking and begins to say approximations of the words heard in the environment. Over time, these approximations begin to become more accurate representations of adult speech. But young children are not just learning to copy what they hear. They are hard at work discovering how the language system works, and so they try out various ways to express themselves, seeking to make themselves understood. Rather than imitating exactly what they hear, they appear to be imitating "people's method for going about saying things" (Britton, 1993, p. 42).

Chomsky posits that infants are born with an inherent capacity to acquire language (a language acquisition device) and that development depends on being presented with ways to use language, all as material to work with in figuring out the rules of the language (Ormrod, 2008, pp. 49–50). Children make charming utterances as they go about this. For example, some children produce the word "amn't," even though they have never heard anyone say it. They are generalizing from learning that one can put "can" and "not" together and get the word "can't" and "should" and "not" together and get "shouldn't," and so they put "am" and "not" together and get "amn't." They'll use it for a while, but it will drop out of their language as they unconsciously discover that other people do not use it. My son created the phrase, "No me don't" when he was about 18 months old. He had not heard anyone say it; he was just using what he had available to him at the time to say he didn't want to do something. In this case, he had not caught on to how "I" and "me" are used as subject and object, so he used "me" as a subject. Several months later, he was able to say, "No, I don't want to," having gained more control over both conventional grammar and syntax.

All these discoveries children make about language in part may involve being corrected by an older person, but mainly appear to be the result of experimenting in the midst of frequent conversational exchanges with people who already know the language. Learning a spoken language, therefore, involves discovering the conventions of the language, including how words are pronounced and how sounds are put into sequences (phonology), the use of certain kinds of words for particular functions (grammar), the meanings of words and word parts (semantics), and word order (syntax). Children who are listening through the benefit of hearing technology go through the same processes of language development as children with typical hearing, although it may take them longer to do so, depending upon the quality of their listening conditions and auditory input. Missing out on speech sounds slows the process, whether the sounds are missing due to diminished hearing or to lack of opportunity to listen. It is not enough just to provide the equipment; the child with hearing loss, even when aided optimally, who does not have frequent spoken interactions will have trouble with spoken language acquisition.

Two Extended Studies of Children's Language Learning and Later Academic Achievement

As I have discussed, deprivation of language results in lesser literacy and other academic achievement. Obviously, such deprivation happens when a child does not hear adequately and does not receive enough auditory training and language intervention. Children in poverty situations often suffer from similar sorts of less-than-optimal language environments when they grow up in chaotic conditions in which they do not have consistent opportunities to converse with and learn from adults and others who use the language needed as the basis for literacy. As you will see below, those of us interested in the language development of children who are deaf or hard of hearing can learn much from studies that have included children in poverty, as the language and academic outcomes of children in these two groups are, on average, similarly low compared to children who develop foundational spoken language capabilities at developmentally appropriate times in their lives.

Dickinson and Tabors

Dickinson and Tabors (2001) reported on the Home-School Study of Language and Literacy Development, their study of the home and preschool environments of 74 children with typical hearing growing up in low-income families. Their particular interest was the children's language and literacy development by the end of the kindergarten year of school, as such development is predictive of later achievement.

The families selected for the study spoke English at home and met certain income requirements, qualification for Head Start, for example. Children were Caucasian ($n = 47$), African American ($n = 16$), Latino ($n = 6$), and biracial ($n = 5$). When the study began, the children were three years old. Twenty-eight lived with their mothers, 40 with two adults, and 6 with as many as five adults in the household. Most had one or more siblings, with 18 being single children at the time (Dickinson & Tabors, 2001, p. 7). Visits were made to the children's homes on a yearly basis beginning at age three and extending to age five. Using audiotape, investigators recorded the mothers and children interacting while reading books, telling stories, and playing games. Interviews were conducted with the mothers during which they were asked about their lives and their family's activities. Mothers were asked to audiotape a family meal, as well. Visits were made to preschools once a year when the children were three and four years old, and audiotapes were made of the children in group meeting time, large group story time, small groups led by teachers, free play, meal times, and transitions between activities (Dickinson & Tabors, 2001, pp. 8–10).

At age five, each child's language and literacy attainment was assessed using the School-Home Early Language and Literacy Battery-Kindergarten (SHELL-K). The SHELL-K includes narrative production (telling a story about three pictures in sequence), picture description, definitions (answering the question, "What's a _____?"), identifying superordinates ("What are tables and chairs?" in order to elicit a word such as "furniture"), story comprehension in response to questions, emergent literacy as determined by five subtests of The Comprehensive Assessment Program, and receptive vocabulary as measured by the Peabody Picture Vocabulary Test-Revised (Dickinson & Tabors, 2001, pp. 10–12).

The results of this study enable Dickinson and Tabors to predict that children achieve more in narrative production, emergent literacy, and receptive vocabulary when they are exposed to a "high home-high preschool language and literacy environment" (pp. 325–328). A low home–high preschool environment is next best, followed by high home–low preschool and finally low home–low preschool. A "high" environment is language-rich; a "low" environment offers little language. For our purposes, these demonstrated differences mean making sure the child with hearing loss is in high preschool language and literacy environments throughout the day and evening.

Notably, Dickinson and Tabors report, "We also found evidence suggesting that children benefit from hearing conversations that other children have with their teachers" (2001, p. 330). This finding suggests that children with hearing loss would benefit by learning from an early age to interact with people of all ages in using spoken language, and provides support for putting these children in school settings with children with typical hearing. For this to happen optimally, it is necessary to provide children the highest quality audiologic technology available and to make sure it is working at its best. Conscious thought and care must be given to creating environments in which children with and without hearing loss need to communicate frequently with each other and with their teachers by using spoken language.

Hart and Risely

Hart and Risely (1995) conducted a frequently cited study in which they sought to find out whether there is anything that parents of children with typical hearing do in the home that influences the future development of their children's vocabulary. Before doing this particular study, they had attempted to increase the vocabularies of preschool children from families in poverty in three ways: (1) setting up a home-like environment in the school and engaging children in talk; (2) taking children on field trips to increase their experiential base; and (3) taking children on field trips and engaging them in small group discussions before and after the trips. In all these situations, they found they could increase the children's vocabularies by teaching them new words, but that the interventions did not influence the children's vocabulary growth after those direct teaching experiences ended (Hart & Risley, 1995, p. 15). They decided they needed to find out what parents and children were doing and saying at home, even before the children's preschool years began.

The study focused on 42 well-functioning families described as professional ($n = 13$), working-class ($n = 23$), and welfare ($n = 6$). Observers visited each family once a month and recorded the talk that took place in the household during the period of one hour. Tapes were transcribed and coded for analysis. In a subsequent publication concerning the study, Hart and Risley report:

> . . . our estimates showed that by the time the children were 4 years old, the average child in a welfare family would have had 13 million fewer words of cumulative language experience than the average child in a working class family. (1999, p. 170)

Thinking about millions of words spoken to a child seems staggering, yet spread over four years it seems possible. In fact, the cumulative number of words used in the professional families was extrapolated to be almost 45 million, based on the assumption that children were usually awake for a 14-hour day. For working class families, the number of words came to 26 million, and for the welfare families, 13 million, yielding an estimated 32-million word difference between the highest and lowest amounts of speaking during the four-year period (Hart & Risley, 1995, p. 198). Hart and Risley expressed the differences among the families in terms of words per hour addressed to children by parents: an average of 2,100 in the professional families, 1,200 in the working class families, and 600 in the welfare families (Hart & Risley, 1999, p. 169). The sheer volume of words, measured in this study as "amount of parent–child interaction per hour," appears to be important to cognitive development, yet judged to be even more important is the amount of talk that goes beyond the talk parents use to control the behavior of the child. Hart and Risley found that parents of all economic levels used about the same amount of controlling language ("initiations, imperatives, and prohibitions," p. 170), but that the talk of the parents in welfare families was often limited to that directive kind of talk ("Look at this . . . Do this . . . Don't do that"). In describing the kind of talk that seems to make the difference for children, they write:

> The extra talk of parents in the professional families and that of the most talkative parents in the working-class families contained more of the varied vocabulary, complex ideas, subtle guidance, and positive feedback thought to be important to cognitive development. (Hart & Risley, 1999, p. 170)

They go on to observe that, "parents who talked a lot about such things or only a little ended up with 3-year-olds who also talked a lot, or only a little" (1999, p. xii). The work of these researchers is of great importance to us in that they have found an explanatory basis for the large and enduring differences in literacy and academic achievement usually seen between groups of children from families in different economic circumstances.

> The data show that the first 3 years of experience put in place a trajectory of vocabulary growth and the foundations of analytic and symbolic competencies that will make a lasting dif-

ference to how children perform in later years. (Hart & Risley, 1999, p. 193)

In general, the literacy outcomes for children with typical hearing who hear and use less spoken language at early ages are lower than the outcomes for children who experience a rich language environment. In one study of children with typical hearing, spoken language ability at preschool age has been found to predict reading ability in second grade (Scarborough, 1989). Oral language skills are regarded by both reading researchers and child language researchers to both predict and cause particular levels of reading achievement. The greater the preschool child's oral language skill, the more confidence one can have that once the child enters first grade, reading will develop normally. Lesser oral language skill predicts and is regarded as causing lower reading achievement (Snow, Scarborough, & Burns, 1999, p. 50).

"Advantaged" and "Disadvantaged" Parents

An interesting question involves the effect of the parent's understanding of his or her role in supporting and stimulating the child's language learning. We could extend this question to ask whether similar effects result from teachers' understanding of their roles. What differences do the parents' and teachers' attitudes make? How do attitudes and beliefs about deafness shape the expectations of the parent? Do they cause a parent or teacher to relate one way or another way with the child? What happens when a parent's or teacher's expectations are low? What are the implications for parents' and teachers' interactions with each other on behalf of the child?

Schlesinger (1988) studied the ways mothers interacted with their children by observing two groups: mothers with typical hearing and their preschool children with profound hearing loss ($n = 40$) and mothers with typical hearing and their preschool children with typical hearing ($n = 20$). The children with hearing loss had "no additional handicaps, had normal intellectual potential, and were from intact English-speaking families" (p. 265). Schlesinger was interested in learning about the language outcomes in children in relation to two frequently observed parent communication styles, observing that some parents try to *communicate* with children by using speech, and some parents try to *control* children by using speech. Furthermore, Schlesinger was interested in parents she labeled as "advantaged" and "disadvantaged." "Advantaged" parents feel they have control over important aspects of their lives; these parents are more apt to use speech to communicate with their children. "Disadvantaged" parents are more likely to use speech to try to control their children's behaviors. Although some of these parental feelings are associated with economic well-being, the descriptor is not limited to the parent's financial situation. Appreciation for education, books in the home, and hope for the future that parents of any income can have add to the security that marks "advantage."

In controlling the child, the "disadvantaged" parent keeps conversation with the child in the "here and now," uses words to issue commands, drills the child on the recitation of colors, numbers, letters, shapes, and so on. Rote memory and certain answers to particular questions are often the goal. "Disadvantaged" parents may be well-meaning as they attempt to equip their children with what they need to know in order to survive, but they are not assisting their children in developing a flexible and wide-ranging ability to deal with the many ways people use language, and they are not equipping their children with the capacity for generating ever more unique utterances. We know this to be the case all too often for children with typical hearing in impoverished situations (see, for example, Hart & Risley, 1995, 1999; Heath, 1994; Snow & Ninio, 1986).

Schlesinger observed that, in trying to communicate with their children with deafness, otherwise "advantaged" parents can become similarly "disadvantaged":

> . . . many parents of deaf (and other disabled) children feel powerless because their children differ from them, because the future of their 'different' children looms uncertain in their minds, and because their usual parenting practices do not result in expected behaviors on the part of their children. (1988, p. 263)

When parents use this frame of reference, they limit themselves to simple statements and commands they are sure will be heard and understood, and so they talk *to*, rather than *with* their children. Consequently, their children do not have access to sufficient spoken language interaction that would foster figuring out how the language works. In this case, the parent is trying to gain control in the situation by attempting to "give" the child useful language, all the while not realizing that it is the child's own developmental work to construct an understanding of the spoken language within a linguistically rich environment. Children, with and without typical hearing, can get stuck in having only one word for an object or a motion, in not being able to categorize and apply labels to categories of subordinate groupings, in not being able to talk about the past and the future, in only being able to label concrete aspects of their environment, and in not having language for feelings and speculations (Schlesinger, 1988, pp. 264–268). The limitations of their environment may result in their not learning effective ways to generate their own utterances.

Schlesinger's study of children and their mothers talking with one another when the children were toddlers and at ages 5, 8, and 16 yielded a positive relationship between "advantaged" talk and reading achievement at adolescence for both children with typical hearing and children with hearing loss. The parents of children with deafness who were able to shake off their "disadvantage" were more capable of providing them with an environment in which to discover and build their language capabilities. Examples of this would involve asking more complex questions than, "what/who/where is this?" The progression to questions of "why?" "when?" and "how?" provides for more complex thought and the necessity for more words and language structures. The importance of this cannot be overstated; according to Schlesinger, "those in our study who failed *why* questions at the age of 8 'failed' reading at adolescence" (1988, p. 285). The child who is an active, thinking participant in learning spoken language is simply more likely to develop the language foundation necessary for learning to read and write.

Conclusion

For our children with hearing loss, the historical difficulty, of course, has been in establishing the hearing that makes listening possible. The pioneers in auditory-verbal therapy had good success in helping many children learn to listen, even though they had primitive technology, but not all children were able to make use of such minimal cues. Over 20 years ago, one successful auditory verbal adult with profound hearing loss who wore only hearing aids told me he thought what he was hearing was probably what hearing people call whispering, and that is how he operated in the hearing world day in and day out. Today's difference is that advanced technology makes it possible for almost all children to hear with relative ease, at least compared to that adult. Such ease translates into learning to listen and learning to speak. With technology and early intervention in the form of natural human conversation, we can give children with hearing loss the access to the millions of utterances they need to hear and the millions of verbal interactions they need to have before age four in order to be ready to learn to read.

References

Adams, M. (1990). *Beginning to read*. Cambridge, MA: MIT Press.

Ball, E., & Blackman, B. (1991). Does phoneme awareness training in kindergarten make a difference in early word recognition and developmental spelling? *Reading Research Quarterly, 26*(1), 49–66.

Beals, D., De Temple, J., & Dickinson, D. (1994). Talking and listening that support early literacy development of children from low-income families. In D. Dickinson (Ed.), *Bridges to literacy* (pp. 19–40). Oxford, UK: Blackwell.

Britton, J. (1993). *Language and learning*. Portsmouth, NH: Boynton Cook.

D'Arcangelo, M. (2000). The scientist in the crib: A conversation with Andrew Meltzoff. *Educational Leadership, 58*(3), 8–13.

Dickinson, D. K., & Tabors, P. O. (2001). *Beginning literacy with language: Young children learning at home and school*. Baltimore, MD: Brookes.

Dollaghan, C. (1994). Children's phonological neighbourhoods: Half empty or half full? *Journal of Child Language, 21*, 257–271.

Goswami, U. (2002). Early phonological development and the acquisition of literacy. In S. Neuman & D. Dickinson (Eds.), *Handbook of early literacy research*, (pp. 111–125). New York, NY: Guilford Press.

Hart, B., & Risely, T. (1995). *Meaningful differences in the everyday experience of young American children*. Baltimore, MD: Brookes.

Hart, B., & Risley, T. R. (1999). *The social world of children learning to talk*. Baltimore, MD: Brookes.

Heath, S. (1994). The children of Trackton's children: Spoken and written language in social change. In R. Ruddell, M. Ruddell, & H. Singer (Eds.), *Theoretical models and processes of language* (4th ed., pp. 208–230). Newark, DE: International Reading Association.

International Reading Association and the National Association for the Education of Young Children. (1998). Learning to read and write: Developmentally appropriate practices for young children. A joint position statement of the International Reading Association (IRA) and the National Association for the Education of Young Children (NAEYC). *Young Children, 53*(4), 30–46.

Mayer, C., & Wells, G. (1996). Can the linguistic interdependence theory support a bilingual-bicultural model of literacy education for deaf students? *Journal of Deaf Studies and Deaf Education 1*(2), 93–107.

Metsala, J. (1999). Young children's phonological awareness and nonword repetition as a function of vocabulary development. *Journal of Educational Psychology, 91*, 3–19.

Metsala, J., & Walley, A. (1998). Spoken vocabulary growth and the segmental restructuring of lexical representations: Precursors to phonemic awareness and early reading ability. In J. Metsala & L. Ehri (Eds.), *Word recognition in beginning literacy* (pp. 89–120). Hillsdale, NJ: Erlbaum.

O'Keefe, C. Personal communication, October 12, 2008.

Ormrod, J. (2008). *Educational psychology* (6th ed.). Upper Saddle River, NJ: Pearson.

Ruddell, R., & Ruddell, M. (1994). Language acquisition and literacy processes. In R. Ruddell, M. Ruddell, & H. Singer (Eds.), *Theoretical models and processes of reading* (4th ed., pp. 83–103). Newark, DE: International Reading Association.

Scarborough, H. (1989). Prediction of reading disability from familial and individual differences. *Journal of Educational Psychology, 81*(1), 101–108.

Schlesinger, H. (1988). Questions and answers in the development of deaf children. In M. Strong (Ed.), *Language learning and deafness* (pp. 261–291). Cambridge, MA: Cambridge University Press.

Snow, C., Burns, M., & Griffin, P. (Eds.). (1998). *Preventing reading difficulties in young children*. Washington, DC: National Academy Press.

Snow, C., & Ninio, A. (1986). The contracts of literacy: What children learn from learning to read books. In W. Teale & E. Sulzby (Eds.), *Emergent literacy: Writing and reading* (pp. 116–138). Norwood, NJ: Ablex.

Snow, C., Scarborough, H., & Burns, M. (1999). What speech-language pathologists need to know about early reading. *Topics in Language Disorders, 20*(1), 48–58.

Snow, C., Tabors, P., & Dickinson, D. (2001). Language development in the preschool years. In D. Dickinson & P. Tabors (Eds.), *Beginning literacy with language* (pp.1–25). Baltimore, MD: Brookes.

Whitehurst, G., & Lonigan, C. (2002). Emergent literacy: Development from prereaders to readers. In S. Neuman & D. Dickerson (Eds.), *Handbook of early literacy research* (pp. 11–29). New York, NY: Guilford Press.

Chapter 5

HEARING, LISTENING, AND LITERACY

> *. . . we may say that the amount of speech a child develops depends not so much on the amount of hearing per se as upon the use he is able to make of his hearing for language-learning.*
>
> Fry, 1966, p. 201

> *. . . even prior to formal reading instruction, the performance of kindergartners on tests of phonological awareness is a strong predictor of their future reading achievement.*
>
> Snow, Burns, & Griffin, 1998, p. 54

Introduction

In looking at the many studies detailed in Chapter 1 concerning children with hearing loss, it should be clear that, historically, the subjects for whom better reading achievement has been reported have been associated with having better hearing, either because they have access to appropriate technology, or because their hearing losses are less pronounced. In fact, the more hearing—or to be more precise, the more listening—the better is the achievement. It is as though a large, natural experiment has been conducted over a period of many years in order to test the hypothesis that the presence of listening is desirable, perhaps even necessary, for reading to develop beyond the lower elementary levels.

For years, people have tried to teach children with hearing loss to identify words without emphasis on their spoken form, the assumption being that the phonological and auditory avenues were closed to them (Hart, 1978, pp. 6–7). Some individuals, even with profound deafness, do develop into skilled readers using this approach. Interestingly, in studies of adults who use sign language as their dominant mode of communication, some reports of "Deaf good readers" have emerged. In some of these readers, phonological processing is evident, but this is not thought to develop until the reader has progressed beyond 4th and 5th grade reading levels, and only as the person requires it for more complex reading (Padden & Hanson, 2000, p. 439). In general, Deaf readers who pay attention to phonology are seen as paying attention to a word's sound elements only after having identified the word using another strategy (Waters & Doehring, 1990, as cited in Padden & Hanson, 2000, p. 438). Padden and Hanson do not specify how this happens, nor do they assert that it happens in a large number of people. They join others in suggesting "more investigation of the use of alternatives to phonological coding by Deaf readers, particularly in the beginning reading of Deaf children" (Padden & Hanson, 2000, p. 439).

I am leaving that thinking and those investigations to others whose assumptions lead them in that direction, as I interpret the research to say the easiest way to learn how to read involves learning to listen to spoken language, learning to interact with people in using it, and thereby acquiring the spoken language to be read. In children with hearing loss, this can happen in much the same way it happens with children with typical hearing. At this point, another caveat is in order: there are people who have excellent hearing and good speech who have difficulty with phonological awareness, phonemic discrimination, and in learning to read and write (Snow, Burns, & Griffin, 1998, p. 55). It would appear, then, that hearing is highly useful, but not sufficient for the development of literacy. This is probably because hearing does not guarantee listening in ways that ensure discrimination among the available sounds of the language. Many who work with children with typical hearing who have reading problems have decided their problems likely involve some combination of undeveloped phonological awareness, lack of print awareness, and deficiencies in oral language (Whitehurst & Lonigan, 2002, p. 12). Problems with word parts are evident in many who lag behind in reading (Stanovich, 1994, p. 267). Although print awareness can be acquired to some extent without listening (through matching signs to whole words, for example), phonological awareness and oral language depend mainly upon listening. Additionally, differences in background knowledge and experience can severely limit vocabulary and language knowledge. This chapter deals with phonological awareness and its development.

Phonological Awareness

Phonological awareness is the ability to isolate and focus on sounds in words and to isolate words themselves. This ability is very important in the process of beginning to read. Yet, it need not be perfect at the beginning; experience with reading helps it develop as the reader has more productive interaction with print (Ehri, 1976, 1979, as cited in Adams, 2000, p. 299; Goswami, 2000). It has been known for a long time that in children with typical hearing, the "phonemic repertory" of their spoken language is complete sometime between the ages of five and seven (Fry, 1966, p. 187). This means they can process all the smallest units of sound that differentiate words from one another both in their receptive and expressive utterances. These small units are known as phonemes. This is not to say the average child has perfect articulation, but it does signal that the listening and phonological foundations have been laid for adding vocabulary and conceptual knowledge throughout life. This listening is entirely possible for children with hearing loss, even without the aid of technology. In 1964, Whetnal and Fry reported on a mother who, having determined early that her daughter was deaf, "had always drawn the child close to her and spoken close to the ear." This child, and others "developed speech spontaneously and understood speech," and none of these children were placed in special schools (p. 18).

Phonological Processing Capabilities

Whitehurst and Lonigan delineate three sorts of phonological processing capabilities: phonological sensitivity, phonological memory, and phonological naming (2002, p. 14).

Phonological sensitivity is seen in children who can recognize rhyming words, put spoken syllables and phonemes together into words, remove syllables and phonemes to create new words, and distinguish among the various phonemes in spoken words. This oral language capability is regarded as a prerequisite for reading that develops through listening. Children move from being able to identify larger sound segments, even phrases, to identifying words and letter sounds within these segments. When they are beginning to learn language, children do not know that the sounds are parts of words and that words are parts of sentences. A phrase such as "up we go!" operates as an utterance that begins to hold meaning. As far as the child knows at this point, it could be one word, "upwego!" Part of learning to read involves discovering where the conventional dividers are between words and what constitutes a word. Over time, the child works toward the discovery that words are composed conventionally of sequences of sounds both in sound and in print.

Phonological memory involves increasing ability to listen to sounds and words, hold them in short-term/working memory, and then repeat them. This is the process we must all use daily as we interact with others in using language. It involves rehearsal and the maintenance of sounds in working memory long enough to be able to make use of them. Children are assessed on their capacity to do this with digit-span tests in which increasingly larger numbers are spoken for them to repeat, but much of this ability shows up in their increasing capacity for carrying on longer conversations.

Phonological naming depends on the successful searching of permanent memory for phonological information. At the easiest level, this could involve naming one picture; at more advanced levels, naming a series of pictures as quickly as possible would be a representative activity. Being able to retrieve multiple names is related to vocabulary size, to be sure, but also to being able to turn to stored sequences of sounds in long-term memory.

In listening, children learn to distinguish syllables, then to differentiate between onsets and rimes (the first phonemes before the vowel and the rest of the word; for example, *wait* can be divided into the onset *w* and the rime *ait*), and finally, they can isolate phonemes. Learning to discriminate among phonemes appears to be helped along by being introduced to reading (Goswami, 2000, p. 252). Children with typical hearing have usually developed both syllable and onset-rime awareness by the time they are in preschool, and many studies have found a strong relationship between rhyming and phonemic awareness and later progress in reading. (See Goswami, 2000, for a long list of such studies.) Learning to listen and speak are the basic building blocks in establishing phonological and lexical (vocabulary) knowledge.

If you have tried as an adult to learn a language other than your first language, you have probably run into difficulty with each of these phonological processes. Think about listening to fluent Spanish if you are not a Spanish speaker. Do you know where the words start and stop? Probably not. Can you repeat more than a few phrases, even words, at a time? This is difficult, because you do not know what constitutes a word, and you do not have much to hang onto. At the beginning, your working memory is overwhelmed by too many sounds to remember at once. Even when you have studied a vocabulary list, you may be tongue-tied when presented with demands for words in the language. After a time, though, the phonological information becomes more settled in your long-term memory, and suddenly you realize that you "know" what the words are. What before had sounded like undifferentiated streams of sound present themselves to you as words and word parts, and you do this now with an unconscious automaticity. Yet, you have had an advantage over a child learning his or her first language: you already know quite a lot about sounds and words. The task for the child who begins with a capacity for language is to make all these determinations without the aid of an already existing language. Completing this amazing task is part of the continuous interpretation of experience that we do from birth, and it is achievable by most human beings (Smith, 2004, p. 2)

It apparently does not matter whether the written language contains a sound-by-sound record of the phonology of the language. In a study of the fluent reading of Chinese symbols, Perfetti and Zhang (1995) find that processing of sounds associated with the symbols takes place in working memory, and they determine this to be a typical language and information process. Furthermore, they assert that learning to read words involves coming to "bind together graphemic, phonological, and semantic constituents," and suggest that once reading mastery has begun for a person, it takes effort to sort out these facets of language (p. 31). They conclude: " . . . there is increasing reason to believe that universal reading processes include phonological constituents as part of word iden-tification" (p. 31). For our purposes in thinking about children with hearing loss, this study suggests that using an approach that by-passes phonology will shortchange them, leaving them only with visual and possibly the semantic constituents of the words to be read.

Fortunately, the phonological can be supplied, even under diffi-cult circumstances. In a fascinating article published in 1966, a long time ago in technologic terms and in a time with little audiologic help for young children and infants, Fry addressed the possibility of the child with deafness learning spoken language. Fry claimed the child needs to learn to hear his or her own speech in order to learn to improve speech and thus acquire "normal speech" (p. 193). Such a self-monitoring feat would have struck most as impossible, particularly at that time, yet he reported " . . . in London, however, no child has been found in whom it was impossible to develop responses to sound . . . no matter how small the amount of hearing the child has initially, this hearing can be used in the development of speech and will in fact show every evidence of increasing in the amount with teaching" (Fry, 1966, p. 200). In his view, children with hearing loss who failed to develop phonologically and learn spoken language had simply not been in the presence of enough spoken language. He held that if the people around those children had presented spoken language in a sustained manner from the children's earliest age, then those children would have developed speech and language according to the ways of children with typi-cal hearing (p. 203). "If this method is adopted, then there is every chance that the child will progress through the normal stages of the development of speech even though he may be slower in doing so than the hearing child" (p. 204). The auditory-verbal approach is a structured way of bringing sound and language to a child by stimulating spoken language in the child.

The Auditory-Verbal Approach

The auditory-verbal approach is designed to promote language acquisition through listening to good, well-formed spoken language and through therapy that helps the child learn to differentiate between and among the many separate phonemes of the language. It has been successful for over half a century and was used before the advent of sophisticated hearing aids and cochlear implants. A lovely book published in 1976 by mothers of children with hearing loss and titled *Learning to Listen* spells out the many ways parents can interact with their children and encourage them to listen and speak. The parent-child interaction becomes the primary facilitator of attention to sound in the child.

Auditory training, as the mothers involved in this book see it, is many things. It is planning and carrying out language lessons with your child on a regular basis. It is talking to your child all day long and making the most of everyday routines to develop his or her language. It is involvement of the whole family. It is, above all an attitude or frame of mind—an attitude that the child is a "listening child," that he or she uses hearing, even though it is imperfect, ALL THE TIME, just as any normal child does (Vaughan, 1976, p. viii).

The *Learning to Listen* mothers describe speaking four to eight inches from the hearing aid, of crawling around to keep close to the ears of small babies, of carrying their children while they talked to them, of spending much time with their children on their laps looking at books and talking about them, and of consistently talk-talk-talking directly into the hearing aid. They found success, even without the advanced technology that assists us today. Daniel Ling, Helen Beebe, Doreen Pollack, and Louise Crawford, auditory-verbal pioneers, worked with children in the 1950s and 1960s who were responding well to spoken sounds they must have heard as whispers.

Of greatest importance, then, is helping the child learn to listen. Today, this means using technology to its best advantage and talk-talk-talking in strategic ways.

The simple premise of the auditory-verbal approach is to use whatever residual hearing a child has available, amplified as well as possible, toward the acquisition of spoken language. Delivering good quality sound to the ear is the goal, because that makes the process easier, and that is now possible with good hearing aids and cochlear implants.

In the auditory-verbal approach, much attention is given to discriminating between and among words. For example, a child might be asked to differentiate between "bat" and "mat," which look the same on the lips. The subtle difference between the sounds of /b/ and /m/ is discernable with extensive practice in listening to the two words. The auditory-verbal therapist builds from simple to complex discriminations, and in doing so, introduces the child to the full range of sounds used in the language. In a very real sense, auditory-verbal therapy is phonological and phonemic awareness therapy that builds both discrimination of and memory for the sounds of the spoken language. It is necessary to blend the listening and spoken language that occurs in the social environment with the coaching parents need. Children who are deaf or hard of hearing need support from everyone in their lives to listen and speak with them; for good progress to result, it is not sufficient to simply provide listening technology and take children to the school (Cole & Flexer, 2007).

Repeated practice and intensity come from the parents in each child's life, and the auditory-verbal therapist (AVT) works in a clinical setting to coach the parents on how to do this with the child. Auditory-verbal educators (AVEds) provide such repeated practice and intensity to the child in a classroom and work with parents so they learn to do the same outside of school.

> To be certified by the Alexander Graham Bell Academy for Listening and Spoken Language, prospective AVTs and AVEds take the same qualifying examination; the difference in their certification designation is the setting (clinic or classroom) of their preparation, mentorship, and practice. (The Alexander Graham Bell Academy for Listening and Spoken Language, 2013)

Descriptions of Listening and Spoken Language Specialists (LSLS Cert. AVT and LSLS Cert. AVEd) can be found in Appendix C. The Alexander Graham Bell Association for the Deaf and Hard of Hearing has established The Listening and Spoken Language Knowledge Center to provide a constant source of information about a large range of issues such as hearing loss, technology, listening, advocacy, and LSLS certification; it also includes ways for people to communicate with each other, lists services, and announces conferences. Two tabs lead to extensive sections for families and for professionals. Everyone is welcome to the Knowledge Center which can be found at: http://www.listeningandspokenlanguage.org/Default.aspx?id=768

Principles of Listening and Spoken Language Specialist Auditory-Verbal Therapy (LSLS Cert. AVT)

The statements below are the now firmly established principles on which auditory-verbal therapists base their work (Alexander Graham Bell Association for the Deaf and Hard of Hearing). In the following pages, I explicate each one in terms of establishing the listening that is foundational to literacy.

1. *Promote early diagnosis of hearing loss in newborns, infants, toddlers, and young children, followed by immediate audiologic management and Auditory-Verbal therapy.*
   Diagnosis of hearing loss should occur as early as possible. Fortunately, 42 states and the District of Columbia and Puerto Rico now require hearing screening of newborns, though only 26 of these states require screening of all infants (National Center for Hearing Assessment and Management). Auditory-verbal therapy and use of appropriate technology can begin as soon as a diagnosis is established, giving the child the best chance of developing according to norms established among children with typical hearing.

2. *Recommend immediate assessment and use of appropriate, state-of-the-art hearing technology to obtain maximum benefits of auditory stimulation.*
   Even today, people sometimes reason that they will provide hearing aids or a cochlear implant when the child is "old enough" to understand what is happening, or they hear advice telling them to wait until the child asks to be able to hear. Such waiting is counterproductive, of course, as such questions

require the knowledge of language that is only gained through hearing and listening.

3. *Guide and coach parents to help their child use hearing as the primary sensory modality in developing spoken language without the use of sign language or emphasis on lipreading.*

   Parents spend the most time with their child and must become the primary communicators with him or her. The auditory-verbal therapist works with the parents to do this in sensitive and continuously ongoing ways. Building listening and then spoken language is the goal, so sign language and lipreading are not the focus, as they could detract from the process of learning to listen and speak. Sign language can be added to spoken language after spoken language is secure and mature, if desired, but it is not used at all during the acquisition of spoken language because when vision is unimpaired, a visual language can become dominant and prevent attention to the spoken language. Auditory-verbal therapists do not focus on lipreading because they want to make sure that listening is being established; most people, with or without typical hearing, depend on some form of lipreading and acquire it naturally without it being taught directly.

4. *Guide and coach parents to become the primary facilitators of their child's listening and spoken language development through active consistent participation in individualized Auditory-Verbal therapy.*

   Participation in auditory-verbal therapy must be consistent. We know very well that children with typical hearing who do not receive constant spoken language input do less well on speech and language tasks than those who do (Hart & Risely, 1995), so it would not be otherwise for a child with hearing loss.

5. *Guide and coach parents to create environments that support listening for the acquisition of spoken language throughout the child's daily activities.*

   All day, every day, parents and other caregivers must interact with the child by providing spoken language that demonstrates and extends experiences with phonology, vocabulary, syntax, and pragmatics, all through using the language in well-formed and meaningful ways. This mirrors the seemingly effortless ways that children with typical hearing are exposed to and acquire spoken language.

6. *Guide and coach parents to help their child integrate listening and spoken language into all aspects of the child's life.*

   There should be no area in a child's life in which spoken language is not being used. Parents can initiate and support conversations with their children about everything that happens. The parent can seek out events and occasions that will offer new words and new ways of expression.

7. *Guide and coach parents to use natural developmental patterns of audition, speech, language, cognition, and communication.*

   Parents do not need to learn new ways to communicate with their child with hearing loss. Instead, they need to learn to speak and interact consistently and intentionally. This involves thinking about using new words and sentence forms and enriching conversations with synonyms so the child is exposed in interactive ways to the richest language possible.

8. *Guide and coach parents to help their child self-monitor spoken language through listening.*

   Parents can learn to respond to their children with well-formed utterances, so the child always has a good model of language available. If the young child says "ba" for "ball," the parent responds with "ball" in its full form, and puts it into a sentence: "Catch the big blue ball!" The parent reminds an older child to listen to all the sounds in a word in order to pronounce it clearly.

9. *Administer ongoing formal and informal diagnostic assessments to develop individualized Auditory-Verbal treatment plans, to monitor progress and to evaluate the effectiveness of the plans for the child and family.*

   The auditory-verbal therapist uses knowledge of typical spoken language development in systematic and regular assessment in order to keep the child and his or her family on track. This involves keeping track of vocabulary, syntactic, and comprehension development in order to find and work toward filling gaps in development.

10. *Promote education in regular schools with peers who have typical hearing and with appropriate services from early childhood onwards.*

    Being with peers and adults with typical hearing promotes the use of spoken language in the child in a way that being with other children who have language delay cannot, and so putting the child with hearing loss together with children with typical hearing is seen as necessary for the achievement of good listening and speaking capabilities. This means placing the child in schools with peers with typical hearing and assisting all of the children in interacting with one another.

It must be noted that an Auditory-Verbal Practice requires adherence to all 10 principles. The term "parents" also includes grandparents, relatives, guardians, and any caregivers who interact with the child. These principles were adapted from the principles originally developed by Doreen Pollack, 1970, and were adopted by the AG Bell Academy for Listening and Spoken Language, July 26, 2007.

Principles of Listening and Spoken Language Specialist Auditory-Verbal Education (LSLS Cert. AVEd)

The AVEd principles are relatively new, having been written in 2007 with the development of the LSLS Cert. AVEd designation for classroom teachers. They parallel the original auditory-verbal principles in large measure (Alexander Graham Bell Association for the Deaf and Hard of Hearing).

A Listening and Spoken Language Educator (LSLS Cert. AVEd) teaches children with hearing loss to listen and talk exclusively though listening and spoken language instruction.

1. *Promote early diagnosis of hearing loss in infants, toddlers, and young children, followed by immediate audiologic assessment and use of appropriate state of the art hearing technology to ensure maximum benefits of auditory stimulation.*
   Technology is the focus for delivering good, well-formed sound to children at all possible times.
2. *Promote immediate audiologic management and spoken language instruction for children to develop listening and spoken language skills.*
   The use of appropriate technology for educational intervention beyond the hearing aids or cochlear implant is emphasized for the classroom (for example, an FM unit and/or a sound-field

system). Teachers must work with audiologists and other hearing professionals to make sure the technology is working so their spoken language instruction is accessible by the children.

3. *Create and maintain acoustically controlled environments that support listening and talking for the acquisition of spoken language throughout the child's daily activities.*

Among the teacher's responsibilities is that of monitoring the listening conditions in the classroom so as to make them as conducive to active listening and speaking by the child as possible.

4. *Guide and coach parents to become effective facilitators of their child's listening and spoken language development in all aspects of the child's life.*

The teacher must work carefully with parents so the parents take on the serious task of monitoring their child's listening and spoken language at all times the parents are with their child. This teacher has greater responsibility to the child's parents than is ordinarily thought to be the case with children with typical hearing.

5. *Provide effective teaching with families and children in settings such as homes, classrooms, therapy rooms, hospitals, or clinics.*

Teaching takes place in a variety of settings, and auditory-verbal educators work in both formal and informal environments in educating both parents and the child.

6. *Provide focused and individualized instruction to the child through lesson plans and classroom activities while maximizing listening and spoken language.*

The teacher teaches in much the same way as with children with typical hearing, planning and carrying out activities whose basis is always listening and speaking.

7. *Collaborate with parents and professionals to develop goals, objectives, and strategies for achieving the natural developmental patterns of audition, speech, language, cognition, and communication.*

The teacher's paramount concern is the natural acquisition of all phases and levels of listening, speaking, thinking, and interacting with others using spoken language.

8. *Promote each child's ability to self-monitor spoken language through listening.*

The child must learn to listen to his or her own speech and language so as to know when it is conventional and when it is not. The teacher helps the child with good models to emulate and helps the child develop the desire to produce clear, intelligible speech.

9. *Use diagnostic assessments to develop individualized objectives, to monitor progress, and to evaluate the effectiveness of the teaching activities.*

   The auditory-verbal educator uses knowledge of typical speech and language development in assessing the achievement of the child in order to determine the extent to which learning is happening and what to present next.

10. *Promote education in regular classrooms with peers who have typical hearing, as early as possible, when the child has the skills to do so successfully.*

   The teacher's role is to move the child into classrooms with children with typical hearing as soon as possible. Because it is recognized that the auditory-verbal educator will at times be working with children for whom later identification and use of technology is the case, this goal differs from the auditory-verbal therapist's goal that children with hearing loss will always be put in classrooms with children with typical hearing.

Conclusion

It should be clear from the principles of auditory-verbal therapy and auditory-verbal education that helping children learn to listen through continuous exposure to well-formed language is a major, achievable goal. Establishing the expectation of frequent, meaningful spoken interactions with these children is paramount. It is as simple as providing access to listening through technology and then making sure that everyone who might interact with the children is aware that they can expect to have increasingly meaningful interactions with them using spoken language. Complexity arises, however, in the larger amount of involvement in conversation the children need compared to children with typical hearing. Technology makes this process easier, but it is not enough; for the development of listening, there is no substitute for extensive and frequent interpersonal interactions using spoken language.

References

Adams, M. (1990). *Beginning to read*. Cambridge, MA: MIT Press.

Alexander Graham Bell Association for the Deaf and Hard of Hearing, the Alexander Graham Bell Academy for Listening and Spoken Language. Retrieved April 14, 2013, from http://www.listeningandspokenlanguage.org/AcademyDocument.aspx?id=563

Alexander Graham Bell Academy for Listening and Spoken Language. Retrieved April 14, 2013, from http://www.agbell.org/AcademyDocument.aspx?id=541

Alexander Graham Bell Association Listening and Spoken Language Knowledge Center. Retrieved April 14, 2013, from ahttp://www.listeningandspokenlanguage.org/Default.aspx?id=768

Cole, E., & Flexer, C. (2007). *Children with hearing loss: Developing listening and talking*. San Diego, CA: Plural.

Fry, D. (1966). The development of the phonological system in the normal and the deaf child. In F. Smith & G. Miller (Eds.), *The genesis of language: A psycholinguistic approach* (pp. 187–206). Cambridge, MA: MIT Press.

Goswami, U. (2000). Phonological and lexical processes. In M. Kamil, P. Mosenthal, P. D. Pearson, & R. Barr (Eds.), *Handbook of reading research, Volume III* (pp. 251–267). Mahwah, NJ: Lawrence Erlbaum.

Hart, B. (1978). *Teaching reading to deaf children*. Jackson Heights, NY: Lexington School for the Deaf.

Hart, B., & Risely, T. (1995). *Meaningful differences in the everyday experience of young American children*. Baltimore, MD: Brookes.

Ling, D. (1989). *Foundations of spoken language for hearing-impaired children*. Washington, DC: Alexander Graham Bell Association for the Deaf.

National Center for Hearing Assessment and Management: EHDI legislation related early hearing detection and intervention. Retrieved July 15, 2008, from http://www.infanthearing.org/legislative/index.html

Padden, C., & Hanson, V. (2000). Search for the missing link: The development of skilled reading in deaf children. In K. Emmorey & H. Lane (Eds.), *The signs of language revisited: An anthology to honor Ursula Bellugi and Edward Klima* (pp. 435–447). Mahwah, NJ: Lawrence Erlbaum.

Perfetti, C., & Zhang, S. (1995). Very early phonological activation in Chinese reading. *Journal of Experimental Psychology: Learning, Memory, and Cognition, 21*, 24–33.

Smith, F. (2004). *Understanding reading* (6th ed.). Mahwah, NJ: Lawrence Erlbaum Associates.

Snow, C., Burns, M., & Griffin, P. (Eds.). (1998). *Preventing reading difficulties in young children*. Washington, DC: National Academy Press.

Stanovich, K. (1994). Constructivism in reading education. *Journal of Special Education, 28*(3), 259–274.

Vaughan, P. (Ed.). (1976). *Learning to listen*. Don Mills, Ontario, Canada: New Press.

Whetnal, E., & Fry, D. (1964). *The deaf child*. London, UK: William Heinemann Medical Books.

Whitehurst, G., & Lonigan, C. (2002). Emergent literacy: Development from prereaders to readers. In S. Neuman & D. Dickerson (Eds.), *Handbook of early literacy research* (pp. 11–29). New York, NY: Guilford Press.

Chapter 6

ISSUES IN CHILD DEVELOPMENT

Gina Dow, PhD

A baby, although helpless and dependent at the beginning, not only learns to affect the behavior of others in his environment through his signals and communications, but is also biased from the beginning toward the development of abilities that will make him increasingly competent. (Caregiver) responsiveness to signals fosters the development of communication. An infant whose mother's responsiveness helps him to achieve his ends develops confidence in his own ability to control what happens to him.

Bell & Ainsworth, 1972, p. 1189

Introduction

The study of human development is by its nature the study of *change over time*. What *causes* the change—the so-called "nature–nurture" question—and the *characteristics* of that change—smooth and continuous or stage-like and discontinuous—have been the source of lively debate for hundreds of years (cf. Crain, 2005). Trends in theory and research for the past 50 to 75 years in the United States and worldwide have shifted many times, and a summary of these trends is well beyond the scope of this chapter. However, on many important points there is good consensus; in particular is that there really *is* no "nature–nurture" question in contemporary developmental science, at least if conceptualized as an "either-or" issue (National Research Council and Institute of Medicine, 2000). As William Greenough rather famously put it, "The interaction of heredity and environment is so extensive that to ask which is more important, nature or nurture, is like asking which is more important to a rectangle, height or width" (quoted in Wray, 1997, p. 79). Development is driven by an irreducible and inseparable transaction between "nature"—the child's biological characteristics—and "nurture"—the child's caregiving and living environment. That is, the effects of biological and genetic factors are only manifested within a particular environmental context.

Another important concept in understanding this irreducible relationship, and more useful than that of the "sensitive period" is that of "experience-expectant development" (Black & Greenough, 1986; Greenough & Black, 1992; Greenough, Black, & Wallace, 1987). In the process of synaptic overproduction and "pruning" back, experiences that have occurred reliably at particular points in development for a particular species are incorporated into the patterns of synaptic connections of the developing brain. For example, the visual cortex "expects" binocular (Timney, 1990) and patterned visual input early in life (e.g., LeVay, Weisel, & Hubel, 1980), and organizes itself around such input. Thus, the same basic, *expectable* experiences would affect development for everyone. Such a process is compatible with Werker and Tees' (2005) concept of "optimal period," with its potentially somewhat variant timing of onset and offset; see Tierney and Nelson (2009) for an excellent brief review on the relationship between early experience and normative brain development.

On the other hand, experience-*dependent* development varies for each individual and is dependent on the particular and unique experiences encountered throughout development. For example, human newborns show a preference for their mothers' voices (DeCasper & Fifer, 1980), as well as for their native languages (Moon, Cooper, & Fifer, 1993), whether mono- or bilingual (Byers-Heinlein, Burns, & Werker, 2010); these specific preferences are clearly based on prenatal auditory exposure to both stimuli and are thus experience-dependent. Finally, experience-expectant and experience-dependent development often operate simultaneously—for example, auditory input from mother and the native language may themselves be seen as "expectable events" in prenatal development.

Developing this further, how is this notion of experience-expectant development relevant for humans and auditory input? Recent research strongly supports the idea that human infants are born with a bias in favor of human speech. For example, human newborns can discriminate between languages when played forward, but not when played backward (Ramus, Hauser, Miller, Morris, & Mehler, 2000); newborns also show a preference for speech sounds over equally complex, acoustically similar nonspeech sounds (Vouloumanos & Werker, 2007); by three months, infants prefer to listen to human speech over even human noncommunicative vocalizations (Shultz & Vouloumanos, 2010). Further, newborns prefer faces in general over equally complex nonfaces (e.g., Valenza, Simion, & Cassia, 1996; cf. Fantz, 1961) and specifically prefer faces with eyes that have a direct gaze—that make eye contact—over faces that do not (Farroni, Csibra, Simion, & Johnson, 2002). These preferences may help orient the human newborn to sources of auditory information that will be become relevant for communication. Finally, auditory experience also serves to narrow the ability to discriminate between phonemes; under ordinary circumstances, young infants can discriminate between speech sounds in any human language, but by the end of the first year of life this ability exists only for the language(s) in which they are spoken to (Werker & Tees, 1984; cf. Werker & Tees, 2005 for an excellent review). Interestingly, research suggests that children who had recurrent otitis media infections in the first years of life, and thus fluctuating and attenuated auditory input, may have less sharp phonemic boundaries (Clarkson, Eimas, & Marean, 1989), and reduced phonological awareness later in childhood (Nittrouer, 1995; Winskel, 2006). Thus, auditory linguistic input, starting prenatally and continuing in the first year, can be seen as an "expectable event" around which the infant's brain can begin to organize language development. It may even be said that, "infants are born with auditory sensitivities that are tuned to human speech" (Gervain & Werker, 2008, p. 1164).

It is important to reiterate, however, that experience-expectant and experience-dependent development occur together (National Research Council and Institute of Medicine, 2000); furthermore, developmental change occurs in all domains simultaneously and interactively—preferences for faces, human speech, and mother's voice are happening in newborns who also are developing socially, cognitively, linguistically, and physically, and are doing so in a caregiving context—that is, with other people who are interacting with them. The *form* that this interaction takes is relevant for development in all of these domains.

Sensitivity in the Caregiving Relationship

Ideally, a caregiver provides care that is both sensitive to and contingent upon the infant's signals; this is generally discussed in the context of the development of the infant's ability to regulate her or his own levels of arousal and attention ("self-regulation"), and in the larger context of the development of the attachment relationship (e.g., Sroufe & Sampson, 2000).

> In studying face to face interactions between young infants and their caregivers . . . researchers have noted that after a period of back-and-forth smiles and vocalization that often build in intensity, babies will look away. Skilled caregivers react by remaining quiet for a moment. The baby then looks back and the two begin to interact again. (National Research Council and Institute of Medicine, 2000, p. 242)

Thus, behaviors and characteristics that might be labeled "caregiver sensitivity" may not be as useful an explanatory construct as that of "caregiver attunement"; the former implies something dispositional on the part of the caregiver, or a one-way transmission of behaviors from the caregiver to the infant. The latter, on the other hand, reflects the transactional nature of the relationship—the caregiver observing and interpreting signals from this particular infant at this particular time, and modulating interactions accordingly (cf. Ainsworth, Bell, & Stratton, 1974; Sroufe & Sampson, 2000). Such attunement exemplifies bidirectional *communication.*

Bidirectional Communication and Infant-Directed Speech

Attunement thus reflects the complex nature of the child-caregiver relationship; far from being a passive recipient of adult attention, the infant is an active *participant* in social and communicative interactions from the beginning. Thus, the adult modification of speech directed to infants—"infant directed speech (IDS)"—that is evidenced cross-linguistically (e.g., Ferguson, 1964, 1977; Fernald, Taeschner, Dunn, Papousek, de Boysson-Bardies, & Fukui, 1989; Sachs, 1977) and infant preference for IDS (e.g., Pegg, Werker, & McLeod, 1992) may be seen as two sides of the same coin.

What function might IDS have in development? Although there is much interest in the relationship between IDS and later linguistic development, of the three functions suggested by Cooper and her colleagues (Cooper, Abraham, Berman, & Staska, 1997) (arousal/attentional regulation, practice in interpretation of emotional signals, and increasing the saliency of linguistic structure in speech), only one of these major functions is explicitly linguistic. For example, IDS has been shown to aid the perceptual learning of phonetic categories, as mothers' speech "enhance(s) the cues distinguishing the linguistic features of the basic combinatorial units of the native language from very early in infancy" (Werker et al., 2007, p. 160). Interestingly, in recent research Singh, Nestor, Parikh, and Yull (2009) have shown that in the first year, infants demonstrate better memory for words introduced in IDS as compared to those introduced in adult-directed speech (ADS)

Overall, IDS attracts infant attention, and positive infant response to IDS may serve as powerful feedback to caregivers, as they learn to become attuned to the emotional and communicative signals of a particular infant. As the child develops in all domains, this back-and-forth of emotional communication in the context of social interaction may be part of her or his developing expectations about relationships (e.g., Sroufe & Fleeson, 1986). Indeed, Emde and Easterbrooks (1985) refer to emotional communication as the "language of infancy."

Part I: Early Identification

Attunement and Early Identification of Hearing Loss

Attunement may be even more important (and predictive of outcomes) when there is a context of developmental risk. For example, positive caregiver–child interaction predicts linguistic development most strongly for children with typical hearing who are at high risk for language delay; similarly, "maternal emotional availability . . . (makes) significantly greater positive predictions for children who are deaf or hard of hearing (D/HH) than for children with normal hearing" (Pressman, Pipp-Siegel, Yoshinaga-Itano, Kubicek, & Emde, 1998 p. 251). This suggests that the earlier children with hearing loss are identified, and intervention is begun, the more likely it is that caregivers' interactions will be sensitive to the child's hearing status and linguistic skills (e.g., Bergeson, Miller, & McCune, 2006). (This is discussed in greater detail later in this chapter.)

Parents also report wanting to know about potential hearing loss as soon as possible. In interviews of parents and other caregivers of 27 early-identified children with moderate to profound hearing loss in England, Young & Tattersall (2007) reported that 22 were unambiguously and strongly positive about having discovered their child's hearing loss so close to birth. Their feelings were mostly attributable to an increased sense of control and agency in caring for their child, as well as prospective relief at knowing that they would not have feelings of guilt or regret for even unintentionally missing an opportunity to help their child. Several also mentioned "being able to tune in appropriately to the deaf child's needs and responses from the earliest time" (p. 213)—attunement—as a notable advantage to early knowledge of their child's hearing loss.

Early Identification and Intervention: How Early is Early Enough?

Although previous reviews have shown equivocal evidence for the relationship between the early identification of hearing loss (defined in earlier research as identification before 2.5 years) and outcomes in language, academic performance, and social interaction, among other areas (cf. Bess & Paradise, 1994), these reviews may be of diminished utility given the drastic reduction in the age of identification that has occurred in many countries with the advent of Universal Newborn Hearing Screening (UNHS). More recent research evidence is clear that better outcomes in language acquisition are associated with early identification, with "early" defined as younger than 6 months (Yoshinaga-Itano and Apuzzo, 1998). In fact, "infants who were identified with hearing loss by 6 months of age and subsequently started receiving intervention were functioning within normal limits of expressive and receptive language when tested at a mean chronological age of 26 months" (p. 381). Other children who either were not identified as having a hearing impairment by 18 months or who did not start intervention by 18 months, did not fare as well; "the later identified children were significantly delayed in receptive and expressive language when compared to the normally hearing population and the infants identified before 6 months of age" (p. 381).

Early Identification in the United States

Over 40 years ago, early identification of hearing loss was urged both for all children (Babbidge report, 1965), as well as for children considered to be at high risk for hearing loss (US Department of Health, Education, and Welfare: National Conference for the Education of the Deaf, 1967). By the later 1980s, consensus was growing that earlier detection was not only desirable but was possible, given advances in technology (American Academy of Pediatrics, Joint Committee on Infant Hearing, 2007). However, due in part to a lack of evidence for the preventative utility of universal screening, earlier recommendations remained focused on screening only infants considered to be at "high risk" (U.S. Preventative Services Task Force, 1996). Thus, screening was offered only to children deemed to be at increased risk due to prematurity/NICU care, family history, or other reasons. It is estimated that assessing only children with known risk factors would miss the 19 to 42% of children with severe to profound hearing loss who have no risk factors (Thompson et al., 2001), including the 90% of infants with congenital

hearing impairments who are born to hearing parents (http://
www.cdc.gov/ncbddd/ehdi/). This increases the risk for those children to be consigned to considerably later identification—even
to early school age for children with mild to moderate hearing
loss. However, as information was gathered from pilot Early Hearing Detection and Intervention Programs (EHDI), it became clear
that newborn screening of all children, and its resultant much earlier detection of hearing loss, is essential (Yoshinaga-Itano, 2004).
Thanks to the implementation of EHDI in more states over time,
as of 2009 approximately 97% of children born in the United States
each year are screened for hearing loss at birth (http://www.cdc.
gov/ncbddd/ehdi/). It is important to note, however, that due to
late-onset sensorineural hearing loss (SNHL) (which may be associated with infections such as bacterial meningitis, or to progressive
loss such as is seen in Usher syndrome and others), hearing should
be regularly monitored throughout early childhood, even for children who pass newborn screening (Batshaw, Pellegrino, & Roizen,
2007; Young, Reilly, & Burke, 2011).

How Screening Is Done

Screening for hearing loss in newborns is conducted with one of
two tests: the otoacoustic emissions test (OAE) or the automated
auditory brainstem response test (AABR). In the OAE test, a probe
inserted into the infant's ear canal produces a series of sounds and
then records the minute sounds made by the movement of the outer
hair cells on the basilar membrane; this tests whether the cochlea is
functioning. For the AABR test, sensors placed on the infant's head
record brain activity that results from sounds presented via small
earphones. Both tests can be done while the infant is asleep and
take less than 10 minutes to administer (Wrightson, 2007; http://
www.cdc.gov/ncbddd/ehdi/).

From Screening to Identification to Intervention

By 2005, every state in the US had started a UNHS system, and the
average age at which children with hearing loss are diagnosed has
declined from 19 to 36 months in 1991 (Mace, Wallace, Whan, &
Stelmachowicz, 1991) to 3 to 6 months currently (American Acad-

emy of Pediatrics, Joint Committee on Infant Hearing, 2007). Ideally, with early identification comes much earlier intervention—for example, the average age for hearing aid fitting in Colorado for children who are early-identified is 5 weeks (Yoshinaga-Itano, 2003)—but as of 2009, 45.1% half of newborns who do not pass the newborn hearing screening test(s) were considered "lost to follow up;" they did not have appropriate follow-up testing to either confirm or disconfirm potential hearing loss (http://www.cdc.gov/ncbddd/hearingloss/data.html; cf. Gaffney, Green, & Gaffney, 2010; American Academy of Pediatrics, Joint Committee on Infant Hearing, 2007); further gains in intervention outcomes will require better follow-up care for these infants.

How Does Early Identification Contribute to Good Developmental Outcomes?

Considerable research is underway nationally and internationally to investigate the potential benefits of this much earlier intervention for development; taken together, the research supports the importance of caregiver-child communication in the context of their relationship for development in multiple domains, including language and speech development (e.g., Yoshinaga-Itano & Apuzzo, 1998; Yoshinaga-Itano, Sedley, Coulter, & Mehl, 1998; Verhaert, Willems, Van Kerschaver, & Desloovere, 2008), as well as social-emotional development (Bat-Chava, Martin, & Kosciw, 2005; Prezbindowski, 2001; Yoshinaga-Itano & de Uzcategui, 2001), and, interestingly, development of "Theory of Mind" (Macaulay & Ford, 2006; Schick, DeVilliers, DeVilliers, & Hoffmeister, 2007).

As mentioned previously, early identification and intervention may enhance sensitive responding to the child's signals (Young & Tattersall. 2007); maternal sensitivity and emotional availability is an important predictor of the development of expressive language in all children, but more so for children with hearing impairment (Pressman et al., 1998). Such sensitivity is seen in the IDS used by mothers of children with hearing impairment who were fitted with cochlear implants. In a recent study, Bergeson and her colleagues (Bergeson et al., 2006) examined IDS of mothers with typical hearing with their infants and toddlers with hearing impairment, who ranged in age from 10 to 37 months; all of the children with hearing impairment used cochlear implants. Bergeson et al. matched these children with two control groups of children with typical hearing; one group was selected to match the children with hearing impairment by chronological age (10 to 37 months), and the other was matched by hearing experience (3 to 18 months). Results indicated that mothers of children with hearing impairment provided IDS that was similar to the IDS provided to the children matched by hearing experience, not age. Bergeson et al.'s results suggest that maternal sensitivity to children's hearing experience and their linguistic abilities is clearly evident for both children with typical hearing as well as for children with hearing impairment who use cochlear implants.

Research also suggests a relationship between early identification and intervention, and social and emotional development (Yoshinaga-Itano & de Uzcategui, 2001). Although expressive language development is an important predictor, the effect on social development appears to be mediated by degree of hearing impairment for children who experienced late identification, in that parents of children *with late identification* who had mild hearing loss report poorer social development of their children, even though the children's language skills were good. The authors make the point that:

> (s)ome have argued that children with mild hearing loss do not demonstrate enough developmental delay to warrant newborn hearing screening. The personal-social skill difference appears to counter this argument. An implication for intervention for children identified later is that a much greater emphasis needs to be placed upon remediation of delays in this developmental area. (Yoshinaga-Itano & de Uzcategui, 2001, p. 21)

Development of Theory of Mind

A "theory of mind" (TOM) is a person's awareness of the mental states of other people, and includes awareness of others' knowledge, intentions, beliefs, feelings, and so forth (cf. Premack & Woodruff, 1978). In children with typical hearing, TOM may play an important predictive role in social development, specifically regarding social relationships with peers (Harris, de Rosnay, & Pons, 2005). Previous research has shown delayed development of TOM in children with hearing impairment, who have parents with typical hearing (e.g., Peterson, 2004; Peterson, Wellman, & Lui, 2005). Given that the children with hearing impairment were significantly language delayed, might these findings be a testing artifact related to language delay? Possibly not; TOM delay was apparent even when the children were tested with tasks that do not require well-developed language to either explain the task or to respond (Schick et al., 2007). However, the language delay itself may have contributed to the delayed development of TOM in these children (cf. Macaulay & Ford, 2006). Peterson and her colleagues (2004; Peterson et al., 2005) note that an important predictor of TOM performance was the child's vocabulary skills; this is consistent with Schick et al.'s (2007) contention that because vocabulary development is predicted strongly by conversational experience (cf. Hart & Risely, 1995), "the vocabulary measure is a proxy for how much rich conversation the children have been exposed to, and hence general conversation will always predict TOM," as "children learn about minds though conversation, even when the topic is not mind talk" (p. 392; cf. Ely, Gleason, MacGibbon, & Zaretsky, 2001). In more recent research, Remmel and Peters (2009) found no delay in TOM development in children with hearing impairment who used cochlear implants; these children had an average age of amplification of just over 12 months (implantation age was about 3 years) and were not language delayed. It is likely, then, that early identification of hearing loss, and concomitant early intervention that results in less delayed or normal language acquisition thus may have both direct (language, vocabulary) and indirect (TOM, social interaction) effects; indirect effects may also affect each other. For example, the improvements over time of children with hearing impairment with cochlear implants to interact socially with peers (Bat-Chava et al., 2005) may be at least partially attributable to improvements in their ability to understand the mental states of others.

Concluding Remarks and Recommendations

The field of developmental psychology began as "child study"; it thus started out as a very "applied" field, with the goal of improving child-rearing practices and education. Since that time, dividing lines have been drawn, to our detriment I believe, between basic research and clinical or applied practice. This brief review makes plain that both basic research and applied work is of great value. We have an obligation to do the best work possible to learn about basic developmental processes, and then to apply what we know to make life better for children and families (cf. Zigler, 1998).

With that in mind, I would like to offer some brief recommendations:

(1) Regarding EHDI: it is clear that early identification of all levels of hearing impairment is of great value, ***but only when followed by early intervention***. Delays in intervention are not only detrimental for the child who is affected, but cause needless stress and anxiety for the child's family (cf. Yoshinaga-Itano, 2003; Yoshinaga-Itano & de Uzcategui, 2001). Equally importantly, we must do a better job of explaining to parents what a "positive screening" test result means—that about 30 in 1,000 babies will have a positive result with a one-step screening test, but of those only 4 will actually have hearing loss; for 26 of those children, follow-up testing will be reassuring (Neault, 2001). Follow-up testing is absolutely essential, however, and given the large proportion of children who may not return for testing—and who then are at risk for very delayed identification—we must do a better job of tracking children who do not return for follow-up. States should also consider mandating a two-step testing protocol, with caregivers either using both OAE and AABR instead of just one method, or simply retesting before discharge (Wrightson, 2007); this has been shown to reduce false positive rates to less than 1% (Clemens, Davis, & Bailey, 2000).

(2) Attuned and responsive caregiving is always important, and may be even more important for children with hearing loss. Parents and caregivers may need enhanced social support and community resources to be able to optimize, as much as possible, their child's caregiving environments.

(3) Given the linguistic, social-emotional, and cognitive outcomes that are predicted by both infant- and child-directed speech and by parent-child conversation, as well as their important roles in relationship building, parents and caregivers should use every opportunity to read with and talk with their children from birth using IDS; children should also have opportunities to overhear more linguistically rich adult-directed speech.

Part II: Typical Development: Birth to Age Five

Newborns come into the world prepared in many ways for the developmental tasks they face. They have reflexes, a variety of sensory capacities, preadaptations to attend to certain stimuli (especially stimuli that are contingent on the infant's actions), and preadaptations for social interaction. In addition, development in all domains occurs together and is mutually interdependent. For example, in infancy, motor development (e.g., self-produced loco-motion) contributes to both cognitive development (development of spatial awareness and object concept), social/emotional development (exploration from a secure base and separation distress) and facilitates and enables autonomy seeking. However, it is still useful to summarize major developmental milestones separately in the various domains of development.

Cognitive Development and Play

Many theories have been proposed to try to account for cognitive development; although they vary in important ways, each is trying to account for rapid and complex cognitive developmental change, and in particular for the developmental milestones that are seen normatively.

From the beginning, infants are active participants in their own development, as they seek out information through their senses. Indeed, for most of the first year and part of the second, cognitive activity seems to be demonstrated mostly through perception and action, rather than internal symbolic representation. Thus, play is the "work" of infants and children. At first, infants explore visually and with their hands and mouths, as they develop visually guided reaching (by about 3 months). Objects become more interesting as they begin to understand that objects continue to exist when hidden; although infants won't search for completely hidden objects until 8 to 12 months, they will show surprise at physically impossible events, such as an object "vanishing" when occluded.

As symbolic representation develops by the middle of the second year, the toddler demonstrates this new cognitive structure behaviorally, in particular, though deferred imitation and pretend play. Imitation itself has been part of the infant's behavioral repertoire since early in infancy, as long as the model was visible; with deferred imitation now possible, however, the toddler can use a mental representation to guide behavior in the absence of a model. Toddlers also begin to engage in pretend play, an astonishing human achievement that entails maintaining multiple versions of reality simultaneously—what something really is, and what one is pretending it is. With development, pretend play becomes increasingly decontextualized; with an increasing "distancing" or differentiation between the symbol and the referent, the child is able to get further and further away from the real.

Pretend play, including increasing complex play and sociodramatic pretending with others (which entails the development of TOM, as discussed above), continues to develop in the three- to five-year-old child. In addition, however, the preschool-aged child is learning more about objects in the world. For example, puzzles and games with rules become interesting, and the scripted nature of events—"how things are supposed to happen"—is of great interest, and by the end of the first year is beginning to help children remember past events and predict future, similar ones. This is also why children as young as 18 months will find silly actions to be funny—they violate the "script" (e.g., wearing a bowl as a hat). In addition, as children gradually become able to separate attributes of objects, many children also become interested in classifying and categorizing based on these attributes (e.g., sorting objects based on size, shape, and/or color). Children's understanding of time, and of numbers and counting also develop in a predictable sequence during this time.

Motor Development

Contemporary research suggests four main principles of motor skill development; the first two parallel the sequence of physical development in prenatal life: cephalocaudal development, proximodistal development, differentiation, and joint roles for maturation and experience. In cephalocaudal development, control over motor skills tends to progress from the head downward to lower body parts. In proximodistal development, control over motor skills tends to progress from the center of the body out to the extremities. Differentiation refers to how whole-body, and later whole-extremity movements become more and more refined to specific sets of muscles. This refinement occurs in the arms before the legs (cephalocaudal) and in the arm before the hand before the fingers (proximodistal). Finally, as in other domains of development, motor development is best understood as a dynamic system in which maturation and experience interact in constantly changing ways. Good examples of the latter principle may be seen in the development of reaching and grasping, as well as in the development of walking.

Early, spontaneous reaching is called prereaching, which declines between 1 and 4 months; intentional reaching, usually visually guided, emerges around 4 months and becomes more refined over time, through physical maturation, active exploration of the environment and the pursuit of particular goals. By 8 months, infants' reaching has been integrated into a complex system of body movements (e.g., leaning and reaching simultaneously) and includes the refined thumb-forefinger pincer grasp.

The complex behavior of walking has its roots in the early stepping reflex; like other reflexes, this one declines early in infancy and a similar behavior reappears later, under voluntary control. The onset of walking depends partly on maturation of the muscles and nervous system and partly on practice, as walking depends on the ability to integrate many systems, including balance. Opportunity for practice may be important; recent research suggests that prolonged restriction of movement in infancy can delay the development of walking, and certain practices appear to modestly accelerate the development of walking.

Finally, although there are well-known "motor milestones" in motor development that involve average ages, there is a great deal of variability around these average ages; both the averages and the variability must be taken into account when assessing whether a particular child may or may not be experiencing a delay in motor development. Current international standards may be found here: http://www.who.int/childgrowth/standards/motor_milestones/en/index.html

Development of Self-Help Skills

The desire to do things for themselves—self-help skills—is partly an expression of normative toddler autonomy seeking, and reflects children's increasingly well developed sense of self-efficacy and executive competence. The actual ability of toddlers and pre-schoolers to perform these skills is usually less than their desires would have it; still developing gross and fine motor control, as described above, often determine just what children can accomplish independently.

Developmental Context

Another important set of factors that affect development in general, and self-help skills among others in particular, are those related to the child's developmental context: the influence of factors extending outward from the child, to the immediate context of the family, to the social and economic context of the community and institutions, and finally to the larger cultural context. Bronfenbrenner's (e.g., 1986) ecological theory outlines the complexity of contextual influences on development by means of a model depicting three concentric rings around the child at the center, with each ring directly and indirectly influencing all the rings inside of it.

The Family Context as the Child's Immediate Environment

The family makes up the majority of the infant and child's immediate environment, and includes parents and siblings, as well as extended family and kin networks. Families represent complex interconnected systems; each member affects others, and is in turn affected by them. These transactional effects are ongoing over time and have cumulative impacts (e.g., Sameroff & Seifer, 1983). At their simplest level, interactive effects are bidirectional, with child characteristics and behavior affecting parents' responses, and parent characteristics and behavior shaping children. Effects can be more complex, such as when marital satisfaction affects parenting behaviors (e.g., Conger et al. 1992, 1994).

The Social and Economic Context

The next "ring" in Bronfenbrenner's model is made up of the social and economic context in which the immediate context is situated;

this includes social, educational, religious, and health care institutions, as well as social and economic conditions in the community and in the larger society. Effects on children at this level are mostly indirect but still may be bi- or multidirectional, as when economic hardship causes increased marital conflict and parental stress, which increases inattentive and insensitive parenting, which may lead to child behavior problems (the nature of which would vary by age and other factors). These behavior problems may then act as another source of marital conflict and parental stress, further exacerbating the problematic situation (e.g., Conger et al., 1992, 1994).

The Cultural Context

The cultural context—the context of the shared system of beliefs, attitudes, values, and guidelines for behavior—has multiple and indirect effects on development. By virtue of our shared humanity, children in all cultures have fundamental needs for care and nurturance, and adults in all cultures prepare children to live and function in that culture by explicitly and implicitly socializing them in the values and standards of that culture. As socialization begins in the family, children's experience of cultural values is filtered through this immediate environmental context.

When Hearing Impairment Co-Occurs with Other Conditions

As of December 2010, there were almost 38,000 children and youth ages birth to 21 with hearing loss in the United States. Of these children and youth, for the approximately 19,000 for whom data is available, 58% are reported to be receiving speech and language services (Gallaudet Research Institute, April 2011). This is consistent with previous reports indicating that most common co-occurring conditions with hearing impairment were speech or language impairments, affecting almost 25% of this population; specific learning disabilities and intellectual disability were the two next most common co-occurring conditions (Gallaudet Research Institute, December 2006). Chapman and his colleagues have found that approximately

31.5% of children identified with hearing impairment at birth had one or more co-occurring medical conditions (Chapman et al., 2011). Over 70 different inherited syndromes include hearing impairment, both stable and progressive, as a common part of the syndrome (Batshaw et al., 2007). For example, children with Down syndrome are at greater risk for conductive hearing loss, due to characteristically small auricles, narrow auditory canals, and frequent otitis media; incidence of hearing impairment estimates range from 35% to 78% (Shott, Joseph, & Heithaus, 2001). There is great diversity among children who have hearing loss and other co-occurring conditions, not only in terms of the specific other condition(s), but also in terms of how both their hearing loss and the co-occurring conditions affect functioning (e.g., degree, age at identification, and intervention of each/all co-occurring conditions). An additional complication may arise when children with hearing loss have a co-occurring condition that is mild or moderate; they may experience delay in fully appropriate intervention due to later identification of the additional condition(s).

Useful Links on Developmental Milestones, Developmental Disabilities, and Hearing Impairment

The Centers for Disease Control and Prevention (CDC)—website for The National Center on Birth Defects and Developmental Disabilities (NCBDDD):
http://www.cdc.gov/ncbddd/index.html

The Centers for Disease Control and Prevention (CDC)—Hearing loss in children:
http://www.cdc.gov/ncbddd/hearingloss/index.html

Zero to Three—Child development information:
http://www.zerotothree.org

Developmental Milestones for Babies (0 to 2 yrs.):
http://nichcy.org/disability/milestones

Growth Milestones:
http://www.kidsgrowth.com/stages/guide/index.cfm

Typical Speech and Language Development:
www.asha.org/public/speech/development/default.htm

Speech and Language Developmental Milestones:
http://www.nidcd.nih.gov/health/voice/pages/
speechandlanguage.aspx

References

Ainsworth, M. D. S., Bell, S., & Stayton, D. (1974). Infant–mother attachment and social development: Socialization as a product of reciprocal responsiveness to signals. In M. Richards (Ed.), *The integration of the child into the social world* (pp. 91–135). Cambridge, MA: Cambridge University Press.

Babbidge, H. (1965). *Education of the Deaf in the United States: The report of the Advisory Committee on Education of the Deaf.* Washington, DC: U.S. Government Printing Office.

Bat-Chava, Y., Martin, D., & Kosciw, J. G. (2005). Longitudinal improvements in communication and socialization of deaf children with cochlear implants and hearing aids: Evidence from parental reports. *Journal of Child Psychology and Psychiatry, 46*(12), 1287–1296.

Batshaw, M. L, Pellegrino, L., & Roizen, N. J. (2007). *Children with disabilities* (6th ed.). Washington, DC: Brookes.

Bell, S. M., & Ainsworth, M. D. S. (1972). Infant crying and maternal responsiveness. *Child Development, 43,* 1171–1190.

Bergeson, T. R., Miller, R. J., & McCune, K. (2006). Mothers' speech to hearing-impaired infants and children with cochlear implants. *Infancy, 10*(3), 221–240.

Bess, F., & Paradise, J. (1994). Universal screening for infant hearing impairment: Not simple, not risk-free, not necessarily beneficial, and not presently justified. *Pediatrics, 93,* 330–334.

Black, J. E., & Greenough, W. T. (1986). Induction of pattern in neural structure by experience: Implications for cognitive development. In M. E. Lamb, A. L. Brown, & B. Rogoff (Eds.), *Advances in developmental psychology* (Vol. 4, pp. 1–50). Hillsdale, NJ: Lawrence Erlbaum Associates.

Bronfenbrenner, U. (1986). Ecology of the family as a context for human development: Research perspectives. *Developmental Psychology, 22*(6), 723–741.

Byers-Heinlein, K., Burns, T. C., & Werker, J. F. (2010). The roots of bilingualism in newborns. *Psychological Science, 21*(3), 343–348.

Chapman, D. A., Stampfel, C. C., Bodurtha, J. N., Dodson, K. M., Pandya, A., Lynch, K. B., & Kirby, R. S. (2011). Impact of co-occurring birth defects on the timing of newborn hearing screening and diagnosis. *American Journal of Audiology, 20*, 132–139. doi:10.1044/1059-0889(2011/10-0049)

Clarkson, R. L., Eimas, P. D., & Marean, G. C. (1989). Speech perception in children with histories of recurrent otitis media. *Journal of the Acoustical Society of America, 85*, 926–933.

Clemens, C. J., Davis, S. A., & Bailey, A. R. (2000). The false-positive in universal newborn hearing screening. *Pediatrics, 106*(1), e7.

Conger, R. D., Conger, K. J., Elder, G. H. Jr., Lorenz, F. O., Simons, R. L., & Whitbeck, L. B. (1992). A family process model of economic hardship and adjustment of early adolescent boys. *Child Development, 63*, 526–541.

Conger, R. D., Ge, X., Elder, G. H. Jr., Lorenz, F. O., & Simons, R. L. (1994). Economic stress, coercive family process and developmental problems of adolescents. *Child Development, 65*(2), 541–561.

Cooper, R. P., Abraham, J., Berman, S., & Staska, M. (1997). The development of infants' preference for motherese. *Infant behavior and development, 20*(4), 477–488.

Crain, W. (2005). *Theories of development: Concepts and applications* (5th ed.). Upper Saddle River, NJ: Pearson/Prentice-Hall.

DeCasper, A. J., & Fifer, W. P. (1980). Of human bonding: Newborns prefer their mothers' voices. *Science, 208*, 1174–1176.

Ely, R., Gleason, J. B., MacGibbon, A., & Zaretsky, E. (2001). Attention to language: Lessons learned at the dinner table. *Social Development, 10*(3), 355–373.

Emde, R. N., & Easterbrooks, M. A. (1985). Assessing emotional availability in early development. In W. K. Frankenburg, R. N, Emde, & J. W. Sullivan (Eds.), *Early identification of children at risk: An international perspective* (pp. 79–101). New York, NY: Plenum.

Ferguson, C. A. (1964). Baby talk in six languages. *American Anthropologist, 66*, 103–114.

Ferguson, C. A. (1977). Baby talk as a simplified register. In C. E. Snow & C. A. Ferguson (Eds.), *Talking to children: Language input and acquisition* (pp. 209–235). Cambridge, MA: Cambridge University Press.

Fernald, A., Taeschner, T., Dunn, J., Papousek, M., de Boysson-Bardies, B., & Fukui, I. (1989). A cross-language study of prosodic modification in mothers' and fathers' speech to preverbal infants. *Child Language, 16*, 477–501.

Gaffney, M., Green, D. R., & Gaffney, C. (2010). Newborn hearing screening and follow-up: Are children receiving recommended services? *Public Health Reports, 125*, 199–207.

Gervain, J. & Werker, J. F. (2008). How infant speech perception contributes to language acquisition. *Language and Linguistics Compass, 2/6,* 1149–1170. doi:10.1111/j.1749-818x.2008.00089.x

Greenough, W. T., & Black, J. E. (1992). Induction of brain structure by experience: Substrates for cognitive development. In M. R. Gunnar & C. A. Nelson (Eds.), *Developmental behavior neuroscience* (Vol. 24, pp. 155–200). Hillsdale, NJ: Lawrence Erlbaum Associates.

Greenough, W. T., Black, J. E., & Wallace, C. S. (1987). Experience and brain development. *Child Development, 58,* 539–559.

Hart, B., & Risely, T. R. (1995) *Meaningful differences in the everyday experience of young American children.* Baltimore, MD: P. H. Brookes.

LeVay, S., Hubel, D. H., & Weisel, T. N. (1980). The development of ocular dominance columns in normal and visually deprived monkeys. *The Journal of Comparative Neurology, 191,* 1–51.

Macaulay, C. E. & Ford, R. M. (2006). Language and theory-of-mind development in prelingually deafened children with cochlear implants: A preliminary investigation. *Cochlear Implants International, 7,* 1–14.

Mace, A. L., Wallace, K. L., Whan, M. Q., & Stelmachowicz, P. G. (1991). Relevant factors in the identification of hearing loss. *Ear and Hearing, 12,* 287–293.

Moon, C., Cooper, R. P., & Fifer, W. P. (1993). Two-day-olds prefer their native language. *Infant Behavior and Development, 16*(4), 495–500.

Nittrouer, S. (1995). The relation between speech perception and phonemic awareness: Evidence from low SES children and children with chronic otitis medial. *Journal of Speech and Hearing Research, 39,* 1059–1070.

Pegg, J. E., Werker, J. F., & McLeod, P. J. (1992). Preference for infant-directed over adult-directed speech: Evidence from seven-week-old infants. *Infant Behavior and Development, 15,* 325–345.

Peterson, C., Wellman, H., & Lui, D. (2005). Steps in Theory of Mind development for children with deafness or autism. *Child Development, 76,* 502–571.

Premack, D., & Woodruff, G. (1978). Does the chimpanzee have a theory of mind? *Behavioral and Brain Sciences, 1*(4), 515–526.

Pressman, L. J., Pipp-Siegel, S., Yoshinaga-Itano, C., Kubicek, L., & Emde, R. (1998). A comparison of the links between emotional availability and language gain in young children with and without hearing loss. *Volta Review, 100*(5), 251–277.

Prezbindowski, A. K. (2002). The quality of mother-child interaction and social competence of deaf and hearing preschoolers: A longitudinal study. *Dissertation Abstracts International: Section B: The Sciences and Engineering* (Vol. 62 [8-B], number AAI3024350).

Ramus, F., Hauser, M. D., Miller, C., Morris, D., & Mehler, J. (2000). Language discrimination by human newborns and by cotton-top tamarin monkeys. *Science, 288*(5464), 349–351.

Remmel, E. & Peters, K. (2009). Theory of mind and language in children with cochlear implants. *Journal of Deaf Studies and Deaf Education, 14*(2), 218–236.

Sachs, J. (1977). The adaptive significance of linguistic input to prelinguistic infants. In C. E. Snow & C. A. Ferguson (Eds.), *Talking to children: Language input and acquisition* (pp. 51–61). Cambridge, MA: Cambridge University Press.

Sameroff, A. J. & Seifer, R. (1983). Familial risk and child competence. *Child Development, 54*, 1254–1268.

Schick, B. DeVilliers, P., DeVilliers, J., & Hoffmeister, R. (2007). Language and theory of mind: A study of deaf children. *Child Development, 78*, 376–396.

Shott, S., Joseph, A., & Heithaus, D. (2001). Hearing loss in children with Down Syndrome. *International Journal of Pediatric Otorhinolaryngology, 61*, 199–205.

Shultz, S. & Vouloumanos, A. (2010). Three-month-olds prefer speech to other naturally occurring signals. *Language Learning and Development, 6*, 241–257. doi:10.1080./154754409003507830.

Sroufe, L. A., Egeland, B., Carlson, E. A., & Collins, W. A. (2005). *The development of the person: The Minnesota study of risk and adaptation from birth to adulthood.* New York, NY: Guilford Press.

Sroufe, L. A., & Fleeson, J. (1986). Attachment and the construction of relationships. In W. W. Hartup & Z. Rubin (Eds.), *Relationships and development* (pp. 51–71). Hillsdale, NJ: Erlbaum.

Sroufe, L. A. & Sampson, M. C. (2000). Attachment theory and systems concepts. *Human Development, 43*, 321–326.

Thompson, D. C., McPhillips, H., Davis, R. L., Lieu, T. A., Homer, C. J., & Helfand, M. (2001). Universal newborn hearing screening: Summary of evidence. *Journal of the American Medical Association, 286*(16), 2000–2010.

Tierney, A. L. & Nelson, C. A., III (2009). Brain development and the role of experience in the early years. *Zero to Three, 30*(2), 9–13.

Timney, B. (1990). Effects of brief monocular deprivation on binocular depth perception in the cat: A sensitive period for the loss of stereopsis. *Visual Neurosciences, 5*, 273–280.

U.S. Department of Health, Education, and Welfare. (1967). *Education of the deaf: The challenge and the charge.* A report of the National Conference for the Education of the Deaf. Washington, DC: Government Printing Office.

U.S. Preventative Services Task Force. (1996). Screening for hearing impairment. *U.S. Preventative Services Task Force to Clinical Preventative Services* (2nd ed., pp. 393–405). Baltimore, MD: Williams & Wilkins.

Valenza, E., Simion, F., & Cassia, V. M. (1996). Face preference at birth. *Journal of Experimental Psychology: Human Perception and Performance, 22*(4), 892–903.

Vouloumanos, A. & Werker, J. F. (2007). Listening to language at birth: Evidence for a bias for speech in neonates. *Developmental Science, 10*(2), 159–171.

Werker, J. F., Pons, F., Dietrich, C., Kajikawa, S., Fais, L., & Amano, S. (2007). Infant-directed speech supports phonetic category learning in English and Japanese. *Cognition, 103*, 147–162. doi:10.1016/j.cognition.2006.03.006

Werker, J. F., & Tees, R. C. (1984). Cross-language speech perception: Evidence for perceptual reorganization during the first year of life. *Infant Behavior and Development, 7*, 49–63.

Werker, J. F., & Tees, R. C. (2005). Speech perception as a window for understanding plasticity and commitment in language systems of the brain. *Developmental Psychobiology, 46*(3) 233–234.

Winskel, H. (2006). The effects of an early history of otitis media on childrens' language and literacy skill development. *British Journal of Educational Psychology, 76*, 727–744.

Wray, H. (1997). Politics of biology: How the nature vs. nurture debate shapes public policy and our view of ourselves. *U.S. News & World Report, 122*(15), 72–79.

Wrightson, A. S. (2007). Universal newborn hearing screening. *American Family Physician, 75*(9), 1349–1352.

Yoshinaga-Itano, C. (2004). Levels of evidence: Universal newborn hearing screening (UNHS) and early hearing detection and intervention systems (EHDI). *Journal of Communication Disorders, 37*, 451–465.

Yoshinaga-Itano, C. & Apuzzo, M. L. (1998). Identification of hearing loss after 18 months is not early enough. *American Annals of the Deaf, 143*(5), 380–387.

Yoshinaga-Itano, C. & de Uzcategui, C. A. (2001). Early identification and social-emotional factors of children with hearing loss and children screening for hearing loss. In E. Kurtzer-White & D. Luterman (Eds.), *Early childhood deafness* (pp. 13–28). Baltimore, MD: York Press.

Young, N. M., Reilly, B. K., & Burke, L. (2011). Limitations of Universal Newborn Hearing Screening in early identification of pediatric cochlear implant candidates. *Archives of Otorhinolaryngology-Head and Neck Surgery, 137*(3), 230–234. doi:10.1001./archoto.2011.4

Zigler, E. (1998). A place of value for applied and policy studies. *Child Development, 69*(2), 532–542.

Chapter 7

LEARNING TO READ

*. . . learning to read and write begins
long before the school years.*

Snow, Burns, & Griffin, 1998, p. 43

*. . . we have to remind ourselves over and over
again that reading means the ability to make sense
out of the print, not sound out of the print.*

Fox, 2008, p. 85

*The progress of children with implants in the
areas of speech perception, speech production,
language, and reading has far exceeded the
expectations of even the most optimistic.*

Moog, 2002, p. 138

*The writer constructs a text with a meaning
potential that will be used by readers to construct
their own meaning. Effective reading is making
sense of print, not accurate word identification.*

Goodman, 1994, p. 1094

Introduction

Essential to our thinking about reading is that the purpose of language is to create meaning, whether we are listening, speaking, reading, or writing. We understand something that we hear or read when we are able to connect it to something we already know about. These connections come in the form of words, word parts, word functions, and general knowledge of the world that we can label by using words. The work that is done by parents, speech-language therapists, and teachers to help a young child who is deaf or hard of hearing learn all facets of spoken language—its sounds, syntax, vocabulary, and conventional uses—counts as helping the child learn to read. We are teaching reading when we speak, read, and write with a child, even though we are not, in the early stages, doing anything that looks like formal instruction. According to Adams (1990):

> . . . the most important activity for building the knowledge and skills eventually required for reading is that of reading aloud to children. In this, both the sheer amount of and the choice of reading materials seem to make a difference. Greatest progress is had when the vocabulary and syntax of the materials are just ever so slightly above the child's own level of linguistic maturity. (p. 86)

With this simultaneous support and challenge, many children with typical hearing simply figure out for themselves how the process works by matching letters to sounds and whole words spoken to whole words in print. I have seen children with hearing loss do this, as well. Frank Smith (1987) writes about this phenomenon as joining the literacy club and explains it in terms of the child learning how to read in the presence of someone who knows how to read, just as an apprentice learns to do a particular process by watching and being guided by someone else who does it. This may seem far-fetched, as our usual mental image of a child learning to read has the child laboriously sounding out words and/or practicing the recognition of a particular set of words. I have come to understand that, regardless of the approach used with them, children learn to read by discovering for themselves how the system works, whether this happens on its own or in a formal instructional setting. Children bring a question to a text, and they work on that question until they feel satisfied they know an answer to it.

I have taught long enough to know that teachers can create an environment for learning and make specific presentations to students, but that learning is not a transference of knowledge from the teacher's head to the student's. It is the learner who constructs an understanding of something. We can hope the student's understanding turns out to be similar to the teacher's, but it will not be because the teacher imposed it on the student in that form. Rather, it will be because the student builds an understanding on foundations similar to those of the teacher. Certainly, some learners simply memorize what the teacher presents, and sometimes such learners at first appear to have mastered the content or processes involved, but memorization is not the same as understanding. It can help to memorize something so that it is in memory to be analyzed, but it is in the active analysis done by the learner that learning takes place. In this active analysis, the learner is seen as creating his or her understanding, rather than just remembering something in the form in which it is encountered. This way of thinking about learning is called constructivism, and it is based on a broad range of thinking including Piagetian, Vygotskian, and other cognitive theory (Kamii, Manning, & Manning, 1991).

Constructivism in Action

In a study of children reading with their parents and then retelling the stories (Robertson, Dow, & Hainzinger, 2006), which is described in greater detail later in this chapter, we observed two preschool children, Rupert and Hallie, in the very moments of learning something fundamental about word identification. Both of the children used cochlear implants, had had intensive auditory-verbal therapy, and had been read with regularly, but had not started kindergarten; neither had received formal instruction in reading, not even from their parents. In the two instances I describe below, Rupert was testing his ideas about the alphabetic principle, and Hallie was coming to the understanding that the same configuration of shapes always stands for the same name.

Here is what happened. Rupert was listening to his mother read *Owen*, by Kevin Henkes, for the third time, with the readings spread over three weeks. There is a point in the story when Owen, a little boy mouse, has his blanket over his head, and he says, "Bet you can't see me!" Rupert listened to his mother read the sentence that, in the book, is suspended above the character's head in cartoon fashion. She had pointed at the picture as she read. Rupert asked her to read the sentence again, which she did. Then he asked for it backward, although he didn't have "backward" in his vocabulary. He said "read it this way" and pointed from right to left at the words. His mother read, "!me see can't you Bet." Then Rupert said, "Read this," and covered the "b" in "bet." His mother said "be." Then "Read this," and Rupert covered the "u" in "you," which elicited "yo" from his mother. They went on this way through covering the "t" in "can't," the "e" in "see," and the "e" in "me," producing "can," "se," and "m." The satisfied smile on Rupert's face showed pure joy. And then, they returned to the story. Rupert was well on his way to using his phonemic awareness to support his newly developing idea that each letter "sounds" a certain way.

In Hallie's case, she was retelling the *Owen* story to her mother by looking at the pictures, when early in the book, she pointed to an instance of "Owen" in the text and said "Owen." Her mother confirmed that the word said "Owen," and they went on with the retelling. Soon, Hallie saw more occurrences of "Owen," pointed to them, and said "Owen." She flipped through the pages, pointing, and exclaiming, "Owen," "Owen," "Owen," "Owen," "Owen," everywhere she saw the name, and her mother said, "Yes, those all say 'Owen.' " At one point, her mother wanted her to stop and to get back to the story, and Hallie said, "I don't want to do that," after which she went on to call out more discoveries of "Owen." Finally, she was satisfied and returned to retelling the story of *Owen* to her mother, with a look of excitement on her face. She knew she was learning to read; in this case, she had discovered something about what a word is and the stability of letter patterns that make up individual words.

These two stories demonstrate well how children pay attention to all sorts of cues as they have experiences and how the parent, teacher, or other adult may not have control over the child's locus of attention. Children set themselves problems to solve and can then be focused and relentless in solving those problems, letting nothing else get in the way until they are satisfied. This is a form of constructivism. Not every child will do this without formal instruction as Rupert and Hallie did, but every child constructs his or her own knowledge in all areas, both of content and procedures, as a matter of course in living. While this is happening, the adult can embrace whatever the child has chosen to attend to and help the child along in coming to understand it.

Children who are read with often ask for the same book over and over again, and then finally there will be a time when they no longer ask for that book, or they let some time pass between requests. Once they have answered their own questions, they have exhausted the book, at least for a time (Kamii, Manning, & Manning, 1991, p. 98). The same phenomenon happens whether the child is learning to walk, to stack blocks, to ride a bike, to ask for a treat, or to play checkers with grandpa (Table 7–1).

Shared Book Reading

A Study of Story Retelling

You may be wondering whether and how the child with significant hearing loss can take in enough of the words, phrases, and

Table 7–1. Factors Predictive of Reading Acquisition

- Phonemic awareness
- Oral language acquisition
- Print awareness
- Semantic knowledge
- Frequent reading and writing practice
- Cognitive organization and categorization
- Parental talk and responsiveness

sentences of a book read aloud to comprehend a story and learn language from it. In a study of shared book reading, my colleagues and I attempted to learn about this (Robertson, Dow, & Hainzinger, 2006). We began with the knowledge that, in children with typical hearing, reading with them has long been associated with their learning to read (Adams, 1990; Durkin, 1966), and that shared book reading leads to oral and written language capabilities in children with typical hearing (Bus et al., 1995). Our original question was, "How many more readings of a book would a child with hearing loss need in order to demonstrate a grasp of it compared to a child with typical hearing?" We hypothesized that, given what can be done to help children with hearing loss to listen, they would be able to listen and comprehend, but that the process with any given book would take longer. We located 21 preschool children, ages 3 to 5, 11 with typical hearing and 10 with hearing loss with whom the auditory-verbal approach had been and continued to be used. We set up a six-week schedule during which their parents would bring them to a central place and read with them. All sessions were videotaped and then transcribed (Table 7–2).

We chose four books for the study and settled on these delightful texts by Kevin Henkes: *Owen, A Weekend with Wendell, Wemberley Worried,* and *Sheila Rae, the Brave.* These books contain well-formed, extended language, complete with descriptions and dialogue. The stories connect to children's experiences, and the pictures illustrate the story well. The vocabulary load of the books appears to have been thought out so as to introduce new words in the midst of words usually known by the children who will have

Table 7–2. Listening to and Retelling a Story Provides Practice in a Variety of Literacy Skills

• Listening	• Speaking
• Thinking	• Selecting and organizing information
• Interacting	• Remembering words and content
• Matching	• Comprehending
• Comparing	• Using language to learn about language

the books read to them; for example, Owen experiences "vinegar," "snipped," and "handkerchiefs," and Wemberley worries about "radiators," "shrinking," and "bolts." Each book has an emotional content that deals with typical children's situations: giving up one's security blanket, getting along with a playmate who always wants to be in control, worrying about things going wrong, and becoming independent.

The procedure was that each parent read the same book with his or her child for the first three weeks. During the next three weeks, three other books were read, one per week. To prevent the possibility that one of the books would be easier than the others, we counterbalanced the presentation of the books, thus giving each child the same chance of getting any particular book during any particular week. Before we began, all children were given the Peabody Picture Vocabulary Test, on which all the children in the study, both with and without hearing loss, scored in the average range. A significant difference existed between the groups on the PPVT, however; the children with typical hearing had a mean score at the 75th percentile, and the children with hearing loss had a mean score at the 50th percentile.

In our analysis of the transcripts, we found that despite having smaller vocabularies, the children with hearing loss remembered and repeated verbatim words from the stories, which we judged to be proof of listening, as often as did children with typical hearing. We also found that three repeated readings did not increase the amount and kind of talking the children in either group did about each story, a result we still wonder about. Perhaps a fourth, fifth, or sixth reading repetition would have stimulated more talking, perhaps not. What we find compelling is that the children with hearing loss did as well in recalling the stories as the children with typical hearing, once their vocabulary differences on the PPVT were taken into account statistically. We had expected them to take longer in coming to a point of demonstrating understanding compared to the children with typical hearing. Interestingly, and perhaps most importantly, we did find a difference in parental behavior; parents of children with hearing loss responded more, used more scaffolding (support in building an idea), and stimulated conversations more than did parents of children with typical hearing. They had learned something that would benefit all children: that parents can be good, intentional language role models for their children, just by conversing with them about a story. Our present understanding is that children with hearing loss who use appropriate hearing technology and who receive auditory-verbal therapy can, indeed, use vocabulary at levels commensurate with their typically hearing peers, and they can listen in ways similar to their typically hearing peers. Parent behaviors with their children with hearing loss contribute to this outcome. We conclude that:

> Parents and teachers of children with hearing loss can feel confident in reading with children often, retelling and talking about the stories, taking turns talking, using words from the stories in meaningful ways, and using synonyms of words from the stories. (Robertson, Dow, & Hainzinger, 2006, pp. 164–165)

This takes care of the question of whether it is possible for children with hearing loss to listen to books read aloud with them with a resounding "Yes!" But, it does not describe exactly how this takes place. For now, we can surmise the process is the same as it is in children with typical hearing. In responding to spoken language, children develop language capabilities that use sounds of words and word parts, phrases, sentences, and extended language, all in the service of making meaning of the world around them. What makes sense enters and remains in memory, and what does not make sense is not retained, so we want to make certain that we initiate and extend meaningful and relevant conversations with our children with hearing loss. This must be done more intentionally and with more forethought than with children with typical hearing, because, however effective our current hearing technology is, it is not equivalent to typical hearing. Much must be addressed to the child directly.

Arnold and Whitehurst (1994) make this point concerning intentionality in their discussion of "dialogic reading." They developed a shared reading program for children with typical hearing based on three general principles: (1) "evocative techniques" used by parents to stimulate their children to be active participants in looking at picture books together; (2) "parental feedback" in the form of "expansions, modeling, corrections, and praise" designed to give children experience with more complex language than they already possess; and (3) "progressive change in adult standards" achieved by pushing the limit of the child's zone of proximal development (pp. 104–105). The "zone of proximal development" is a concept developed by Vygotsky who defined it as:

> . . . the distance between a child's actual developmental level as determined through independent problem solving and [his or her] potential development [level] as determined through problem solving under adult guidance or a collaboration with more capable peers. (Vygotsky, 1978, as cited in Harris & Hodges, 1995, p. 288)

The idea is that the child adds to his or her current capabilities in the company of someone who can demonstrate a more advanced level of competence and mentor the child while he or she constructs new knowledge.

In this spirit, the goal of dialogic reading is that, having had the parent as a model storyteller, the child gradually takes over the role of telling the story seen in the pictures, and the parent becomes the listener. In this program, parents are taught to do the following with two- and three-year-olds: ask "what" questions, follow up with more questions, repeat what the child says, help the child as needed, praise and encourage, and follow the child's interests. Next, the parents learn to ask open-ended questions and to expand the child's language. Most important, parents are urged to have fun by making a game of looking at the pictures and taking turns talking (pp. 106–107). In an experimental application of this program, randomly-assigned parents of middle to high socioeconomic status learned the approach in two half-hour training sessions and practiced it with their children. Another randomly assigned set of parents and children served as a control group. After four weeks, the experimental group produced statistically significantly longer utterances on two expressive language measures, the Expressive One-Word Picture Vocabulary Test and the Illinois Test of Psycholinguistic Abilities, and these results were maintained at the end of the next nine months (p. 108). Taking this as evidence that it is possible to intervene in order to influence the growth of children's expressive language, the research turned to an experimental and a control group of parents and children of low socioeconomic status using the same experimental approach, and they recorded similar results (pp. 112–113). It is clear that parents from all backgrounds can learn to enhance their children's language abilities.

A Conclusion: What Can Be Learned Through Shared Book Reading?

Weaver (2002, p. 283) provides a helpful list of what can be learned through experiencing books alongside an older reader, and I have adapted it here:

1. The way to handle a book is by starting from the front and turning the pages until the book's end is reached.
2. Words are read from left to right and top to bottom on a page, and they begin to understand what constitutes a word and a letter.
3. Book language is different from spoken language, and there are differences of vocabulary, dialect, and dialogue descriptions. An example in which dialogue is written includes: "'Isn't he getting a little old to be carrying that thing around?' asked Mrs. Tweezers" (Henkes, 1993, p. 4). This usage of language is found only in writing.
4. Word identification can be done in context, both of whole words and word parts.
5. Listening to a book involves using what one already knows both about the world (the child's schemata) and about the way spoken language is written on paper.
6. It helps to predict what might come next within the story line, as well as in a particular sentence.
7. Listening involves "making connections, drawing inferences, asking questions, determining importance, creating visual (mental) images, [and] monitoring meaning and comprehension." (p. 283)
8. There is a vocabulary for talking about books, letters, and words.

The totality of this knowledge becomes the basis for responding to formal instruction when the child enters school. Certain content and processes will be in the child's repertoire, and then formal instruction contributes more instances in each category.

Sharing Constructions and Negotiating Meaning

In work with older children in classrooms, Brown and Cambourne (1987) gave story titles to children, asked them to write a prediction of what the story would contain, and then had them share their ideas with each other. Next, the children were given the actual story to read and asked to think about their original prediction in terms of where their ideas came from and how they differed from the story. Finally, the children were directed to reread the story until they felt comfortable to retell it in writing and then to do that writing and share it with other students. This extended process causes children to read and think about text very carefully and to use multiple language processes in doing so. In sharing their comprehension with others, students must refer to the text at all its levels as they discuss the overall meaning of the story. This results in their examining letters, words, phrases, punctuation, and sentences, and it leads to discussions of literal details as well as inferences and judgments made during the numerous readings that led to writing about the text. The children with whom Brown and Cambourne worked learned about comprehending text and adding to their vocabularies through active engagement individually and with each other. They came to durable understandings by negotiating meanings with each other and reported they had learned:

- to "understand more,"
- to spell and punctuate better,
- to get "lots of ideas for [their] own writing,"
- to know about how others come to understand something,
- to figure out the meaning of an unfamiliar word,
- to think about what they already know about a subject, and
- to enjoy positive feedback from other children. (pp. 10–11)

The children became flexible in their reading and displayed good willingness to read and reread particular texts as they developed their understandings of them (p. 11). Above all, they learned for themselves about how listening, speaking, reading, writing, and thinking intertwine with one another, and how they all involve using a spoken language. Brown and Cambourne term this "linguistic spillover" (p. 23) and believe the reading and retelling process is "an opportunity to use language to learn about language" (p. 115).

Listening and/or reading and then retelling is important for children with hearing loss as these activities lead them through the steps of examining language meaningfully at all levels and in all its facets. Children can and do make many discoveries for themselves and have many opportunities to compare what they think with others, including their parents, teachers, and peers. Capability with language and then with reading and writing develops through use of the language, and this requires patience and consistent willingness to interact with the child through spoken language, whether actually spoken or written. It is clear that literacy development depends upon the interdependence of vocabulary, syntax, discourse, and phonological sensitivity (Dickenson, McCabe, & Essex, 2006, p. 13).

Establishing a Rich Literacy Environment

In Chapter 4, we looked at the levels of spoken language used in the home and how greater quantity and quality of spoken language benefit children. This is one component of establishing a rich literacy environment. Such an environment includes frequent and varied opportunities to converse with adults who use a mature form of their spoken language as well as access to explanations of many forms of written material. Numerous studies have found that children who lag behind in reading have had far less access at home to books and other reading materials. One study found that middle income children in a particular community had an average of 199 books at home and 392 in their classroom library compared to 2.6 books at home and 54 in the classroom for lower income children. For the lowest income children in the study, the numbers were 0.4 and 47, respectively (Smith et al., 1997, as cited in Allington, 2006, p. 74). Another study in another community found an average of only 1 book per 300 low-income children compared to 13 books for each middle-income child (Neuman & Celano, 2001, cited in Neuman, 2006). The same researchers discovered that even when low-income children have access to materials in a public library, they often do not have the help of an adult to make sense of them (Neuman & Celano, 2001). Access requires, therefore, the presence of a facilitator who explains the significance of writing wherever it is present: books, menus, magazines, newspapers, catalogues, signs, and so on. One example of this is found in Adams (1990), where she describes her son John as a typical middle-class child who by age six years, three months would have spent 1000 to 1700 hours in one-on-one story book reading which began when he was six weeks old. At age five when she described him, he was not yet a reader, so she was writing at that point about his positive prospects for learning to read. Adams estimated that by his entrance into first grade, he would have also spent 1,000 hours watching *Sesame Street* and about the same amount of time playing with magnetic letters and crayons and reading and playing in a variety of ways with others who know how to read and write (p. 85). Compared to John, the typical child from a low-income family at school entry has had only 25 hours with storybooks and about 200 hours with other sorts of print (p. 90). Discrepancies of this magnitude matter.

The differences in reading achievement and time spent reading by the time a child is in fifth grade demonstrate both the cause and the effect of lack of reading practice. Among fifth graders keeping a log of their reading, those scoring at the 90th percentile read for an average of 40.4 minutes each day, which translated into 2,357,000 words per year. Those at the 50th percentile read an average of 12.9 minutes per day and 601,000 words per year; at the 10th percentile, the children were reporting 1.6 minutes per day and 51,000 words per year (Anderson, Wilson, & Fielding, 1988, as cited in Allington, 2006, p. 37).

Children who listen and talk only a little, and then read with others and later by themselves only a little are less likely to develop high levels of literacy. Practice is that important.

Reading Comprehension and the Child

Comprehension is, of course, the goal of reading *from the beginning*. Some suppose that children learn how to "sound out" words and then later learn to comprehend what they are reading, but children want their world and their actions in it to make sense, and they are unlikely to be drawn to an activity that produces sounds that hold little or no meaning for them. Listening comprehension is a prerequisite for reading and underlies the ability to predict what comes next either in a conversation, a message, or a reading passage. Especially when beginning to read for themselves, children ought to be reading what they can listen to with successful comprehension. This way, the text will be meaningful, and when it comes time to match words stored in auditory memory with words printed on a page, the child will be in a good position to do so. Of course, the child should always be learning to say and use new words. "The easy way to learn words is to experience lots of them in meaningful text" (Smith, 2004, p. 154). These come to the child in shared book reading, as well as in meaningful conversation with others who know more words. I have adapted the following guidelines from Marie Clay's advice for helping children build their background knowledge (schemata) and comprehension capabilities (Clay, 1991, p. 27):

- Provide many learning experiences for the child, include all the senses (hearing, sight, taste, smell, feeling), and talk about each experience with the child, using new vocabulary and new ways of using words embedded in words and usages the child already knows.
- Talk with the child about what he or she finds interesting. Find out what piques the child's interest, provide for experiences that help the child learn more, and ensure that the child hears and sees both old and new words appropriate to the subject.
- Think about talking with the child as getting him or her to think. Take the time to listen to a child's response in a conversation, and use your next response to expand on the topic at hand.
- Pose well-formed questions to the child and notice what she or he does with them in an effort to understand the child's view of the world. Think about where the child would benefit from adding to that worldview, and lead the child into talk about those areas.
- Provide the sort of information to the child that allows the child to add to his or her existing knowledge and interactions with the world.

Practical Ideas for Helping Children Learn to Read

How to Read Aloud with the Child with Hearing Loss

Children with hearing loss probably need more contact with literacy materials in the presence of a knowledgeable adult than the average middle-class child entering first grade. Teachers, parents, and others should read with them and talk about the stories, characters, and pictures in the book. I stress reading *with*, rather than reading *to*, because it is important to think about the child as being an active participant, rather than as a vessel to be filled up by the adult reader. Reading *with* includes reading aloud by the adult, talking about the story or information, and playing games with language. Practice is vital to any kind of learning, so it is important for children to be read with regularly, more than once a day, if possible. A typical recommendation is to read for a total of forty-five minutes each day and to read three books each day to a young child, one that is a favorite, another that is familiar, and a third that is new (Fox, 2008). Teachers should share this information with parents in order to teach them what they can be doing at home while the teacher is also reading with the child at school.

Reading with a child with hearing loss is similar to reading with a child with typical hearing, and it can begin at the earliest possible moment in the child's life. It is not advisable to wait until you think the child can understand what is being read, *as it is the reading itself that builds such understanding*. As I described above, the child will learn something during each reading session, and you will not always be able to specify what that something will be. That will depend on the child and what catches his or her interest during that particular session.

We have ample evidence that reading aloud with children from an early age and continuing to do so over the years results in wide knowledge of the world; excellent comprehension, problem-solving skill, and critical thinking ability; and solid—often exemplary—academic achievement (Trelease, 2006; Ozma, 2012). Most important, reading aloud creates in the child a desire to read and learn. Trelease quotes a college admissions director as saying he has "never met a student with high verbal SAT scores who wasn't a passionate reader" (p. xii). Ozma, a high-achieving student and excellent writer, describes how her father read aloud to her every night without fail for 3,218 nights in what they called "The Streak." Her father had always read aloud to Alice, but not necessarily every night. When Alice was in fourth grade, they made a pact to read for 100 straight nights and extended the challenge they set for themselves, only stopping when her father, Jim Brozina, took her to college. An additional effect of an adult reading regularly with a child is the relational bond they build together, a bond that provides the child with security, confidence, and the ability to speak for him or herself.

Chapter 8 provides more information about reading aloud, as well as practical suggestions for doing so.

Language Experience Books and the Language Experience Approach

Helen Beebe introduced me to what she called experience books. She had parents get a notebook or composition book and make a daily entry that dealt with something their child had experienced during that day or very recently. An entry could include a drawing or a bit of something, a ticket to the zoo, for example, pasted prominently on the page with a few words or a sentence or two written below the image or artifact. Before the child is talking, the parent or teacher thinks about a recent experience of the child's, provides words to represent it, writes them on the page, and draws a picture or pastes in a souvenir or a snapshot. At this point, the words should mainly be words the child has heard spoken in the environment. The adult can also choose a new word or phrase, or even a new bit of information to introduce in the context of the known words. Parents are to read this with their child as often as possible and to use it as a jumping off point for conversation. After speech is well enough established that the child can provide some of the words to write on the page, the process becomes one of dictation in which the child says the words to be written on the page, as in the Language Experience Approach, described below. Parents' active involvement in this fascinating process should extend over many years during which they move from providing all the language to a long period of sharing the writing and reading, and finally to independent writing and reading by the child. The experience is

Table 7–3. When Reading with a Child, Think About Building

• Vocabulary	• Life experiences
• Conversational language	• Thinking
• Textual language	

twofold: the parents and child talk about and remember events in their lives, and they spend time on the activity of conversing, constantly building language in the process (Table 7–3).

I think of this practice primarily as *language* experience and am influenced by the Language Experience Approach to reading that I learned about in my early graduate school work, and so I call these books "Language Experience Books." In the Language Experience Approach to teaching reading, the focus is on the child's language and on giving the child multiple opportunities to read his or her own language (Durkin, 1993; Dorr, 2006; Ivey & Fisher, 2006; Weaver, 2002). The principle involved is that one can best read what one knows: the vocabulary, syntax, and schema will be highly familiar to the young reader, and thus highly predictable, because the words to be read were spoken to the child in the child's normal environment and then chosen, composed, and uttered by the child.

> What I can think about, I can say. What I can say, I can write or someone can write for me. I can read what I have written or what someone has written for me. I can read what others have written. (Van Allen, 1982, cited in Dorr, 2006, p. 139)

Predictability is important to fluent reading and comprehension because it allows the reader to move smoothly from each word to the next. Predictions may be based on verbatim memory of one's own words, and as more time passes between uttering the words and then reading them, predictions may be based on a general memory of what one meant in saying the words. The child learns to pay attention to the *word meaning* (vocabulary) that ought to come next within the schema the child used in making the sentence(s), to the *kind* of word (syntax) the child thinks ought to come next, and to the set of words the child usually associates with the concept (schematic network) at hand. Initial letters and other parts of each word give further cues for children as children learn letter sounds, which works well when the words are spelled in phonemically regular ways.

The Language Experience Approach to reading assumes a child who is using a spoken language. The child tells a story to the parent, teacher, or other person who can listen and write. That person prints the words of the child somewhere on the next blank page of the language experience book and draws a picture that in some way represents the story. In time, the child will begin doing the printing and drawing, which I address in Chapter 8 in a discussion of writing. The stories are used as reading material for the language learner and then the beginning reader, and, of course, they will be interesting and accessible to that particular child, as they come directly from his or her experience. Children love to pore over stories about themselves, and when they do this, they learn much about language and concepts, and how these are recorded on paper.

The stories and their pictures can be done on separate pieces of paper that are bound together, but it is easier to keep it all together if a language experience book starts as a blank book or notebook of some sort. This book should not be elaborate; a plain school notebook will do. If the book starts looking like a fancy scrapbook decorated beautifully by the adult, the point of it being the child's creation is lost altogether. The adult who wants to document the child's life in a beautiful scrapbook should do so, but such a scrapbook is not, properly, a language experience book. The language experience book's purpose is to become the child's own personal reading book, put together in such a way that the child can imagine him or herself making such a book. The book also can be shared by parents and teachers to inform each other about experiences in the child's life, and it can be used as a starting point for delightful, extended discussions with the child that enrich the child's vocabulary and give him or her models for new sentence structures.

Sample pages from a Language Experience Book I did with my daughter before she could supply the language can be seen in Figures 7–1 through 7–8. We read the entries often and pored over the pictures to make sure she was able to hear and attend to the vocabulary, sentence structure, and background knowledge she needed in her daily activities. As time progressed, she began to provide the words for the language experience entries.

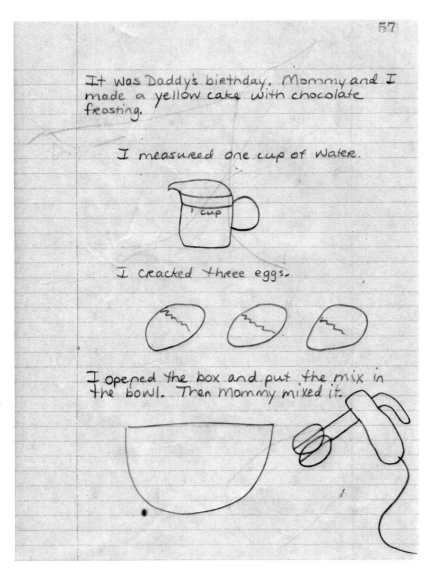

It was Daddy's birthday. Mommy and I made a yellow cake with chocolate frosting.

I measured one cup of water.

I cracked three eggs.

I opened the box and put the mix in the bowl. Then Mommy mixed it.

Figure 7–1. This story offers new vocabulary (frosting, measured, electric mixer), the concept of measuring, and a chance to count to 3.

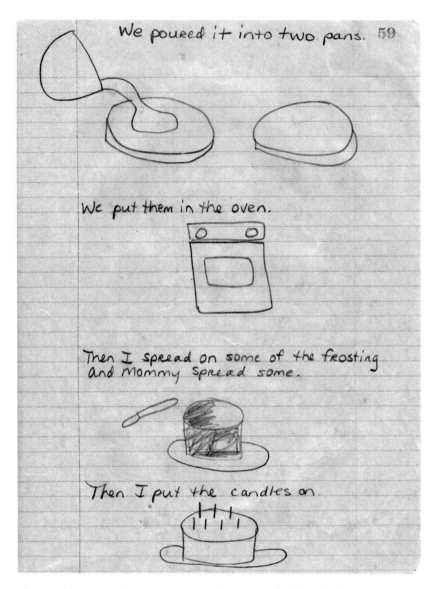

Figure 7–2. The cake story continues the sequential steps in the cake-making process and presents many objects to name (pans, oven, spreader, candles). (It's not clear how the cake got out of the oven, out of the pans, and on the plate!)

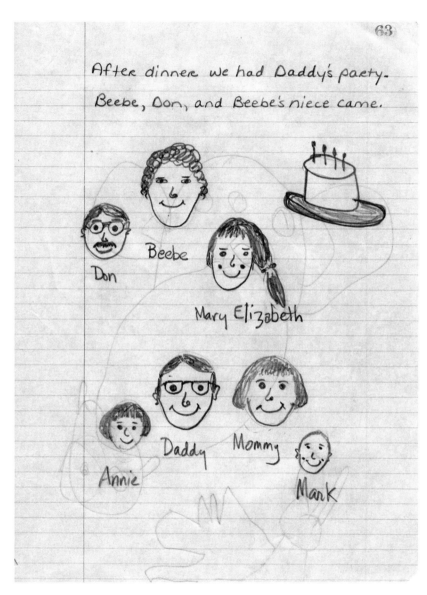

Figure 7–3. This page presents the concept of a party and an opportunity to remember the names of the new people she met.

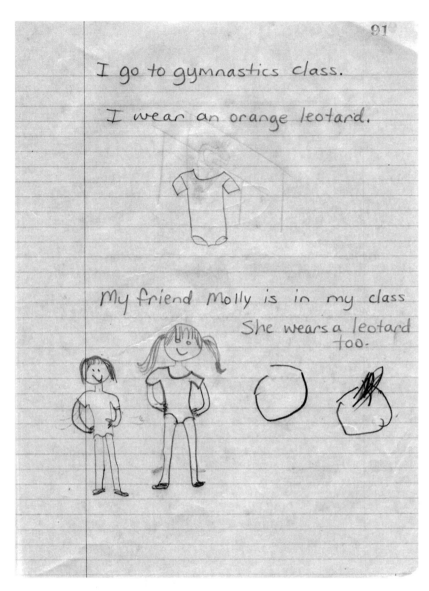

Figure 7–4. This page stimulates talk about going to gymnastics class with a friend. New vocabulary presented includes: gymnastics, orange, leotard.

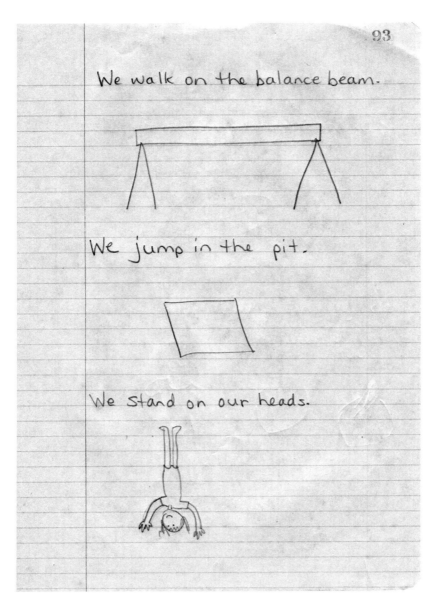

Figure 7–5. Here is a way to practice the names of the various activities at gymnastics class: balance beam, the pit, head stand.

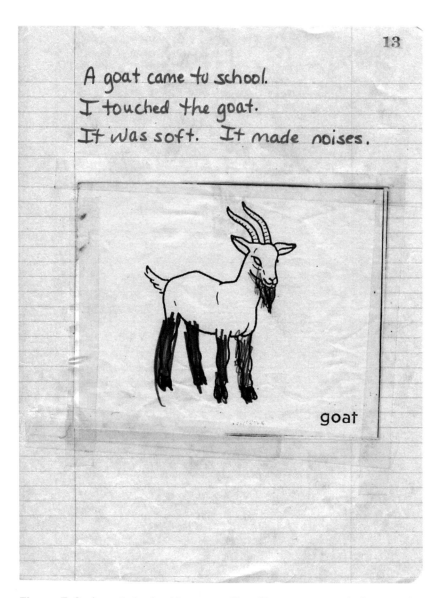

A goat came to school.
I touched the goat.
It was soft. It made noises.

goat

Figure 7–6. A goat at school is very exciting. The page presents the opportunity to ask, "How did the goat get to your school? In a car? In a van? In a farm truck?" "How did the goat's fur feel when you touched it?" Vocabulary includes: horns, eyes, ears, long legs, soft fur.

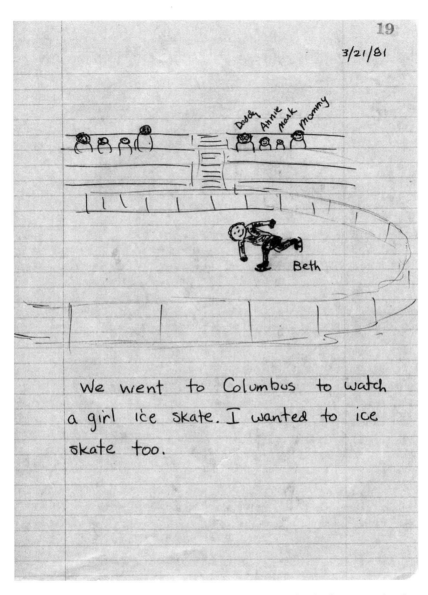

We went to Columbus to watch a girl ice skate. I wanted to ice skate too.

Figure 7-7. This page offers a way to talk about getting in the car and going on a short trip to watch a performance. New words include: skating, skating rink, bleachers.

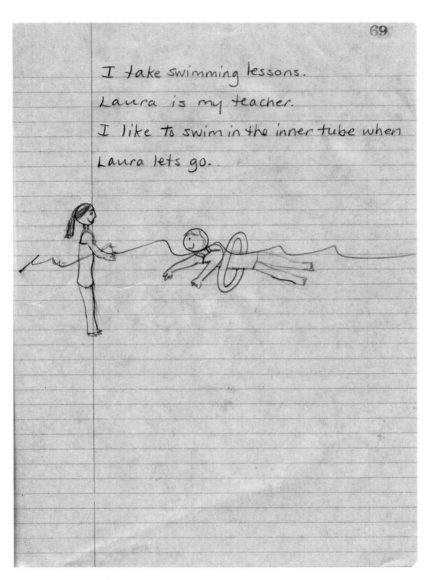

I take swimming lessons.
Laura is my teacher.
I like to swim in the inner tube when
Laura lets go.

Figure 7–8. Talking about an activity is a good way to build memory of the teacher's name and related vocabulary: pool, water, teacher, inner tube.

Conclusion

We must help the preschool child with hearing loss develop spoken language proficiency, knowledge of as many words and kinds of words as possible, and broad background knowledge of the world. This is what should be happening for all children, regardless of their hearing status. Daniel and Agnes Ling (1978) point out that it can appear to be a good idea to teach children with hearing loss to memorize and identify written words and their referents; most children can do this, and they look as though they are making progress in reading. Children with hearing loss who are as young as 3 or 4 can learn such associations easily: "A vocabulary of 50 to 100 nouns and 10 to 15 verbs may be taught quite quickly in this manner" (p. 242), but the problem is that those words may represent the child's entire spoken language vocabulary. The child in this situation does not know enough about language to truly learn how to read. That we can see the negative effects academically of depriving children with typical hearing of access to sufficient language development makes a strong argument for intervening as effectively as possible in the language development of children with hearing loss. The goal is to deliver the child who wears hearing aids or a cochlear implant to the first grade classroom where he or she can enter into the regular curriculum for beginning reading. Children who have much experience with shared reading and with language experience books have an excellent chance of learning to read and write alongside their peers with typical hearing when formal instruction is begun. I hope you have noticed that the discussion in this chapter is not about drilling children in letter and word identification or the sounding out of words. When such information is needed in the course of constructing meaning with a child, it should be given, but these are not the starting points. When the focus is on meaningful uses of language, the child learns to read in the company of one who knows how to read. Please see Chapter 10, "Creating and Using Language Experience Books" for practical information and application of using this approach.

References

Adams, M. (1990). *Beginning to read*. Cambridge, MA: MIT Press.

Allington, R. (2006). *What really matters for struggling readers: Designing research-based programs*. Boston, MA: Pearson.

Arnold, D., & Whitehurst, G. (1994). Accelerating language development through picture book reading: A summary of dialogic reading and its effects. In D. Dickinson (Ed.), *Bridges to literacy: Children, families, and schools* (pp. 103–128). Oxford, UK: Blackwell.

Brown, A., Palinscar, A., & Armbruster, B. (2004). Instructing comprehension-fostering activities in interactive learning situations. In S. Neuman & D. Dickinson (Eds.), *Handbook of early literacy research* (pp. 780–809). New York, NY: Guilford Press.

Brown, H., & Cambourne, B. (1987). *Read and retell*. Portsmouth, NH: Heinemann.

Bus, E., van Ijzendoorn, M., & Pellegrini, A. (1995). Joint book reading makes for success in learning to read: A meta-analysis on intergenerational transmission of literacy. *Review of Educational Research, 65,* 1–21.

Clay, M. (1991). *Becoming literate: The construction of inner control*. Portsmouth, NH: Heinemann.

Dickinson, D., McCabe, A., & Essex, M. (2006). A window of opportunity we must open to all: The case for preschool with high-quality support for language and literacy. In D. Dickinson & S. Neuman (Eds.), *Handbook of early literacy research* (Vol. 2, pp. 11–28). New York, NY: Guilford Press.

Dorr, R. (2006). Something old is new again: Revisiting language experience. *Reading Teacher, 60*(2), 138–146.

Durkin, D. (1966). *Children who read early*. New York, NY: Teachers College Press.

Durkin, D. (1993). *Teaching them to read* (6th ed.). Boston, MA: Allyn and Bacon.

Fox, M. (2008). *Reading magic*. Orlando, FL: Houghton Mifflin Harcourt.

Goodman, K. (1994). Reading, writing, and written texts: A transactional sociopsycholinguistic view. In R. Ruddell, M. Ruddell, & H. Singer (Eds.), *Theoretical models and processes of reading* (pp. 1093–1129). Newark, DE: International Reading Association.

Harris, T., & Hodges, R. (1995). *The literacy dictionary: The vocabulary of reading and writing*. Newark, DE: International Reading Association.

Henkes, K. (1987). *Sheila Rae, the Brave*. New York, NY: Green Willow Books.

Henkes, K. (1993). *A weekend with Wendell*. New York, NY: Green Willow Books.

Henkes, K. (1993). *Owen*. New York, NY: Green Willow Books.

Henkes, K. (2000). *Wemberly Worried*. New York, NY: Green Willow Books.

Ivey, G., & Fisher, D. (2006*). Creating literacy-rich schools for adolescents*. Alexandria, VA: Association for Supervision and Curriculum Development.

Moog, J. (2002). Changing expectations for children with cochlear implants. *Annals of Otology, Rhinology, and Laryngology, 111*, 138–142.

Neuman, S. (2006). The knowledge gap: Implications for early education. In D. Dickinson & S. Neuman (Eds.), *Handbook of early literacy research* (Vol. 2, pp. 29–40). New York, NY: Guilford Press.

Neuman, S., & Celano, D. (2001). Access to print in low-income and middle-income communities: An ecological study of four neighborhoods. *Reading Research Quarterly, 36*(1), 8–26.

Kamii, C., Manning, M., & Manning, G. (1991). *Early literacy: A constructivist foundation for whole language*. Washington, DC: National Education Association of the United States.

Ling, D., & Ling, A. (1978). *Aural habilitation: The foundations of verbal learning in hearing-impaired children*. Washington, DC: Alexander Graham Bell Association for the Deaf.

Ozma, A. (2012). *The reading promise*. New York, NY: Grand Central.

Palincsar, A., & Brown, D. (1987). Enhancing instructional time through attention to metacognition. *Journal of Learning Disabilities, 20*, 66–75.

Robertson, L., Dow, G., & Hainzinger, S. (2006). Story retelling patterns among children with and without hearing loss: Effects of repeated practice and parent-child attunement. *Volta Review, 106*(2), 147–170.

Smith, F. (1987). *Joining the literacy club: Further essays into education*. Portsmouth, NH: Heinemann.

Smith, F. (2004). *Understanding reading* (6th ed.). Mahwah, NJ: Lawrence Erlbaum Associates.

Snow, C., Burns, S., & Griffin, P. (1998) *Preventing reading difficulties in young children*. Washington, DC: National Academy Press.

Trelease, J. (2008). *The read-aloud handbook* (6th ed.). New York, NY: Penguin.

Weaver, C. (2002). *Reading process and practice* (3rd ed.). Portsmouth, NH: Heinemann.

Chapter 8

READING ALOUD
WITH CHILDREN

*Children who haven't been read to don't expect
print to make sense. And if children don't expect
sense, they'll find learning to read very difficult.*

Fox, 2008, p. 97

*The single most important activity for building the
knowledge required for eventual success in reading
is reading aloud to children . . . it is a practice
that should continue throughout the grades.*

Anderson et al., 1985

Introduction

Yes, it seems like a leap of faith to read aloud with a baby, toddler, or child with whom you cannot yet converse, and it's natural
to ask questions such as these: What is the point of talking if the
child can't understand what I'm saying or reading? Doesn't the
child need to know all the words before what I'm reading can
make sense to him or her? Don't I need to "preteach" vocabulary in
order to read to the child? As the child with hearing loss is already
behind, aren't we wasting precious time by not teaching the child
more directly about how to read?

Such questions are important and understandable, and the answers they imply follow a certain kind of logic. But another kind of logic that begins with knowledge of spoken language acquisition helps us understand why and how we can make progress toward language and reading acquisition by reading with a child with hearing loss. Fortunately, the interaction the adult and the child experience when reading and talking together solves the problems inherent in such questions. Infants and young children learn spoken language by having spoken language addressed to them in their environment and having frequent and continuous opportunity to use the language to interact with adults and others, at first by using novel approximations of the language, and then by refining the ability to speak and converse in the language over time. The important reality is that we cannot expect a child, especially a child with hearing loss, to be able to skip essential steps in this developmental sequence. The Listening and Spoken Language approach makes clear that parents and others in the child's life need to interact with the child using spoken language at every possible moment, and this includes both conversing with and reading aloud with the child.

When Should Reading Aloud Begin?

As soon as the child can hear by using technology, the child can begin learning to listen and to use listening to learn. As a parent or teacher, you can be assured that conversing and reading aloud with the child stimulates the language growth and development that lead to reading, writing, and communicating with others using proficient spoken language. Reading aloud with a child begins, ideally, when the child is an infant and even before birth, if possible.

It has been established for many decades that children with typical hearing begin listening in utero, and at birth are "sensitive to rhythmicity, intonation, frequency variation, and phonetic components of speech" (DeCasper & Fifer, 1980). In an interesting study, expectant mothers were audiotaped reading Dr. Seuss books aloud during their third trimester; when tested shortly after birth, their infants demonstrated recognition when presented with the same taped readings (DeCasper & Spence, 1986). Although infants born with hearing loss are already behind in developing their listening capabilities, knowledge of how listening begins in children with typical hearing is helpful to us in thinking about how to begin reading aloud with children with hearing loss. Because of this gap in listening experience, parents of the child with hearing loss have no time to lose and should begin talking intentionally and reading aloud as soon as possible.

How—and Why—Should Reading Aloud Begin?

Logically, then, we need to begin with passages that provide the "rhythmicity, intonation, frequency variation, and phonetic components of speech" referred to in the DeCasper and Fifer study. In a delightful book about setting children on the path to reading, Mem Fox (2008) emphasizes that the "rhyme," "rhythm," and "repetition" built into children's books serve as the building blocks for learning how to read on one's own. Listening to and learning rhyme, rhythm, and repetition stimulate the proficient listening and speaking foundational to reading.

Reading aloud with a child provides ample examples of rhyme and rhythm, along with the frequent repetitions that build the memory structures that strengthen the capacity to make predictions and then to confirm or disconfirm them. It's important to begin with whole stories so as to introduce the child to extended language. Of course, at first, the infant or child who hasn't developed expressive spoken language doesn't understand the story as a whole, but he or she will grasp it bit by bit over multiple readings by focusing at different times on various elements of language including sounds, word order, phrasings, meanings, and contexts. Such repeated encounters with book language and the conversational language of the adult about the book and whatever else comes up as they converse build the capacity to listen and to concentrate on sounds, words, ideas, and language structures that aid the development of spoken language. Without this spoken language base, it is hugely difficult to learn how to read. At the same time, reading aloud with a parent or teacher helps a child know he or she is special and valuable, it develops bonds between the adult and the child, and it spurs on the desire in both to encounter more books together.

Reading Aloud Is an *Indirect* Way of Teaching a Child How to Read

We are happy that, many children, even children with hearing loss, begin to pick up on reading all on their own as they begin hypothesizing about connections between the spoken language they know with what they begin to notice on the page. As described in Chapter 4, learning the spoken language isn't mainly about imitation, but about learning to construct meaning in the presence of sounds through a complex series of hypotheses and approximations within a setting in which others are using the language. The best way to learn language is from a proficient user of the language, and this includes *hearing* the language in books, which explains why we should choose books with more language than the child already has, and not just books for which the child already knows all the words. It's a good idea to think of the book as a vehicle for great discussions that give the child extended practice in using language.

Consequently, reading aloud with a child is not about directly *teaching* the child to read, but about *providing the rich language experience and interactions* that make the child ready to learn to read (see Table 8–1 for important elements of such language experience). Elementary school teachers are prepared to teach children how to read. They help children by providing them models of written language, and children go through hypothesis testing, predicting, and approximating, just as they did in learning spoken language. Therefore, the proper goal of the parent is to deliver to the teacher a child who has the language and experiential knowledge that makes him or her ready to learn to read. The more spoken language experience children have, the better.

Reading Aloud Is Also a *Direct* Way of Teaching a Child How to Read

When reading with a child, you can also direct his or her attention to the print itself, though I would caution that you keep the fun of the story itself in the forefront. A recent study (Piasta, Justice,

Table 8–1. When Reading with a Child, Think About Building:

- Conversational language
  - Turn-taking
  - Question asking
  - Staying focused
  - Attunement
- Connecting to the child's life experience
- Vocabulary
  - New words and phrases
  - New ways to use known words
- Sounds
  - New combinations of sounds and syllables
  - Enjoyment of linguistic and environmental sounds
- Textual language
  - Longer sentences
  - Series of items
  - Story structures (story grammar)
  - Descriptions
- Thinking
  - Predicting
  - Problem solving
- Emotions
  - Identifying and naming emotions in the characters and in the child
  - Helping the child talk about how she or he would feel in the situation of the character

McGinty, & Kaderavek, 2012) suggests that during the preschool year when a child is four years old, several simple strategies aimed at developing print knowledge can contribute to the child's literacy achievement once the child reaches school and direct reading instruction. By print knowledge, Piasta et al. mean "emerging knowledge of the specific forms and functions of written language" (p. 810). Such knowledge encompasses letters, reading from left to right, and the understanding that a word can be both spoken and written. Strategies for bringing a child's attention to print and its relation to sound include:

1. Talking about and pointing to words and letters
   - "Do you know this letter?"
   - "Can you find an 'm' on this page?"
   - "How many b's can you find?"
   - "This word is 'Owen'"
   - "Do you know this word?"
   - "Let's follow the words with your finger while I read"
   - "What direction do we go in?"

2. Talking about how a book "works"
   - "Where is the title of this book?"
   - "How do we turn the page?"
   - "Where should I read on this page?"
   - "Look at the words in the illustration" (adapted from Piasta, Justice, McGinty, & Kaderavek, 2012, pp. 813–814).

One of Marie Clay's important contributions to the teaching of reading involves the understanding that children need to develop particular concepts about print in order to navigate text. These include:

1. names for the parts of a book (front, cover, back)
2. print tells a story (apart from the pictures)
3. letter sequences make up words (concepts of first and last)
4. letters can be in upper and lower case
5. spaces are where they are for a reason
6. punctuation carries meanings
7. books are read from left to right and top to bottom (Clay, 1993, p. 47).

Teachers sometimes use Clay's Concepts About Print Score Sheet (Clay, 1993, p. 52) in order to keep track of a beginning reader's knowledge. I include the categories here for the purpose of suggesting what a parent, teacher, or therapist can bring a child's attention to in talking about books and reading.

How to Read Aloud with a Child with Hearing Loss

Begin by making sure the infant's or child's hearing aids or cochlear implant(s) are working. Checking the child's equipment should be a daily procedure performed when the child awakes in the morning, but things can go awry, so it's important to check before reading aloud. This could involve using the Ling 6–Sound Test in which you present the following speech sounds to the child to find out if his or her equipment is providing access to the fundamental sounds of spoken language:

ah (as in father)

oo (as in moon)

ee (as in key)

sh (as in shoe)

s (as in sock)

m (as in mommy) (Estabrooks, 1994, pp. 30–31)

Before reading aloud, attend to the equipment if it is not working optimally.

Next, think about what you want to accomplish with the child, both during this reading session and over a period of time. Table 8–2 provides an overview of the purposes of reading aloud with a child.

Sit in a comfortable chair with the child on your lap, or sit next to the child in bed for a bedtime story. In a classroom with a few children, make sure the FM system or sound field system is working optimally, and sit on the floor with the children gathered around.

Table 8–2. Preparation for Learning to Read Includes Read-Alouds That:

- help a child learn to listen, speak, and converse
- engage a child's attention about as much content as possible
- help a child understand multiple experiences and stories about the world

If there are many children, make sure the child with hearing loss is next to you so that you are speaking as near to the better ear as possible. If you have many children with hearing loss, arrange for volunteer readers to read individually with each child. Always aim to deliver the clearest sound possible to the child or children.

The principle here is that the child be able to hear the story, see the pages in the book, and converse with the person reading the book. Dickinson (2001) suggests reading at least three times a day for a minimum total of 45 minutes in an all-day preschool classroom designed for children with typical hearing (p. 201). For children of preschool age who are not attending preschool, a minimum total of 45 minutes daily spread over several sessions would be the goal for the parent at home. Children with hearing loss need at least this much time. A suggested guideline for what to read specifies at least three books each day to include a favorite book, a familiar book, and a new book (Fox, 2008, p. 17).

Hold the book in front of both of you so that you and the child are looking easily at the same pictures and text. Speak into the microphone of the hearing aid or CI of the better ear in order to deliver the clearest sound possible. Begin by saying something welcoming or exciting, such as, "It's time to read together! I've waited for this all day!" or "This is a book about what fire fighters do!" Read the words on the page expressively and with enthusiasm. Use your voice in many ways: loud and soft, high and low, fast and slow—and build in pauses (Fox, 2008, p. 42). Make up voices for different characters and point to the pictures to help the child connect language and image in meaningful ways. This may mean that you'll need to practice reading a book aloud by yourself or with others before you read it with your child.

Concentrate on understanding what you are reading aloud in order to convey with your voice the meaning you are creating while you read and the pleasure you are experiencing with the story. Monitor what your voice is doing while you are reading and make sure you are not just saying one word after another in a monotonous way. When you are making sense of the words and the story for yourself as you read it aloud, you will be helping your child comprehend the words and the story. Abandon your inhibitions—get excited, and be dramatic. Resist the impulse to use shared reading primarily to teach the child to identify letters and words, unless he or she asks for that, and trust that just reading and talking about the books is a valuable learning experience for the child. Stop to point to pictures and to make explanations. For example, point out instances of words in the pictures in order to reinforce a word or words you know the child has encountered recently or to introduce a new word or words.

Here's an example:

> "Look. Mrs. Tweezers is standing on *six stacked-up flower pots.* Let's count them!" and "Owen takes his blanket with him to the *barber* and to the *dentist.*" These can be read in this way: . . . signifies a pause and **bolding** and *italics* signify reading with more emphasis to bring attention to a name, a new word, or a concept: "Look . . . **Mrs. Twee**zers . . . is standing on *six* . . . *stacked-up flower pots.* Let's **count** them!" and "**Owen** . . . takes his blanket **with** him . . . to the *barber* . . . and to the *dentist.*"

Focus on new words in print, use new words in your own talk, and give synonyms or explanations for them. Point to clarifying pictures when possible. Ask both explicit (literal) and implicit (indirect) questions, and interact about the story. Be patient, make it fun, and make sure you are using an inviting tone of voice.

Formulate real questions and use them as a way into the story, rather than as a checkup or quiz. Literal questions help with concentration and build memory. They help a children know what they're working with in their thinking. But, it's very important not to stop with such questions, because remembering is not the same as comprehending. More complex questions involve using what one remembers in order to think logically and emotionally. Children need adults to model such thinking for them, so at the beginning, the adult can pose a more complex question and then answer it out loud for the child. As such thinking progresses, the adult can pose follow-up questions designed to help the child get to a more complex answer. If you as the adult show that you love doing all of this, your child will grow to love it, as well.

Sample Literal Questions

■ "What color is Owen's blanket?"
  Sample follow-up: Let's find all the yellow things on this page.

- "Where did Owen hide his blanket?"
  Sample follow-up: Show me the picture of Owen hiding the blanket in his pajama pants.
- "What did Owen's mother do to his blanket?"
  Sample follow-up: Do you remember when she put something on it to make it stinky? What smelled so bad?

Sample Implicit Questions

- "Why does Owen want to keep his blanket?"
  Sample follow-up: I know you like your blanket. What makes it special for you?
- "Why did Owen put his blanket over his head?"
  Sample follow-up: Why is Owen hiding?
- "What do you think they should do about Owen's blanket?"
  Sample follow-up: Why do Owen's parents think the blanket is a problem?

Sample Emotion Questions

- "How does Owen feel about giving up his blanket?"
  Sample follow-up: Why does Owen like his blanket so much? Why does he call it "Fuzzy"?
- "Is Owen excited to go to school?"
  Sample follow-up: I know you like school. What do you like about going to school?

Sample Application Questions

- "Do you remember what we did with your blanket?"
  Sample follow-up: Your blanket is safe in the blanket place. What do you like about getting it out now and then?
- "What would it be like to be invisible?"
  Sample follow-up: What could you do if your brother couldn't see you?

Most important is that you share language, treat each reading time as important and meaningful, and make the experience enjoyable for the child and for you. This will result in the child learning the spoken language and the comprehension of stories necessary for future direct reading instruction to make sense to him or her. Parents and teachers should share with each other information about what the child is encountering in books. It is helpful to review the guidelines in Table 8–3 periodically to keep yourself on track.

Dealing with an Uncooperative Child

I often hear from parents something like, "But my boy won't sit still long enough to pay attention to a book. He squirms out of my lap and runs around, and I give up." Yes, children will do this, especially if we expect it and especially if we let it happen. There is no point in getting into a tussle with the child, and there is even less reason in letting the child avoid this wonderful process that she or he needs so much. It can take time and persistence to establish that the person reading with the child is doing so as a leader who expects the child's attention. Think about possible distractions, and eliminate them before beginning. If the child is having trouble paying attention, try to find out why. Is something uncomfortable? Itchy? Tight? Is there a distracting toy tantalizingly close? Can the child see and hear? Let the child choose the book,

Table 8–3. A Few Guidelines to Remember

- Read for several short periods for a total of 45 minutes each day.
- Read a favorite, a familiar, and a new book each day.
- Read with expression; use your voice to emphasize rhyme, pitch, rhythm, new words, emotion.
- Converse about the pictures, the story, the characters, and anything that catches your child's attention.
- Concentrate on reading for meaning.
- Enjoy reading with your child!

perhaps offering two or three possibilities. I have seen parents of children with hearing loss quickly answer a question, adjust how they are sitting, whisk away a toy, and then just go on reading in order to make it possible—and necessary—for a child to pay attention. Usually, making it a low-pressure, pleasant activity in which the child gets some choice is enough. Only occasionally is it best to forgo a reading session because of a child's behavior. In the face of uncooperative behavior, it is best to try to understand the situation from the child's point of view and to see what you can do to help the child enjoy listening and interacting about the book. In time, the adult and the child will be able to share the lead during reading sessions, asking and answering each other's questions and talking easily about the reading. It is important that the adult keep in mind what the child already knows about and point out where new words and information connect with that knowledge.

An Extraordinary Example of Reading Aloud: The 1,000-Day Reading Streak

In March of 2010, I saw a heartwarming story in the *New York Times* about a father and daughter who read together every day without fail for 3,218 nights. They had read together regularly before that, but their "Reading Streak" started when the daughter was in third grade, and they decided to read *every* night for 100 nights. Jim Brozina, the father, did the reading aloud, and he practiced what he intended to read beforehand. He didn't teach his daughter to identify words, but to love stories and language. Her memory and background knowledge increased, and she became an expert reader and capable thinker. Once they reached the 100-night goal, they tried for 1,000 nights, and then just kept on reading, only stopping in 2006 when Kristen Alice left home for college.

But, this isn't just a nice story that makes me feel good; it's also a story of an exceedingly healthy and strong parent–child bond and of the outcomes realized from their consistency in reading and using language together. Kristen Alice, who now goes by "Alice," excelled throughout school, both academically and emotionally. In college, she majored in English, earned a 3.94 grade point average, "won two national writing contests, was Resident Assistant of the year, an editor of the humor and literary publications and won the annual English department award" (Winerip, 2010). She was accepted to a prestigious graduate school, and has now written *The Reading Promise*, a beautiful book about "The Reading Streak" (Ozma, 2011).

Such success is not unusual among students who have been read with consistently from an early age. Jim Trelease (2006) begins the fifth edition of his classic, *The Read-Aloud Handbook*, with this story:

> Of the four hundred thousand students taking the 2002 ACT exam with Christopher Williams, only fifty-seven had perfect scores—he was the fifty-eighth. When word got out that this kid from Russell, Kentucky (population 3,654), had scored a perfect 36, the family was besieged with questions, the most common being "What prep course did he take? Kaplan? Princeton Review?" It turned out to be a course his parents enrolled him in as an infant, a free program, unlike some of the private plans that now cost up to $250 an hour . . . Theirs is a house brimming with books but no *TV Guide*, Game Cube, or Hooked on Phonics. Even though Susan Williams was a fourth generation teacher, she offered no home instruction in reading before the boys reached school age. She and her husband, Tad, just read to them. (Trelease, 2006, pp. xi–xii)

The lesson is this: once you ensure that your child with hearing loss can hear, you can help him or her learn to listen, and the spoken language, thinking, and reading open to any other child are open to your child.

The rules for a "Reading Streak" are simple, and they can apply from birth through high school:

1. Read for at least 10 minutes.
2. Read every night, before midnight, with no exceptions.
3. Read from whatever book you are reading at the time, but if that isn't possible, anything—a program, a magazine—is all right.
4. Read in person, but in a pinch, reading on the telephone is permissible.
   (Ozma, 2011, p. 5)

Not surprisingly, Alice and her father usually read for more than ten minutes, and as Alice grew older, the reading—and the conversations they had—became more complex. In Jim's words:

> If you want to start your own reading streak, you should begin by taking your child to your local public library, where the two of you can look through the stacks for books that would fit your reading desires. When either of you find something, show it to the other. Let your child overrule your choices if he or she chooses, but be hesitant about rejecting those your child is excited about. Remember, this is being done *by* you but *for* him or her. (Ozma, 2011, p. xix)

Conclusion

You may be thinking that such a reading streak is amazing! Of course it is. It's an unusual example, which is why Alice's book about it has received so much attention. But it's a proper goal for attending to the spoken language needs of a child with hearing loss. The salient point here is this: reading aloud and conversing about the meaning of text are important components of language development. Luckily, reading and talking are also fun, which will keep you doing them often, whether you are a parent, teacher, or therapist. Consistency and frequency in using spoken language in extended reading and conversation with your child matter greatly in your child's linguistic, cognitive, and literacy development.

References

Anderson, R., Hiebert, E., Scott, J., & Wilkinson, I. (1985). *Becoming a nation of readers: The report of the commission on reading* (p. 23). Champaign-Urbana, IL: U.S. Department of Education, Center for the Study of Reading.

Clay, M. (1993). *An observational survey of early literacy achievement.* Portsmouth, NH: Heinemann.

DeCasper, A., & Fifer, W. (1980). Of human bonding: Newborns prefer their mothers' voices. *Science, 208*(4448), 1174–1176.

DeCasper, A., & Spence, M. (1986). *Infant behavior and development, 9*(2), 133–150.

Dickinson, D. (2001). Book reading in preschool classrooms. In D. Dickinson & P. Tabors (Eds.), *Beginning literacy with language.* Baltimore, MD: Paul H. Brookes.

Estabrooks, W. (Ed.). (1994). *Auditory-verbal therapy for parents and professionals.* Washington, DC: Alexander Graham Bell Association for the Deaf.

Fox, M. (2008). *Reading magic.* Orlando, FL: Houghton Mifflin Harcourt.

John Tracy Clinic. (2003). Retrieved from http://www.jtc.org/uploads/docs/The-Ling-Six-SoundTest.PDF

Ozma, A. (2011). *The Reading Promise: My Father and the Books We Shared.* New York, NY: Hatchette Book Group.

Pennsylvania State University. (2009). *Can babies learn in utero?* Retrieved from http://www.rps.psu.edu/probing/inutero.html

Piasta, S., Justice, L., McGinty, A., & Kaderavek, J. (2012). Increasing young children's contact with print during shared reading: Longitudinal effects on literacy achievement. *Child Development, 83*(3), 810–820.

Winerip, M. (2010). *A father-daughter bond, page by page.* Retrieved from http://www.nytimes.com/2010/03/21/fashion/21GenB.html?pagewanted=all&_r=0

Chapter 9

LEARNING TO WRITE

First graders . . . are beautifully positioned for writing:
They can write all the words they can say.

Elbow, 2004, p. 9

Introduction

Writing is often regarded as the productive side of reading. People who do not learn to read well also do not write well, as the same processes and skills are involved. Searches of the literature on literacy and children with hearing loss do not turn up many reports concerning their writing achievement. One researcher reported that children with hearing loss performed much less well than children with typical hearing, but that rule acquisition for writing seemed to take place in a predictable way similar to the way children with typical hearing progress (Taylor, 1969). Conway (1985) focuses on children in an auditory/oral class, and Ewoldt (1985) reports on 10 children with deafness ages 4, 5, and 6, all of whom used a signed language, with a few also using some "voice." They concurred that children like to write for meaningful purposes and that they make progress when they do so. Another study describes immersing six kindergarten children with hearing loss using ASL in authentic literacy activities including reading predictable books and using environmental print, read-alouds, and language experience stories.

These authors report growth in written language from scribbling to printing one random letter and then a series of random letters, to printing whole words, with some children progressing to printing phrases and sentences and even whole stories (Andrews & Gonzalez, 1992). Ruiz (1995) recorded her own daughter's progress, much of which paralleled that of children with typical hearing, though, perhaps because she used Signed English, she differed from them in her dependence on visual strategies. "I did not ever observe Elena to use a sound-based strategy as she wrote, that is, to say or 'stretch out' the word as she wrote letters down" (p. 211). Elena made connections between finger spelling words and writing them on paper. By the time she was in third grade, she scored at the 90th percentile on an achievement test designed for children with typical hearing, causing her mother to question the necessity of a well-developed phonemic system in the development of reading (p. 216). It would be interesting to know about this child's subsequent progress.

Williams (2011) investigated interactive writing in a group of six kindergarten children with hearing loss, one of whom used a cochlear implant, and began with the observation that many children with hearing loss enter school behind in language development. She describes interactive writing as "an instructional approach that embeds learning to write within an authentic writing activity; thus, children learn this ordinary practice of the culture by doing it" (p. 24). Such writing instruction makes use of scaffolding by the teacher, social interaction, and collaborative learning and problem solving, all of which can help children develop the conceptual knowledge they need to express themselves in writing (p. 24). Williams concludes that children with hearing loss can learn to write more easily through the use of this approach with appropriate adaptations, including making English phonology visible, and suggests that the approach be tried with children with hearing loss who have more access to spoken language than did the children in this study (p. 33).

A recent discussion describing the writing of college students with hearing loss cites problems with syntax, grammar, and factual knowledge, and describes the great difficulty college instructors have in attempting to bring such students to even average levels of language use in their writing (Biser, Rubel, & Toscano, 2007). These researchers queried 81 alumni of NTID (National Technical

Institute for the Deaf) and received replies that they perceived their writing strengths to include "clarity, organization, and creativity," but with 57% reporting grammar as a major weakness (p. 363). Interestingly, when the researchers surveyed employers, employers reported that "grammar, clarity, organization, and spelling" were "the most serious problems for deaf employees" (p. 364).

Writing and the Auditory-Verbal Approach

In my study of literacy development in individuals who had learned spoken language through the auditory-verbal approach (Robertson, 2000, discussed in Chapter 1), I had everyone in my study in fourth grade and above produce a writing sample after completing the standardized Gates-MacGinitie Reading Test. This was not an elaborate task; I simply asked these children, adolescents, and a few young adults to "write about something that interests you." If they wanted to discuss their choice of topic with me before writing, we did so, but most simply responded by saying, "Is it all right if I write about _____?" and I accepted all suggestions. Representative choices were "My Best Friend," "The Roller Coaster," and "Science Fiction." In doing this study, there was not time to give each writer time to make notes and plan the writing or to revise the writing, and so each writing sample was a first draft. I was concerned that since standard tests of writing give students such opportunity, these writers might not be able to produce their best work.

In having these writing samples evaluated, I wanted to have them compared with writing samples of children, adolescents, and young adults with typical hearing, just as I had given the students a standardized reading test on which their achievement would be compared to students with typical hearing. So, I submitted them to an assessment process being used in the public schools in my home county at that time. That process recognized that in looking at writing, it is clear that there are no "right answers," in the sense that there are not certain words, phrases, sentences, or organizational structures that must be present in order for a written piece to be judged "excellent," "good," "average," or "poor." Instead, this process included criteria set up in the form of rubrics that enabled a team of evaluators to determine scores for students' written work.

In setting up their scoring system, teachers from schools throughout the county had come together to read papers written by students in each grade level and then to choose sample representative papers, known as "anchor papers," for each grade at levels "4," "3," "2," and "1." A "4" presents careful organization; good and varied vocabulary; a sense of audience (a demonstration of purpose and understanding of what is necessary to say to be understood); good sentence structure; few errors in mechanics, usage, grammar, and spelling; and creativity and originality. Levels "3" and "2" show lesser, but not unacceptable achievement in those areas, and Level "1" rates the sample as poor in those areas and is regarded as a failing score.

The teacher-evaluators had set up a system used across their public school districts whereby their judgments were standardized by testing their placements of each paper at each level and establishing a high level of interrater reliability. Teachers had to demonstrate that they could place a particular student paper at the same level other teachers would place it in order to be part of the evaluation team, and then this team evaluated the writing of the students in all the schools in the county school districts. I turned to this system to find evaluators of the writing samples I had collected.

I typed each writing sample precisely the way it was written so that handwriting would not be a factor in the evaluation. All misspellings, misuses of words, and unconventional word orders were preserved, although for the children from Toronto I changed their Canadian spellings to reflect United States usage and deleted geographic references so they would not distract the teacher-evaluators. Then, for each grade level for which I had samples, I mixed at random the papers of the writers with hearing loss with two established "anchor papers" from each of the levels 1, 2, 3, and 4 that were not marked as such, reasoning that if they were assigned those same scores, the other judgments would be accurate, as well. Two experienced evaluators from each grade were recruited to read the papers representing the grade level they taught currently. I simply asked them to score the papers as they usually did, on a scale from one to four. They did not know they were reading the work of children with hearing loss; as they were teachers of children with typical hearing, they may not have had any preconceived ideas, but I did not want to influence them in any way.

The teachers-evaluators' identification of their own system's anchor papers' levels was accurate, and so I had confidence in the scores they assigned the papers in question. Of the 23 writing samples evaluated, only three were judged as "1" and thus not acceptable for their grade levels. One of the three was by an elementary student and two were by high school students. Only students in grades 9 to 14 produced samples that scored at "4," but every grade level had at least one student scoring at "3." All scores can be seen in Table 9–1.

To experienced readers of writing by students with typical hearing, writers in this study did not look different from students in the public schools of one county in central Ohio. I was curious about how the writing appeared to them and gave them a checklist that asked whether each paper had:

1. Phrasings and/or tone characteristic of the conversational style of the writer's age group;
2. Phrasings and/or tone characteristic of the writing style often used in books read by the writer's age group;
3. Phrasings and/or tone characteristic of the writing style often used in schoolbooks read by the writer's age group;
4. Use of language or punctuation that indicates the writer is beginning to use more sophisticated language but that he or she hasn't quite mastered it yet; and

Table 9–1. Writing Scores for 23 Students, Grades 4 to 14*

	Grade Level			
Score	4–5	6–8	9–14	
4			3	
3	1	3	3	
2		6	4	Passing
1	1		2	

*The first two years of college are included as Grades 13 and 14.

5. Use of language or punctuation that indicates the writer is not a mainstream user of English.

Of all the age groups, more middle school teacher-evaluators commented that the papers they read reflected the conversational style of that age group. Papers included statements such as, "He is really cute!"; "I am totally crazy about animals"; and "Well, that's alllll [sic] about me!" This may reflect good listening behavior in those students, as these are statements we can all identify as coming from 6th through 8th graders.

Teacher-evaluators found examples of book language and of schoolbook language across the grades. Examples of book language included, "I like them because they are interesting" (written by a 5th grader) and "Before I go any further, let me . . . " (written by a 6th grader). Such examples suggest that these students were reading carefully and storing in memory some of the ways books use language. At the high school level, the highest praise from evaluators included, "very sophisticated for 11th grade, in terms of style, organization"; "very formal tone"; and "the vocabulary is sophisticated." This teacher cited this passage by a student writer: "On the other hand, there are those who deserve the title of professor/teacher, and so forth. These teachers are open to new ideas and methods of fostering maximum student/teacher interaction." The capability of using reading to inform one's own language, both in speaking and in writing, is important, especially for the individual who does not hear everything uttered in his or her environment. Reading fills in the spaces that gaps in hearing or listening create and prepares the person for future listening, speaking, reading, and writing. These students were demonstrating they were capable of using reading to learn more language.

The teacher-evaluators noted instances of student writing that seemed to be just on the verge of growing in its sophistication and mastery of language. This is a common phenomenon recognized by teachers of writing. Awkwardness of expression can signal the writer's understanding that more can be done with words. The writer may be trying to express something in a more elegant or more efficient way, and he or she may be on the brink of developing a higher level command of language. In these cases, we can see development in process. In the students with hearing loss, such awkwardness can be caused by a limited vocabulary, lesser experience with challenging talk, and less knowledge of prose that provides models of more complex structuring of language. Additionally, it can be hard to hit on just the right word or phrasing, especially in a first draft. Sentences of this type referenced by the teacher-evaluators included, "Another trail called Parsenn Bowl, is, too located in Winter Park and is new to the area, because it is challenging" and "Graduation leads on to better things in life and therefore going onwards with your life." The writers of these sentences were trying to convey many thoughts, but became a bit tangled up in their words. Perhaps these sentences reflect gaps in language; perhaps if the students had had time to revise, such sentences would not have appeared in their writing. In any case, these oddly crafted sentences demonstrate a desire to say something in a more complex way. They appeared to the teacher-evaluators to represent normally developing language usage for students in their age groups.

At some point, reading should begin to inform spoken language use. The person who is deaf or hard of hearing is often at a disadvantage, even when residual hearing is well-amplified by good technology. Not hearing every word in a sentence or every sound in a word can hamper spoken language use which, in turn, can disrupt reading. Children who achieve sufficient language proficiency to begin to learn to read learn to look at all the language cues on the page and begin to use such cues to support both speaking and writing. For example, the child who does not always hear /s/ may not know that people are using it in certain expressions. Learning to look for /s/ markers on the page can translate into listening for them, speaking them, and then writing them. Examples in this study include, "He love to ride" and "he ride" (grade 5), which struck the teacher-evaluators as perhaps being from a student whose first language was not English. Other sorts of examples represented a lack of English knowledge: "In the park, they were so crowded in this park because the weathers hasn't been warming enough in these seasons" (grade 6); and "she say that next week it will be the test Tuesday" (grade 7). The samples written by students beyond grade 8 did not contain such sentences, suggesting that more facility with language, especially among those who read regularly, may be developed by about that time.

Not one teacher-evaluator indicated that he or she thought any of the samples was from some special population of students for whom expectations might be lower, and I came away from this study confident that I had found at least one group of children and adolescents with hearing loss who were making progress in written expression commensurate with their hearing peers. Their progress can be explained using a theory of literacy that regards reading and writing as simultaneously depending on and creating an increasingly complete process of spoken language acquisition. Higher levels of reading and writing achievement could become the norm for children with hearing loss, if learning to listen to the language spoken in their environment were more widespread. In view of the small number of investigations that have been done on writing achievement and hearing loss, I concur with Williams (2004) that much more research is needed in this area.

A Word About Development

Listening, speaking, reading, and writing are all ways to use language. On the surface, it looks as though one must first listen in order to speak, speak in order to read, and read in order to write. Developmentally, though, once learning begins, all are growing and influencing the others to grow. " . . . children show signs of knowledge of written language in oral delivery form and show signs of oral language in written delivery form" (Sulzby, 1986, p. 50).

Peter Elbow (2004) argues for getting children writing actively right from the start. Having repeated experiences in putting the words one knows on paper helps children reach for making ever increasingly better meaning: "Most students can see how writing is a process of slowly constructed meaning, often socially negotiated through feedback. They have learned that clarity is not what we start with but what we work toward" (p. 13). Writing is a social activity prompted by wanting to communicate with others. It is also an active process, perfectly suited to children. Pairing writing with reading, rather than waiting for reading to develop before introducing writing, has a good effect on reading development as children come to see firsthand that materials for reading come from real people who "think up" the words.

Practical Ideas for Helping Children Learn to Write

Pay Attention to the Child's First Attempts

Long before a child has fine motor coordination, he or she will want to participate in drawing and writing on paper (and other surfaces!). Drawing and scribbling are important stages in beginning to write, and the parent's and teacher's responses to this expression can be very helpful in supporting the processes involved. Writing should be about meaning making from the very first, and the adult can help by taking the child's written expression seriously. When a child brings a picture or some scribbles to the adult, the best response from the adult is, "Tell me about what you have drawn [or written] here." This kind of question prompts the child to talk about the content he or she put on the page. It does not matter if the child gives different accounts of the same page on different occasions. At this point, he or she is just beginning to learn about how the system works. The adult should simply engage the child in a conversation about what the child says the marks are about. As time goes on, the child will begin to provide more stable accounts and will begin to make certain marks representative, for him or her individually, of certain meanings. These ordinarily will be in the form of shapes, as the child begins to draw pictures. Ordinarily, these pictures are not recognizable to anyone else, but over time the child may begin using the same expressive form for the same content, and the adult will recognize it. This could involve the increasingly consistent way a child draws a house or a dog, for example. Next, the child begins to explore drawing letters, if they have been introduced to him or her. At first, they will be drawn, just as a picture of anything else could be drawn. As the repertoire increases, letters will be written at random, and in any direction on the page. At this point, the child is trying to do what he or she sees others doing, and that is to write a message. The child is learning how to think of something to communicate and then to represent it on the page. Gradually, and usually with the assistance of someone who knows how to write or with formal instruction by a teacher, the child learns to write letters in conventional order and direction and understands the relationship between words spoken and words written. Although the child can learn the alphabetic principle through reading, he or she can further comprehend it by learning to write the language in this way. Figures 9–1 and 9–2 are examples of two of my son Mark's pages from a trip diary he started when he was 6 years old during March of the first grade. They show phonemic awareness and a grasp of the alphabetic principle.

The Language Experience Book

The Language Experience Book's first use is to stimulate spoken language learning and then reading, as laid out in Chapter 7. At first, the adult supplies the language, writes it beneath the picture, and reads it with the child. Gradually, and over time, but as soon as possible, the activity of creating the language moves into the child's realm. As the child becomes more verbal and vocal, he or she begins supplying some of the language, and the adult writes exactly what the child says, reads it with the child, and invites the child to read it, too. Writing the child's dictation on a page of the experience book is a preliminary step in the child's learning about how to write, as the child learns that he or she can think of something to say, say it, and then see someone write it. It does not take long until the child begins to discover how what he or she can say is written. As development takes place, the child will begin to get control over producing letters, and the adult can help the child get them going in the right direction, in the right order, and with spacing between the words.

Sulzby (1986) lists six areas in which writing develops, with each successive stage building on the previous one: drawing, scribbling, letter-like forms, well-learned units, invented spelling, and conventional orthography (pp. 68–69). Mark's examples show the emergence of learning to produce each letter on paper using both conventional and invented spelling, as well as the beginnings of good control over conventional forms in writing. Using invented spelling is a natural phase during which the child learns to record the phonological and visual memories he or she holds for words. Sometimes people worry that children will get "stuck" in a habit of misspelling words, but that is not the final outcome for children in rich literacy environments (Richgels, 2002, p. 142).

Encouraging children to write down what they want to say helps them understand that conveying a meaning is the point of writing.

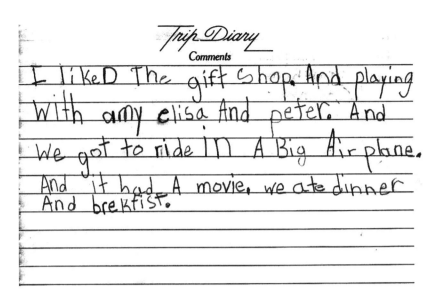

Trip Diary
Comments

I likeD The gift Shop. And playing
With amy elisa And peter. And
We got to ride In A Big Airphne.
And it had A movie, we ate dinner
And brekfist.

Figure 9–1. The language in these sentences approaches conventional language, although capitalization is still in the experimental stage. Names of people are not capitalized, whereas "Big Airplane," perhaps, is suggesting a hypothesis that big things should be marked by "big" letters. "Breakfist" is written just as it sounds in the midwestern United States. There are no commas, but each sentence has a period at its end.

Trip Diary
Comments

on the way we stopped at Stalkhome
sweeDin. I had A Roast beaf
Sandwich to eat

Figure 9–2. "Stalkhome sweedin" looks mainly like it sounds with some indication in "stalk" of having seen this word part somewhere else and plugging it in here.

The more they understand this, the more they will want to learn the conventional ways of writing so their messages can be understood by others. The achievement of conventional writing will come, as long as children are continuously acquiring more knowledge about the spoken and written forms of the language used in their environment. Focusing on meaning is the important matter in shepherding a child through the steps in a language experience book. It should not be a forced activity, and the adult should give the child all the help necessary in getting words down on paper during the sequential stages from scribbling to conventional writing. Stopping frequently to get a child to "sound out" sounds to write down can detract from the message the child is trying to produce. Children using invented spelling have been found to write more, spell more words correctly, read more real words, and decode more nonsense words than children who do not use invented spelling (Clarke, 1988, as cited in Weaver, 2002, p. 344) Instead of focusing on spelling at the expense of meaning, the adult can ask the child what he or she wants to say and keep it in memory while the child labors over producing it, in case the work of writing makes the child forget the message. This is definitely a time for teamwork.

About the time children are capable of talking enough to tell a story, they are beginning to have experiences away from their parents, and, of course, they have experiences away from their teachers. So, they have stories to tell and information to give to people in their lives who have genuine interest in what they have done while apart from them. Such experiences are perfect for the language experience book; they will spark good dialogue as the adult asks sincere questions in trying to understand the story or information being told. For example, the child may say, "Went water," and the teacher can respond in an enhanced way, with more complex language, "Oh, did you go in the water? Did you go swimming?" And the child might say, "I went in the water. I went swimming," which the teacher then writes down in the language experience book. The teacher might ask, "What did you wear when you went swimming?" and the child might respond, "Wore red suit," giving the teacher the chance to respond with, "You wore your red swimming suit?" "Yes, I wore my new red swimming suit," which the teacher writes down. And so on. The point is that the adult elicits more language from the child and then is in a position to write down statements with more detail that are the child's authentic language to be in a book the child will then learn to read. The child is in the position of making continuous discoveries about both spoken and written language, as well as about negotiating meaning in a real conversation in which new information is passed from one person to another.

Keep in mind that purposes for writing vary from communicating with others via letters, notes, stories, and essays, to communicating with oneself. Writing for oneself includes writing anything a person wants to remember, and so we write lists, directions, and descriptions, as well as diary and journal entries. Writing for oneself also involves writing to solve a problem and to find out what one thinks or believes; sometimes the written result is shared with others, sometimes not. Being able to write in such fashion is a higher-level kind of writing because it is writing in the service of thinking. Such writing can help prepare one to communicate with another in clear fashion, whether in speech or in print. All these kinds of writing are especially useful to children, adolescents, and adults with hearing loss, as they make it easier for them to make their way through the world. What cannot be heard with clarity can be read, and having notes can aid memory for specific language that might not have formed in a phonologically complete way.

Please see Chapter 10, "Creating and Using Language Experience Books" for practical information and application of using this approach.

Authentic Written Communication Activities

Children can participate in many actual written communication functions of the home and classroom (Table 9–2). Adults should make sure that children see them reading and writing and that they talk with children about why they are doing so. Such actions provide a model, as well as scaffolded (structured) support for the child to learn about how to write in a particular situation. A parent might involve a child in making a grocery list, for example. The involvement of the child depends on the child's language capabilities, of course, so at first, the parent could have the child help look in the pantry or the refrigerator and ask what they need to get. After some practice for the child in listening to and saying the names of items needed, the parent writes them down on the shopping list: "peanut butter," "apples," and "eggs," for example.

Table 9–2. Writing Activities for Children

- Labeling drawings
- Making lists
- Writing letters and thank you notes to family and friends
- Writing notes to mom, dad, the teacher
- Making a treasure hunt with written clues to follow
- Role-playing activities (pretending to be a server in a restaurant, a clerk in a store, a mail carrier, a doctor, a reporter . . .)
- Making a family tree
- Making books

The progression of this authentic activity could move through having the parent ask the child, "Please look and see if we need any peanut butter" and the parent writing it down on the list when the child reports the jar is almost empty, to the child writing "peanut butter" on the list in response to the question, all the way to an older child discovering on his or her own that peanut butter is needed and writing it independently on the family-generated shopping list.

Children can be involved from a very early age in writing that is sent to grandparents and other important people in their lives. The parent can make a family tree complete with pictures and names of family members so the child can begin to understand the relationships. Children should see parents writing letters or electronic messages and can be asked what they would like to say. At the beginning, this could be a few scribbles on a sheet of paper; later on it can be a drawing or a note left for Mom or Dad. As with the language experience book, the parent can ask the child to tell about what is on the page, and the parent can write the words on the page, with the child assisting. As the child's spoken language develops, the parent can write down a story or some information dictated by the child, and over time, the child can take on doing the writing him or herself.

At a real meal, a child could take the role of a server, ask each person at the table what he or she would like to drink, write it down on a notepad, and then bring each "order."

In the classroom, even young children can see teachers write messages and then carry them to others in the room or building, and children can learn to help with taking attendance by putting a mark next to each child's name on a list. Children can make scribbles and pictures about which the teacher inquires and writes on them what the child says about them. Stories and information-giving come next, and the process moves from the teacher doing the writing to the student doing the writing. Such papers can be hung on the wall or assembled into a book for all to see, giving the child evidence that writing is important. One wise teacher I know kept a box on her desk with a slot in it. Children in her class could write notes to her; she responded to them on the same paper, and sent each note back to the child who originated it.

Pretend Activities

Children love to pretend to be a mommy or a daddy, a teacher, a mail carrier, a waiter/waitress, a store clerk, a doctor, a person meeting someone new, and so on. Think about when and how each of these individuals needs to read and write, and all kinds of activities will come to mind. These activities offer children opportunities to try out and play with the roles of the adults around them. For example, a child could make a list and pretend to go to the grocery or hardware store, write "letters" and then become the mail carrier who picks them up, set up a restaurant and take orders from mommy and daddy or others and then serve a snack, write out a receipt when someone in a pretend store buys something, write a prescription, and take down someone's address. Children can have great fun in making a treasure hunt and writing clues to hide at each stop along the way. At first the child does these activities in scribbles and later in real words.

Conclusion

Children with hearing loss can learn to write in natural ways, and in doing so, they make many preliminary discoveries about the process, paralleling the meaning-making process in which they learn to read. The determining factor in whether they do so is how much they learn of the language spoken with them and around them. Learning to write begins with observing people write and hearing about what and why they have written, and extends from making seemingly aimless scribbles through drawing pictures and letters to arranging letters randomly and then into words, with the endpoint being a good level of mastery over conventional means of setting thoughts down on paper or computer screen. Writing and reading are intrinsically intertwined; experiences with each enrich the performance of the other.

References

Andrews, J., & Gonzalez, K. (1992). Free writing of deaf children in kindergarten. *Sign Language Studies, 73*, 63–78. Retrieved as ERIC J443039.

Biser, E. Rubel, L., & Toscano, R. (2007). Bending the rules: When deaf writers leave college. *American Annals of the Deaf, 152*(4), 361–373.

Conway, D. (1985). Children (re)creating writing: A preliminary look at the purposes of free choice writing of hearing-impaired kindergartners. *Volta Review, 87*(5), 91–107.

Elbow, P. (2004). Write first! Putting writing before reading is an effective approach to teaching and learning. *Educational Leadership, 62*(2), 8–13.

Ewoldt, C. (1985). A descriptive study of the developing literacy of young hearing-impaired children. *Volta Review, 87*(5), 109–126

Richgels, D. (2002). Invented spelling, phonemic awareness, and reading and writing instruction. In S. Neuman & D. Dickinson (Eds.), *Handbook of early literacy research* (pp. 142–155). New York, NY: Guilford Press.

Ruiz, N. (1995). A young deaf child learns to write: Implications for literacy development. *Reading Teacher, 49*(3), 206–217.

Sulzby, E. (1986). Writing and reading: Signs of oral and written language organization in the young child. In W. Teale & E. Sulzby (Eds.), *Emergent literacy: Writing and reading* (pp. 50–89). Norwood, NJ: Ablex.

Taylor, L. (1969). *A language analysis of the writing of deaf children: Final report.* (ERIC Document Reproduction Service No. ED039684). Retrieved from ERIC (Educational Resources Information Center) database.

Weaver, C. (2002). *Reading process and practice* (3rd ed.). Portsmouth, NH: Heinemann.

Williams, C. (2004). Emergent literacy of deaf children. *Journal of Deaf Studies and Deaf Education, 9*(4), 352–365.

Williams, C. (2011). Adapted interactive writing instruction with kindergarten children who are deaf or hard of hearing. *American Annals of the Deaf, 15*(1), 23–34.

Chapter 10

CREATING AND USING LANGUAGE EXPERIENCE BOOKS

Listening is the first step and the last step.
(Cantus Fraggle) Henson, 2005, p. 17

Introduction

This chapter is a practical step-by-step guide to creating and using language experience books (LEBs). I know it can be daunting to read about an approach and then to try to apply it without having a set of directions and a range of examples, and so this chapter is my attempt to provide enough to get you started in using the LEB approach. That said, I want to emphasize two points. First, there is no *one* way to use LEBs, and second, it's critical to remind yourself frequently about the purposes for using LEBs and how these purposes are built upon literacy theories discussed in previous chapters. Whether you're a parent, teacher, or therapist of a child with hearing loss, it's a good idea to work with others in the child's life in creating and using these books. Talk with each other about how you and the child are using the books, and use the books to learn more about how the child is progressing in language use and literacy acquisition. It is vital that you use the books with regularity and frequency, as otherwise the child won't grasp their importance or have the practice that results in learning to rely on reading and writing for authentic purposes.

Reading and writing with a child can be incredibly rewarding for both of you, and it can also be beautifully messy as you work toward using words, ideas, images, and diagrams to create meaning together. By "beautifully messy," I mean that this kind of reading and writing doesn't follow a particular pattern. Instead, it follows the interests and curiosity of the child, with the adult providing the knowledge of how spoken and written language work. I realize this is both liberating and frightening. All of us, children and adults, learn deeply when we care about something. We make connections and create meanings that matter to us. We remember this kind of learning as opposed to the superficial, fleeting learning produced by rote processes. I hope that by the time you have read this chapter, you'll feel confident in helping children become authors of their own ideas.

Start and End with Listening

A language experience book is based on listening. The adult listens to the child in the child's environment, pays attention to the language the child is using, uses that language, and adds to it. The child listens to the language the adult uses, supplies some of his or her own, and listens to the result. As all this is taking place, the child has many opportunities to connect the listening with what the adult puts on the page and to what the child wants to put on the page. The LEB approach is appropriate for all children, regardless of their hearing or learning status, because it's about using and learning language for meaningful purposes.

A Spiral Progression Through Using Language Experience Books

Think of a process of spiraling up and around through increasingly complex processes in which you learn something and return to it later, newly able to handle it in a more nearly complete or a more complex form, and you will have an idea of how you can begin using LEBs with a child and over many years help the child become an adult who reads and writes for him or herself. Jerome Bruner, an educational psychologist and theorist proposed a spiral curriculum (Bruner, 1961), and we can use his thinking here.

Remembering that I'm not proposing the following as a "lock-step," invariant process, you might have in mind this developmental sequence of ways to use the LEB approach:

1. The adult creates or supplies a drawing, picture, or souvenir and writes words or sentences about it for the child while the child is present. The adult and child look at the page together, the adult reads the words aloud, and they talk about it together each day for a while. Such talk includes linking the image or souvenir (a ticket to a ball game, for example) to the words and may involve using synonyms and/or antonyms to expand upon the child's language knowledge.

2. The child creates or chooses a drawing, picture, or souvenir, and the adult asks the child for words or a story to go with it. The child responds, and the adult uses the child's language, at times expanding it in order to introduce the child to some new words, word forms, or new ways of using known words. The adult writes words or sentences for the child while the child watches. Each day for a while, the adult and child look at the page together, the adult reads the words aloud, and they talk about it, with the adult concentrating on linking language with the drawing, picture, or souvenir in ways that provide new words and phrases in an attempt to expand the child's language a bit more each time.

3. The child creates or chooses a drawing, picture, or souvenir and supplies words or a story without being prompted by the adult. The adult acts as a scribe and writes the child's words and/or sentences in the child's presence. Each day for a while, the adult and child look at the page together, the adult reads the words aloud, and they talk about it, with both the adult and the child concentrating on linking language with the drawing, picture, or souvenir in ways that add to the child's language and understanding.

4. The child creates or chooses a drawing, picture, or souvenir and writes words and sentences with the help of the adult. The

adult may also do some of the writing. Each day for a while, the adult and child look at the page together, with both the adult and child reading the words aloud, taking turns as they wish. They converse about the words and ideas with both feeling free to prompt each other and to bring in new interpretations, ideas, and questions.

5. The child creates or chooses a drawing, picture, or souvenir and writes words and sentences without the help of the adult. The adult asks questions and for expansions from the child, and the child writes more with the adult's help. Each day for a while, the adult and child look at the page together. The child reads the words aloud, and they converse about the words and ideas, always seeking more complexity.

6. The child creates or chooses drawing, picture, or souvenir and writes words and sentences without the help of the adult. The adult asks questions and for expansions from the child, and the child writes more. Each day for a while, the adult and child look at the page together, the child reads the words aloud, and they converse about the words and ideas. The adult asks questions for editing purposes and helps the child make the changes.

7. The child keeps a journal on subjects of his or her choice and writes on his or her own for school and other purposes. The child shares the writing with the adult who acts as a sounding board and peer editor, and at times the child simply uses the journal to reflect on his or her experiences and to think things through without sharing the writing with anyone.

I hope you noted in this sequence that the adult initiates and carries out the process at the beginning, and gradually—and intentionally—the ownership of the process shifts from the adult to the child. The adult working with the child keeps in mind Vygotsky's zone of proximal development by assisting the child with the next step for which she or he is ready. Such assistance helps the child grow with little resistance, because the adult provides support as the child needs it. This process is done well when adults are mindful of their role as guides, rather than directors, though the adult can ask the child what he or she wants to know how to do and provide direct instruction when the child wants it.

Deciding on the Content for an LEB Entry

The focus for any page might be:

- A concept
- A part of speech: noun, verb, pronoun, adjective, adverb, preposition, conjunction, interjection, article (note: some people define words such as "a," "the," "an," etc. as articles, and others call them adjectives)
- A key phrase
- A metaphor
- Something about word or sentence order
- A story
- Adult models of words, phrases, sentences
- Child's words
- Poetry
- Music

An Example

In the First Years Program at the University of North Carolina, the students drew from many LEBs they had made and put together a language experience book that functions to explain language experience book. Their work can be found at: http://tarheelreader .org/2009/12/22/language-experience-books/

Conversations About Making and Using Language Experience Books

The following represents several exchanges I've had with teachers and therapists about the practice involved in using LEBs. The inquiries and comments from different individuals appear in italics, and my answers and comments are in plain type.

*How do you do the LEB with a child early in her language develop-
ment? She is not yet speaking with words.*

Before the child can supply the language, you need to supply the language. You say it and write it, and then you read it and
talk about it with the child. The reason for the LEB is to stimulate
language development in the child. This can be hard to understand
until you start seeing the child responding and adding to his or her
language knowledge. The LEB gives you a concrete place for your
focus, and it helps you maintain a record of the child's language
development.

*My child with hearing loss "wrote" her own text on the second page
we worked on. She is 4.9 years, and it is squiggles across the page
without anything resembling a letter. While she scribbled, she nar-
rated perfect sentences to accompany her writing. When we review
her page in the future, do I have her recall what she wrote, or do I
add her text in myself now so that we both remember what she said?
I was leaning toward leaving her page alone so that she doesn't feel
self-conscious about her "writing."*

Either way will work, but each produces something different.
Whatever you choose, remember that the child should be immersed
and surrounded with language in its spoken and written forms. Her
squiggling is perfectly normal writing development, but it won't
serve as a record of what she said, and it's doubtful she'll remember
her own exact words. I would lean toward writing down under the
squiggles what she said after she squiggled, as the goal is that she
come to understand that what she says can be written down in a
way that everyone else can read.

*It seems as if we are not supposed to correct the spelling, the gram-
mar, and so forth, but rather let the creative process for the child
take over. Even if we are reading it back to the child and writing it
for him or her, we are not supposed to correct the grammar. Well, I
found this VERY difficult and had one of the parents question me
about it.*

This can be hard for parents to understand, because they may
be thinking about the disagreements people have about invented
spelling versus traditional spelling. This needs to be set aside in
the case of the LEB, as the LEB is not *direct instruction* in reading
and writing; instead, it's an approach that helps children use language and learn about communicating using spoken and written

language by demonstrating the relationship between spoken and written language. So, it's not so much about the creative process as it is about your getting a chance to interact with the child using language in increasingly meaningful ways. It's also a chance for you to see how the child makes meaning and uses language. Keep in mind what you know about language acquisition. Children move toward mature language use by approximating it. Using the LEB really isn't about correcting grammar and spelling, but about making meaning, so that children will come to understand conventional grammar and spelling and care about producing language that communicates with others.

In order to really use this technique in a therapeutic way, I feel as if I have to help guide the child toward goals we are currently working on. For example, we used one in past tense as that is a current goal. So, she told her story in the past tense, but when she got to writing it she did most of it in present tense. So, I wasn't sure if I was supposed to correct her or not.

No, for this purpose, you don't need to worry about that. Remember that children don't get stuck using just one tense. They learn new tenses as they get better at using language and at thinking about time in relative ways.

So, I guess I need some clarification about the underlying goals of the experience book and what we are trying to accomplish.

The LEB is about experiencing language by using it for communicative purposes. Please allow yourself to abandon ideas about "correct" language in these early stages!

The other difficult part was that sitting and letting a child spell out an entire story takes some time and I felt like we were twiddling our fingers waiting for her to finish this part of it.

Yes, whether you are parent, teacher, or therapist, you need to be patient while this happens in the child. If you are a teacher or therapist, you need to be a role model for the parents for how to do this. The parents should see how you do it (patiently!), and then they'll understand they can do this, too! While you're sitting there being patient, observe what the child is doing and think about the growth and gaps in the child's language so that you can feed into the child's zone of proximal development when you work with the child.

General Comments from Teachers and Therapists About Using Language Experience Books

My Early Intervention babies range from 6 months to 2.11 years and seem to be demonstrating typical development in scribbling and early drawing skills. They all seem interested in getting a pen or crayons and trying to put marks on the paper. They see adults writing and want to do the same. They have experienced writing and have a schema for how to go about it.

Seeing adults and other children writing provides important motivation. Children need models for what they will be learning to say and do.

Wonderful job. You can see them making sense of their experience and feel the excitement that comes through . . . it's exciting to watch as they put their ideas together.

This is part of the power of the LEB. You can see the child's understandings and capabilities grow.

"Writing should be about making meaning from the very first" (Robertson, 2009, p. 160). Our students can spot busy work. They know when an assignment is just another attempt for control or time filler.

Yes. The LEB is about "real" life, so it carries meaning for the child.

"H" has great artwork and ideas. You can almost imagine this on her mamma's refrigerator so that she can show everyone that comes into their house as a reminder. And it's sad that there are not enough experiences like this in life where you get to be creative about something that you care about.

Caring about something is the first part of making it meaningful. Creativity is important for the reason that we care about what we create. Promoting creativity is not a "frill." Putting what the child creates in a book or on the refrigerator tells the child that his or her thinking is valuable and leads to more such learning of all kinds by the child.

I was involved with all of the stories the children did, which was a great experience for me. A child with normal hearing and autism has really progressed with his spoken language over the past 6 months, but surprisingly he typically speaks in one or two words at a time. The language experience books really caught me by surprise at the amount of detail he could provide. It seemed to tap into an area that was otherwise not being drawn out from him.

Children often know more than they can express, regardless of the reason for that being the case. Parents, teachers, and therapists need to try many ways of helping children express themselves.

"Listening, speaking, reading, and writing are all ways to use language" (Robertson, 2009, p. 159). That's what I see in students regardless of their grade, ability, or handicap.

Yes! These comments demonstrate that the LEB isn't just for children with hearing loss.

One student in middle school wrote about his aunt who went on a shopping trip for one item. Apparently she was frying chicken in her kitchen and needed one more ingredient, so she decided to run up to the local store while the chicken was still on the stove. The fire department was there when she got back and the kitchen was full of smoke. That, in my opinion, was an excellent opportunity for this student not only to explain what happened, but also to take a look at the experience to see what it meant.

That situation must have provided endless opportunities for discussion and expansion of vocabulary and language!

I've seen the same process at work with high school juniors who were writing fiction. One girl ended up with the top average in that room and it was an honors class, but her story was about a girl with a deep emotional problem. There was something going on for her to work with a topic like that. I never learned if it was about something in her own life or among her friends, but I saw that the writing process helped her to explore the idea on a personal level.

The LEB and related processes of reading and writing work for all ages. The seventh item in the spiral of development was at work for this girl as she was using writing to think about her own life or someone else's.

Similarities and Differences Among Children With and Without Hearing Loss

I have asked teachers and therapists what they have seen in the writing of children with hearing loss that is in the realm of typical writing development and what differences in writing they have seen between children with typical hearing and children with hearing loss.

My students with hearing loss like to write when given a chance to explore something that is meaningful. They may be behind in syntax or punctuation, but I've seen similar problems in students with normal hearing who come from homes where the television is always on and there are no books or conversation. All students need opportunities to write. It needs to be every day. Journals work well because they're flexible. You can list what happened in your life, respond to something you read, question the logic of rules or events in the news. They're also an opportunity to experiment with language. Our students need that regardless of their disability. Writing is an effort to make sense of life. Our students need more of that—especially with all the changes that they will face in the culture now.

Making sense of one's experiences is the making of meaning about them, and that's precisely what language helps us do.

While doing the language experience books with two students, one with hearing loss and one with typical hearing, it has been eye-opening to see how complex and rich the child with typical hearing's language is vs. the simple language and sentence structure of my child with hearing loss. Although they are too young to be writing, I have been doing the written part for them. But to see what they are able to remember from the experience and have the ability to express is quite profound.

Doing something with an experience, whether it's talking, reading, or writing about it, makes it more memorable, and if the child with hearing loss has ample opportunity to talk about his or her experiences, the child's ability to create rich, complex language will develop in ways similar to the child with typical hearing.

Memory for sequence and detail should grow through repeated opportunities for expression.

It is interesting to see the various stages that children go through while learning to read. I think that these aspects give us a real understanding about development happening in a sequence as well as across domains at the same time, and that children's attempts in writing are preparing them for the rules and instances they will learn next. Although our children with hearing loss may be behind linguistically, we can follow a sequence and guide them when they are learning to write just as one would do with a child with typical hearing.

This is a realization in action that children with hearing loss can and do develop within a sequence similar to the development of children with typical hearing.

I see my auditory-verbal students drawing pictures and telling what they have drawn while someone writes the words. I also see some of my students making scribbles for the words depending on their age, language ability, and other disabilities. I am seeing creative, well-written stories with both conventional spelling and words spelled by how they sound from one of my second grade students who is on grade level in reading and language. I also see another second grader struggling with writing. He can dictate wonderful stories to me; however, his confidence or focus keeps him from finishing writing activities in his mainstream class.

Children differ from each other, of course, so we can't expect literacy to unfold at the same pace in every child; if we pay attention to what a child *can* do and help the child build upon that capability, we can be confident that the child's literacy achievement will advance.

I'm seeing these examples of typical development:

- *Awareness of letters within environmental print (e.g., "I see a "J" for Jamie")*
- *Movement through the stages of writing*
- *Lots of invented spelling*
- *Initial confusion between letter names and letter sounds*

- *Use of phonics to sound out or segment words when writing*
- *The ability to develop a paragraph with a topic sentence, supporting details and a conclusion sentence.*

I'm seeing these differences:

- *Prolonged confusion of sound-letter association*
- *Confusion over segmenting a word in order to write it down*
- *Lack of proper word endings (plurals or subject verb agreement)*
- *Misuse of articles*
- *Misuse of prepositions*
- *Simple sentence structure (contains only noun + verb)*
- *Limited knowledge of irregular past tense verbs*
- *Poor sentence structure that reflects poor spoken language structure*
- *Limited vocabulary (lack of general knowledge vocabulary, multiple meaning words and pop culture vocabulary trends).*

This is an excellent list of strengths and areas where growth is needed. As such, this list provides useful information about where to focus next with the child. For example, the teacher, parent, and/or therapist may decide to begin using longer sentences in speaking with the child so that the child has models for them. Remember that the language used in the child's meaningful environment will become the language that the child uses.

I see my students assuming that the reader knows about what they're writing, so the writing is at times vague and leaves the reader confused. I have noticed this so much while doing the language experience books with older kids. I can now see how helpful the LEBs are in getting the child to try and take the reader's perspective in order to help him figure out what he needs to write down. Very interesting insights have come from doing the LEB!

Developmentally, young children expect that the person on the other end of a communication knows what they're trying to convey, especially when that person is one of their caregivers or teachers. With enough experience, children begin to understand they need to provide background information so that the person they're speaking to and writing to will understand their message. In making an LEB entry, the adult can ask questions that elicit that information (and more language!) from the child. This is one of the ways the LEB helps children expand their linguistic repertoires.

The student that I am doing my experience stories with constructs her stories from background knowledge. She has a lot of support with language at home and at school. Another student that I work with has a lot of background knowledge and creates stories, but they usually have to be pulled out of her brain. She seems to also still need a lot of good literacy activities one-to-one with an adult.

Children differ from each other, and they differ in their responses from one time with an LEB to another. Sometimes we watch a child create an entry, and sometimes we need to help.

Using Background Knowledge

I have also asked teachers and therapists about the kinds of reliance on background knowledge they are seeing in the children with whom they're interacting, about what they see as the significance of this, and whether they have seen a child construct a story or an idea in writing.

Clay (1991) discusses the importance of background knowledge with writing from a cultural perspective and how some kids will be more prepared for reading and writing simply by being exposed to this in the home through books, magazines, and watching others read and write. I have seen an 8-year-old child construct a story in writing. She uses invented spelling and has good control over directional behavior, ways to represent ideas in words, and letter forms. She consistently asks, "How do you spell _____?" and has been encouraged lately to try to spell it herself; I tell her that we will review it at the end of her writing. Clay (1991) states, "A powerful strategy for teachers to encourage is for children to use the sounds they hear in words they are trying to write, and finding letters for those sounds they don't" (p. 111). Clay (1991) also states that "integration is the heart of early reading success" (p. 105). She is describing the integration of remembering the ideas, re-telling them,

*finding them in print, and then moving across the print" (p. 105).
I see that this little girl is beginning to construct ideas more independently and is on her way to reading and writing independently.*

This is a lovely description of a child learning to use spoken
and written language to express herself in an increasingly integrated way. She is developing certain understandings about how
language works, and she asks for help when she decides her own
understanding is incomplete. Over time, continuous work of this
sort results in the ability to use language in mature ways.

*One of my students had normal hearing and it was interesting to
see the themes in the stories that she told. She's in first grade and
has an older sister who is 11. Apparently, they sit around and tell
stories to one another at times, so this student was good at developing plots on the spot. We worked together for several sessions and all
of her stories were about a pet that was lost and needing its mother
or a young girl who wanted a pet and her parents (or grandparents) wouldn't let her because "we already have enough." She wrote
several different stories around this and then went into detail with
the drawings as if she had thought about it. At one point, she told
me one of the stories was something that she already discussed with
her sister the day before. Later she got to talking about one of my
other students (who is her same age). "Joe lives in my apartment
complex," she said. "We were in the same pre-K class." "Oh, that's
nice," I said. But I got to thinking about that. This girl lives around
other people. She writes about pets or the sensation of feeling lost
and wanting comfort. There's some background to this combination. The emotions come through in her work. I don't know if she
wants a pet but can't have one because of her life in the apartment.
I also don't know if she feels isolated and wants her mother. But
why else would she write about that in several different contexts?
Ferreiro (1991) would tell me that children come to school with the
ability to construct and interpret schemas and then act on the reality that they experience. It was clear that this girl had thought about
pets and the feelings of being left alone. That's why she told stories
about it. Even if she encountered those themes from other stories (in
school even), those ideas were meaningful to her and she wanted to
express them. Clay (1991) would advise me to use this opportunity
from the girl's writing as a chance to "attend" to the ideas in print
since what she wrote can now be used to help with reading. Either
way, the girl benefits. She brings a meaningful experience from her*

own life, explores that in her own writing and then can learn to read better from it. In my mind, education doesn't get better than that since the personal meaning now holds everything together.

This child is demonstrating that she is thinking about what's happening in her environment. It doesn't matter for our purposes that she has typical hearing; this account could just as well describe the progress of a child with hearing loss who is learning to listen and speak.

I think background knowledge plays a significant role. Children are better able to comprehend information about a topic they have some experience with. Children also tend to write about what they know; background knowledge is a source of inspiration.

This observation that children write better about what they know about is important. Knowing about something involves both knowing and wanting to know the words and language structures for talking and writing about it. We should always start with what the child knows and then help the child add to that.

The following story expresses this well:

I have a student who is seven, but has pretty minimal expressive language (due to being profoundly deaf and unaided for five years in a refugee camp.) She does have background experiences. (Just imagine, five years in a refugee camp she could tell me things that would probably blow my mind!) However, she does not have the language to do so. At this point, we are working collaboratively on her language experience book, and I am filling in the gaps for her. She'll often gesture to show me what something is, and I'll help her to get that word. A couple of weeks ago, she wanted to write about crossing the monkey bars on the playground. We went outside and played around. I took her picture by the bars, and told her they were called "monkey bars." She laughed hysterically about them having the "monkey" label. I think she even suspected that I had made it up! She dictated that in her language experience book and read it back perfectly. Essentially, I think kids bring SO much background knowledge with them, and as their language progresses, they're able to better express their experiences.

This teacher was very helpful to the student by providing her more experience and the words she needed to label the experience. The teacher is correct in surmising that the child has a lot of knowledge but does not yet have the vocabulary with which to describe that knowledge. This is a primary aim of the LEB.

Clay (1991) would say to let my student start with a picture and then give her the words she needs. This teaches her that a picture is "a rough guide to the message and the print carries the precise message" (p. 96). If students are not able to supply the print themselves, then we supply it for them to build language.

This is a good example of scaffolding student learning in ways that are sensitive to the student's experiences and background knowledge.

I feel that my students with more diverse background knowledge and experience related to reading and sharing books:

- *have a larger and more diverse vocabulary;*
- *create/write their own stories more easily;*
- *include "book talk" in their own writing; and*
- *generate writing for different purposes and use the appropriate vocabulary for these purposes (e.g., letters, informative, descriptive, persuasive).*

I have seen students with hearing loss construct an idea in writing. This past week I was working with two students and asked them to "tell me about something that happened in your life that you will never forget." I gave just a few examples like a vacation, the first time they flew on a plane, or the day they got their dogs. I wanted to see what they would come up with, or what was really important to them, without giving too many hints. One student used my example of vacation and wrote about going to Hawaii for the first time. The other student surprised me by choosing something that dug a little deeper. She talked about the day she met her best friend in kindergarten (they are now in fifth grade). She got the point that "something you'll never forget" had to have an emotional component. I think Clay's (1991) idea of making reasons to write meaningful could apply here. Clearly this was something she was excited about, and she was inspired to write. Writing is a struggle for her and this was probably one of the longest pieces of writing I've gotten from her. The girls also knew that they'd share their writing with each other, so perhaps that was a motivating factor, as well. This student can clearly connect meaning to print. She has mastered the "code" or gone through the stages of writing development.

This teacher shows an understanding of the *process* of student learning; she has taken the time to observe what students can do and to learn about her students' thoughts and experiences.

My son (with typical hearing) is very into superheroes . . . recently, he came to me and wanted to write his own book so that he could read it to his daddy later. His entire story and characters were named and modeled after stories that he is familiar with and places that he has either been or seen in books. The significance of this to me is that children need to experience the world and gain appropriate vocabulary and knowledge of it so they can expand their learning from that starting point. Wanting to write his own book about superheroes is connected to his daily exposure to print (he reads about superheroes ALL the time!) and he tries hard to use written language to convey meaning.

This is a great example of how a child uses his background knowledge to start the new task of book writing.

Experiences of Teachers Who Have Been Trying Language Experience Books

Britt Petro: *My experience with language experience books has been very positive, especially with one student in particular. "John" is in first grade now, but we started the books informally during his last year of preschool. He is very creative. He loves to color, cut, and turn his creations into books. At first, I just went with his preference for these types of activities because it kept him engaged. Then last year, I really started revisiting his books and reading them together. I could see how it boosted his confidence, kept him engaged, and allowed him to explore writing in a nonthreatening manner. The books allowed him to practice letter-to-sound association, segmenting words, and identifying sight words. We just started a new book this school year and he is still just as interested. In general he is a CI superstar, meaning that he has age-appropriate language or above. He uses funny phrases and slang all the time, but he has struggled with early reading skills.*

Two of his pages can be seen in Figures 10–1 and 10–2. *One demonstrates the concept of rhyming, which we were talking about that day. When reading his sentence he stated, "Ape in a cape." His picture is of Super Ape in a cape, saving a cat. The second page of his is a little chaotic! It is a story about him and the super hero Blue Ear. That day, in his book, he decided to sequence his pictures. I thought it showed his concept of a story, and also his concept of book language that's used in comics. He loves super heroes and comics and I started to see little word bubbles appear in his books saying things like "Pow" or "Crash!" Frame number 4 says "Boom" and frame 7 says "me help!" which he read as "Help me!" He read the sentence in frame 6 as "Blue Ear has a bad guy."*

Dara Ellen Breitkopf: *I have found that the excitement surrounding the reading of these books invigorates both the child and parents. The fact that my guy saw his own words on the page made the entire experience much more meaningful for him. Personally, I truly believe that his fluency increased with his experience books, because we were using his own language in them! He enjoyed seeing the familiar pictures and reading the familiar words. He even enjoyed showing others the book and reading it to them. He would add comments during reading to further elaborate on what was already written. I think that because we already wrote a lot about each picture, he had to go above and beyond what he would usually say because he had already said it! In other words, the experience books helped him stretch his linguistically expressive muscles. It's like when we tell stories over and over. We remember more detail. We add little bits and pieces. He would add to his stories as well, and that made our language experience when reading the books that much richer. I have also found that when Jason gets the book, he'll often turn to a favorite page and begin reading or just narrating what he sees. On one of the pages in one of the books, you can see Dunkin Donuts munchkins in the background. One day when we began to read his experience book, we had a long discussion about munchkins and how much he likes them! It made the whole linguistic experience that much more meaningful for him.*

Tammy Croak: *I began using the LEB with my preschoolers with hearing loss after learning about them in my First Years courses.*

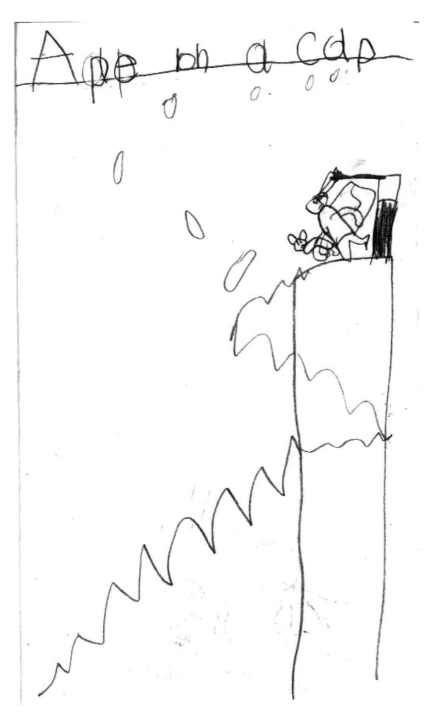

Figure 10–1. Ape in a cape.

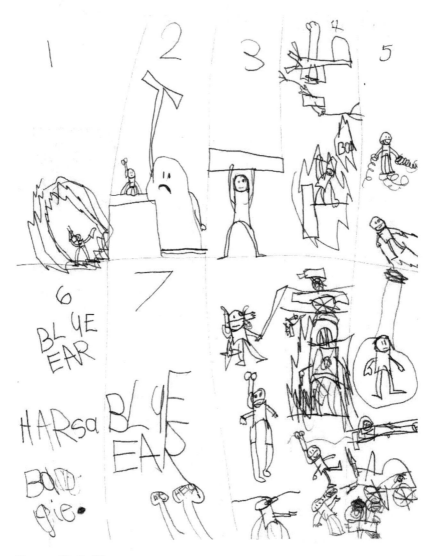

Figure 10–2. Blue ear sequence.

I expanded its use to my students with autism and childhood apraxia of speech. For the past two years, I have also been using the LEB with my school-aged students with a wide range of speech and language impairments. Basically, now I use it with ALL students, and it is without a doubt the most effective tool in my toolbox to access my entire communication goals for my students and their families.

Figures 10–3, 10–4, and 10–5 represent some of the LEB entries collected by Croak. Note that they are simple drawings done by children accompanied by words written mainly by an adult and supplied by the child or an adult.

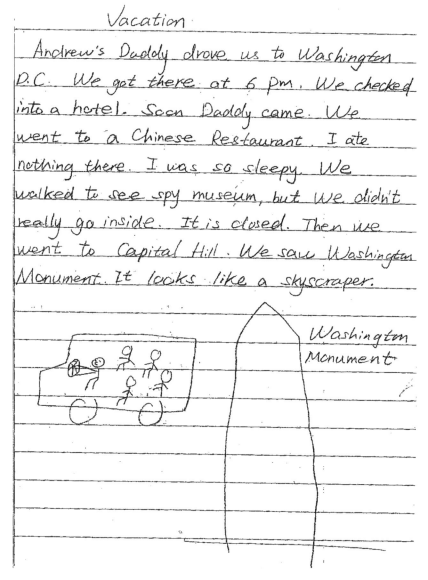

Figure 10–3. Vacation.

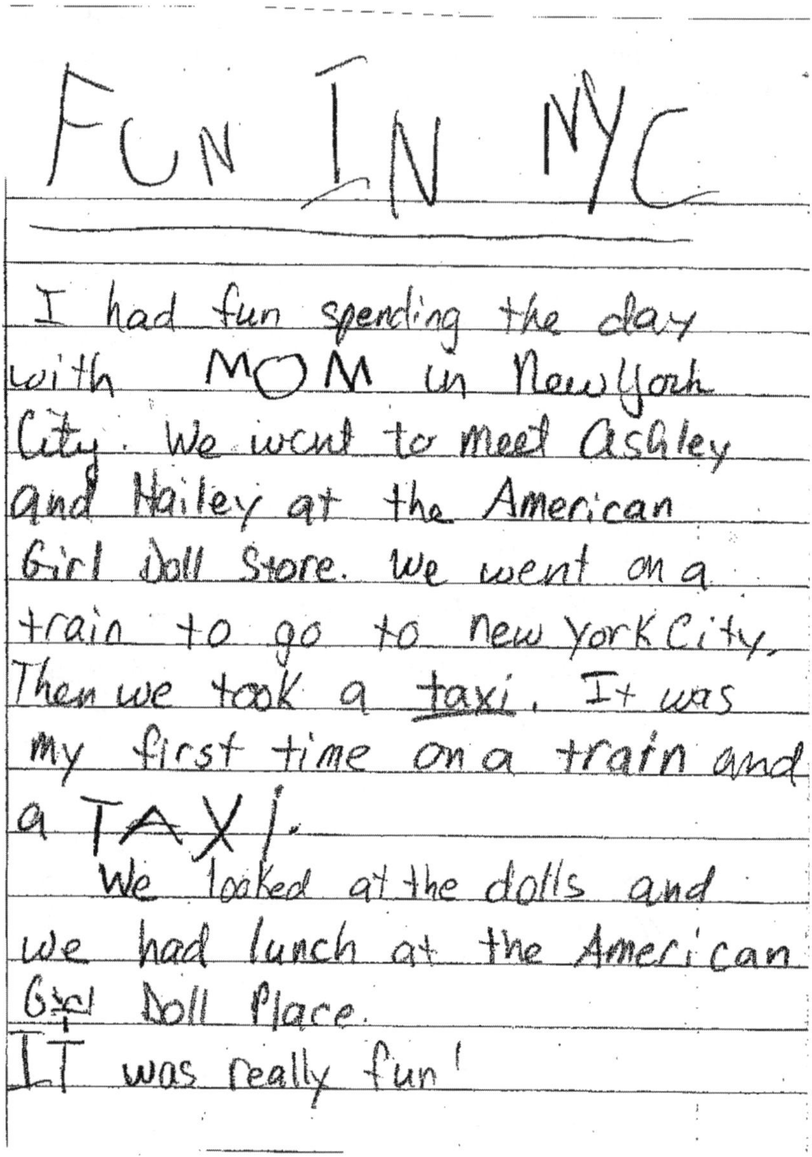

FUN IN NYC

I had fun spending the day with MOM in New York City. We went to meet Ashley and Hailey at the American Girl Doll Store. We went on a train to go to New York City. Then we took a taxi. It was my first time on a train and a TAXI.

We looked at the dolls and we had lunch at the American Girl Doll Place.

IT was really fun!

A

Figure 10–4. A. Fun in NYC.

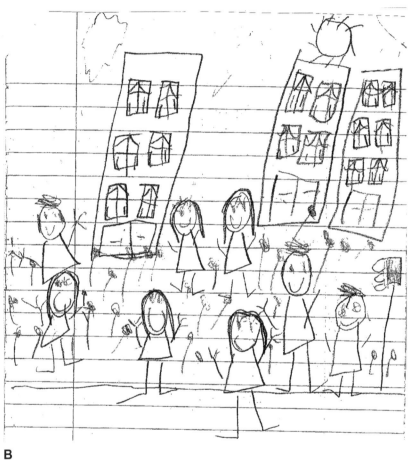

B

Figure 10–4. B. Fun in NYC drawing.

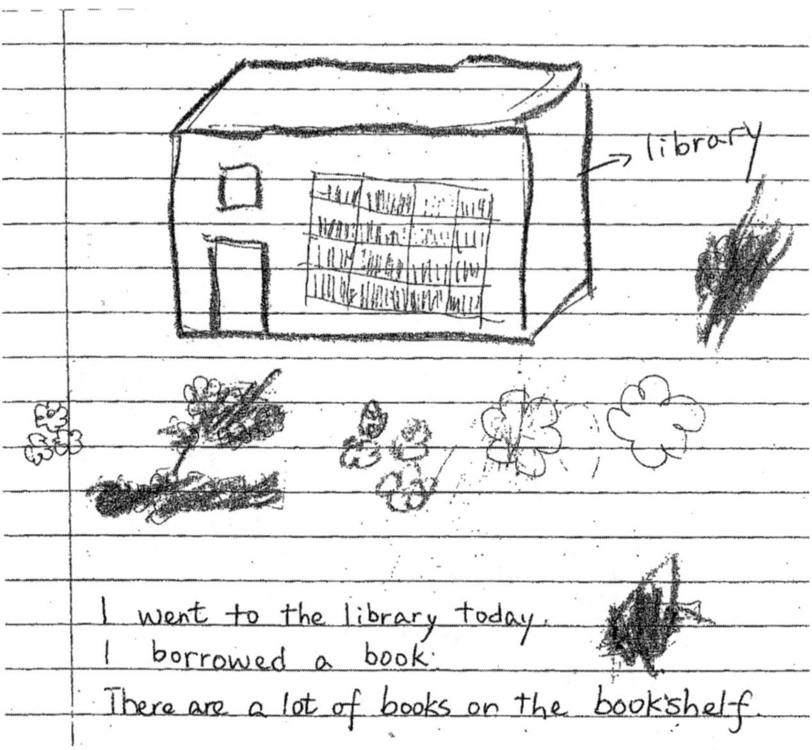

Handwritten text in figure:

I went to the library today.
I borrowed a book.
There are a lot of books on the bookshelf.

Figure 10–5. Library.

A Mother's Experience with Language Experience Books

Gloria Fan is the mother of a son who received hearing aids at 16 months and two cochlear implants, the first at 2½ and the second at 3 years of age. As she has worked with her son, she has created books to support learning particular words and types of words. To illustrate the concept "beside," she took photographs of him in situations where he was next to someone important to him (for example, a picture of their neighbors captioned, "Our neighbors live **beside** us," and pictures of the baby, mommy, and daddy sitting **beside** him, captioned, "The baby is sitting **beside** me" and so on).

They read the book over and over together, and Gloria would make sure to use the words in conversation with him. She reports that she poured the target word into her son and that developing a good understanding of each word conceptually took at least a week. Then, she notes that he would start using it, often tentatively at first, until he had mastered it. The preschool therapist worked along with them, charting the words he knew receptively and expressively, comparing these to language development in children with typical hearing, and suggesting words and concepts to work on. They focused intentionally on words her son was having trouble picking up (for example: "catch," "catch**ing**," "catch**er**," and other forms of "catch"). Gloria made books in which she:

- Highlighted the word in a color that made it stand out
- Used the word in many ways (example: "**catching** scarves is really fun"—after an activity with juggling at a museum)
- Presented the word in different ways, always putting the word in context.

After her son showed that he knew a word by using it meaningfully, Gloria moved on to new words and concepts, allowing two to four weeks for experience with the word and for setting up opportunities to use the word.

Gloria's practical advice for creating language experience books includes:

- Go back through photos you have already to find illustrations of particular words.
- Be ready with your camera.
- Set up situations so you can take illustrative pictures.
- Use card stock, tape a photo to it, write a description, use different colors to write, and then tie the pages together.
- Make each book for a targeted purpose, and then use it immediately.
- Think ahead about possible scenarios based on the upcoming week's schedule and make a list, so as to be ready with words and camera.
- Be attentive to the child's interests.
- Draw what you can't photograph.
- Link the auditory with the visual.

As her son is growing and developing more language, she is learning about letting him follow his own interests, and often lets him choose books for them to read together.

Conclusion

The language experience book is a dynamic approach that starts and ends with listening. In between, the child encounters the words of his or her experiences and, over time, learns to attend to and produce language in its spoken and written forms. Each page is a model for the child of how to use language to make sense of the world. This simple approach with its many variations supports the complexity of spoken and written language.

References

Bruner, J. (1961). *The process of education*. Cambridge, MA: Harvard University Press.

Clay, M. (1991). *Becoming literate: The construction of inner control* (pp. 91–112). Portsmouth, NH: Heinemann.

Ferreiro, E. (1991). Literacy acquisition and the representation of language. In C. Kamii, M. Manning, & G. Manning (Eds.), *Early literacy: A constructivist foundation for whole language* (pp. 31–56). Washington, DC: National Education Association.

Henson, J. (2005). *It's not easy being green* (p. 17). New York, NY: Hyperion.

Vygotsky, L. (1962). *Thought and language*. Cambridge, MA: M.I.T. Press & Wiley.

Chapter 11

PROCEEDING THROUGH SCHOOL

. . . learning is the making of meaning.
Elbow, 2004, p. 10

Introduction

So far, we have been considering the very young child, which is of vital importance, because many school and learning difficulties can be prevented by beginning intervention at the earliest possible time. In fact, the earlier intervention occurs in the form of listening technology and language therapy and education by highly qualified professionals, the greater the possibility—even the likelihood—that children with hearing loss will be schooled alongside their peers with typical hearing and will achieve at levels commensurate with them (Daya et al., 2000; Dornan et al., 2007; Geers, 2003; Moog, 2002). This is not to say that every child with hearing loss will be "at the head of the class," but that the child can be prepared so as not to have the problem of not hearing, listening, and acquiring spoken language that is a primary hindrance to achievement. We must keep in mind that the academic achievement of children with typical hearing spreads itself widely and, in the case of achievement in reading, writing, and math, and other activities and areas of study, often unevenly within a given individual. A student may earn high scores in reading, but low scores in math, or do well in math, but much less well in writing, and so on.

The "Fourth-Grade Slump"

Some children, both with and without typical hearing, make good progress in literacy during the early years of elementary school, and then their achievement levels out at about the fourth-grade reading level, with slow progress being made thereafter. This happens often enough that the phenomenon has a name: "the fourth-grade slump." Various explanations have been offered. One is that the slump is reflected in the way testing is set up; it is possible that the fourth-grade tests do not assess the next step in reading growth and are assessing something else, or that what is tested at third grade is not relevant to fourth-grade development. Second, some early reading instruction focuses too much on word identification and thereby implies to children that comprehending is not the aim of reading; in this case, comprehension problems can go unnoticed until testing begins to include more on comprehension items of various sorts (Snow, Burns, & Griffin, p. 77). A third possibility is that other problems existed at the first, second, and third grade levels that are finally being uncovered through testing during fourth grade (Snow, Burns, & Griffin, p. 78). A fourth hypothesis is that at fourth grade, children are given more informational texts to read. They may have difficulty adapting to a new kind of text, having read stories primarily up to this point. The informational texts may not be written well enough, or the children may lack the requisite background knowledge with which to comprehend the texts (Allington, 2006, pp. 173–174). A fifth idea is that fourth-grade books begin to use more "big words." Such words cannot be decoded easily by children who are still looking at words in a letter-by-letter fashion, and such words need to be in the reader's listening vocabulary in order to be identifiable and pronounceable when encountered on the page (Cunningham, 2003, as cited in Allington, p. 174). Children whose vocabularies have not been growing all along will be at a distinct disadvantage by the fourth grade. In any case, it is clear that reading fourth-grade materials and scoring at the fourth-grade level involves more demonstration of comprehension than at the previous levels. Comprehension does not necessarily accompany being able to pronounce the words on the page; instead, comprehension is the result of thinking actively (Allington, 2006, p. 120).

Leach, Scarborough, and Rescorla (2003) report on numerous studies that identify "weakness in higher order comprehension," sometimes in the presence of "strong word-level skills," and deficiencies in oral language, background knowledge, metacognitive awareness, strategy use, and memory capacity as being associated with the "fourth-grade slump." They observe that either or both text comprehension and word-level processing deficiencies can be responsible (p. 212).

It is important to note that some students sail through all the elementary years, only to stall in the middle school or high school years when reading demands heighten even further. As a preventative, Allington recommends that the teaching of reading be done intentionally throughout the school years (2006, p. 175). There is evidence that teaching higher level reading skills and strategies does not take place consistently (Farber, 1999) and that teachers must concentrate on helping students prepare to read the texts that come their way. Learning to read must make way for students to learn more about reading from reading itself. Children make many important discoveries about words and ideas through inspecting the ways words and sentences are constructed when written. For example, the word "sign" is pronounced "sine." The "g" in "sign" shows up in "signature" where it is pronounced, thereby demonstrating a meaning-related connection between the two words.

Readers Who Are Deaf or Hard of Hearing and the Fourth Grade Level

In view of "the fourth-grade slump," and the ideas concerning why it happens, I find it interesting that the fourth-grade level has been so frequently cited as the median functioning level for persons who are deaf or hard of hearing. It is easy to see that each of the hypotheses discussed above may hold some explanatory power in the case of children with hearing loss, as these ideas have their roots in language, word, and world/background knowledge. Although Paddon and Hanson (2000) do not reference "the fourth-grade slump," they associate reaching the fourth- or fifth-grade level with the need for phonological knowledge:

> In the case of Deaf children, early reading may not use pho- nological mediation at all. It may only be when the reader passes a critical level of difficulty, perhaps above the fourth- or fifth-grade reading level, that evidence for use of phonological information can be found. It would be in the case of reading complex material that the Deaf reader might need to learn to use phonological information. (p. 439)

Some of the fourth-grade ceiling effect may be attributed to the technical reasons that testing may not reveal adequately what someone knows about reading, that tests at lower levels mask dif- ficulties a person has with reading, and that harder tests begin to pick up on those difficulties. For our population of interest, it makes sense to pay attention at least to the following potential reasons for their leaving elementary school, or even high school or college, with measured reading achievement stalled at an elementary level:

- Problems with oral language
- A limited listening vocabulary
- Lack of phonological information
- Lack of background knowledge
- General comprehension problems
- Word-level processing deficiencies
- Lack of ability to deal in reading with words of more than one or two syllables
- Treatment of each word as an identifiable whole
- Lack of metacognitive awareness
- Poor strategy use
- Limited memory capacity
- Lack of practice with informational reading.

Phonological Awareness, Vocabulary, and Reading Achievement

In a discussion of lexical restructuring, Metsala and Walley (1998) argue that younger children identify and remember words holisti- cally, as separate entities, but that this only works up to the point when vocabulary growth begins to require a "segmental restructuring" that facilitates word processing. They suggest that such restructuring of words held in memory develops across early and middle childhood, which in most children is a time of huge vocabulary growth (p. 100). Being able to segment words and store the parts in memory within categories assists with identification of old and new words in listening and reading, and then retrieving them from memory to use in writing. In typical fourth grade materials, the child must begin to deal with words in parts and by analogy with other words, simply because at this point there are so many words that they cannot be remembered one by one. Individuals who are making good progress may hold categories of word parts (sounds, prefixes, root words, suffixes, plural endings, etc.) from which to assemble, disassemble, and then reassemble words flexibly during the word identification process. The related words are called "neighborhoods" by a number of researchers. At first, a neighborhood may be composed of phonemic variations that signal the difference between "bag/bug" or "bib/bit," (Metsala & Walley, 1998), but as vocabulary grows, word parts become recognizable in other words, and a neighborhood might contain "cartoon" and "cartilage" (p. 101). High-frequency words and word parts in well-populated neighborhoods are more easily recognized than words and parts the child sees and uses less frequently, and over time, the child learns to recognize them by their phonemic differences represented in letter form. This corresponds with Padden and Hanson's (2000) suggestion that phonological information is needed in order to read the more complex writing encountered in the fourth or fifth grade, as this cannot be done easily without the phonological support that assists memory storage and retrieval. A growing listening vocabulary is necessary to this endeavor, as it is not very useful to a child to figure out how to pronounce a word encountered in reading for which there has been no prior experience and thus no knowledge of what the word stands for conceptually. Growth in reading achievement beyond the fourth grade may well depend on capitalizing on a developing ability to be more flexible in identifying words by analogizing their parts with other known words, both in listening and in reading. Any sort of deprivation that results in the child not listening to enough spoken words and not seeing enough words in written form will hinder this process. The sensitive teacher who is aware of the child's vocabulary, thus knowing what the child does and does not know, can design instruction for growth beyond the fourth grade level; the child's success will depend on him or her being able to listen to the teacher and to interact with others in order to build language facility. Parents can help facilitate this, too, and the teacher should be talking with the parents about this.

Metsala and Walley (1998) describe studies that link vocabulary knowledge and phonemic awareness, and that describe the ability to segment words as affecting vocabulary development (pp. 110–111). They conclude, "There appears to be a direct link between spoken word recognition and reading performance" (p. 112). In sum, listening drives the ability to distinguish phonemes (phonemic awareness), which in turn drives vocabulary growth. Vocabulary growth and flexible memory storage for words of all kinds, both high- and low-frequency words and those that sound and look both similar and dissimilar to each other, are necessary for growth in reading and writing achievement. This holds true for children with typical hearing, and is perhaps even more important to keep in mind for children with hearing loss. Expecting children to learn to recognize each word holistically without regarding the phonemic qualities of each word is to leave them with a small vocabulary that does not equip them to generate recognition of more complex words. The process of becoming a reader and writer is based on language knowledge, including spoken word forms, vocabulary, and phonemic knowledge; this interactive process spurs on more learning about spoken words, vocabulary, and phonemic patterns.

Vocabulary Growth

As should be clear from the above, as children progress through school and through life, an enormous amount of their ability to get along and then to thrive hinges on their knowledge of and growth in vocabulary. Simply put, it is necessary to know many, many words—what they sound like, what they look like in print, and above, all, what they mean and how they work relative to other words. Estimates for the number of spoken words known by children with typical hearing are instructive for those working and living with children with hearing loss: 2,500 to 3,000 for 4-year-olds in preschool, 7,000 to 10,000 for first graders, and 39,000 to 46,000 for fifth-graders (Anglin, 1989, cited in Metsala & Walley, 1998,

p. 100). These goals are not unrealistic for children with hearing loss, as long as they are using hearing technology consistently and are expected to interact using meaningful spoken language with people of all ages. Too often, not enough is expected, and low levels of vocabulary knowledge are taken for granted. This is also related to becoming stuck at the fourth grade reading level.

Teachers and parents have the huge responsibility to help students make progress in developing their vocabularies. In order to engage in conversation or to read about something, a person needs to know the words being used. When an unknown word comes up, the person needs to become aware of the gap, identify and focus on the word, and employ strategies for learning what the word means. This means that, from childhood on, the person needs to expect to know what is going on and to take an interest in being fully informed. Having a curious, questioning attitude is vital to the process. In the normal course of events, a very young child begins by acquiring words useful in his or her environment: "mommy," "daddy," "go," "more," and so on. New words enter in as they become useful in the child's life: "more" becomes "want more," which after a while turns into "I want more milk, please, Mommy." This sort of addition to language and vocabulary happens easily for the child when hearing and listening are established, especially in an environment where words are valued, and it happens over and over again in the child's daily interaction with people who know what the child knows and who lead the child along by offering new words as they are needed and enjoyed by the child. This seems to take place without particular intention, especially at the beginning when it just feels like good fun, but parents and teachers can and ought to become more intentional about vocabulary and seek multiple ways to offer new words and concepts to the child, particularly to the child with hearing loss, in order to help the child build a vocabulary in a continuous, meaningful fashion.

For vocabulary learning to take place optimally, it is important that the child be in a rich language environment where word learning is encouraged and enjoyed. Fostering a curious attitude in the child is important, because an active learner comes into contact with more, makes more sense of his or her surroundings, and makes more progress than a passive learner.

The following exchange is drawn from a conversation related to me that took place between a mother and a preschool-age son at the *Tyrannosaurus rex* exhibit in the Natural History Museum in London. It is an example of acting as a model for the child by introducing something new for the child in terms of what the child already knows. Note that the adult repeats, elaborates, explains, amplifies, and rephrases, all in the process of introducing the child to two new words that mean *very big* and getting the child thinking about what this dinosaur looked like.

> Mummy: That's a picture of a dinosaur. Can you say *dinosaur?* Let's say "*dinosaur.*"
>
> Child: Dinosaur
>
> Mummy: Yes, that's a dinosaur. This one is called "*Tyrannosaurus rex.*" He was a *very, very big* animal. He was *tremendous*! But, look—he had very short arms. Do you think he could reach his mouth to brush his teeth? [The exhibit had a sign next to a picture of *T. rex* with a toothbrush that said *T. rex's* arms were too short for him to brush his teeth.]
>
> Child: No—too far.
>
> Mummy: He would need a *very, very long-handled* toothbrush. It would have to be *gigantic*! It's a good thing dinosaurs didn't have to brush their teeth!

In this exchange, the adult takes the opportunity to introduce the words "tremendous" and "gigantic" by putting them into context. The *Tyrannosaurus rex* isn't just big; he is *very, very big*, but his arms are so short that he needs a *very, very long-handled* toothbrush. Repeating "*very*" adds to the image of the extreme size discrepancy. Putting "*tremendous*" and "*gigantic*" in the place of "*very, very big*" supplies a definition for these words the adult thinks the child might not know. Observing that *T. rex's* arms are so short that they don't reach his mouth connects to what the child knows from his own daily experience and supplies context and images that help in fitting the new words in with words the child knows already.

Semantic mapping and semantic webbing are established approaches for incorporating new words into one's repertoire (Blachowicz, 2000, p. 505; Vacca & Vacca, 2002). For the above instance, a map could look like this:

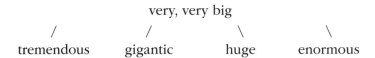

Semantic mapping attempts to mirror the memory organization a person carries around in the form of a schema, in this case, several labels for the concept of being exceedingly large. The newer labels are more memorable because of their connection to the labels the child already had. Such mapping is relevant for young children, as well as for older students and adults, because it presents a visual demonstration of the relationships between and among various words. The semantic map can be presented to the learner, or the learner can be helped in producing the semantic map, beginning with his or her own prior knowledge. Any one of the words that mean *very, very large* could be at the top of the semantic map or at the center of the semantic web, depending upon the learner's prior vocabulary knowledge.

In the process of picking up new words in the spoken environment, the child begins to learn strategies for learning word meanings. When the child holds sufficient strategies, he or she is capable of being independent in seeking out and learning new words from the environment. Teachers and parents can teach children to use context by providing explicit instruction, scaffolding, practice, and feedback (Blachowicz, 2000, p. 506). Returning to the *dinosaur* example, we can see how this works:

Mummy: That's a picture of a dinosaur. Can you say dinosaur? Let's say "dinosaur." [practice]

Child: Dinosaur

Mummy: Yes, that's a dinosaur. This one is called "*Tyrannosaurus rex.*" He was a *very, very big* animal. He was *tremendous*! [explicit instruction] But, look—he had very short arms. Do you think he could reach his mouth to brush his teeth? [scaffolding]

Child: No—too far.

Mummy: He would need a *very, very long* toothbrush. It would have to be *gigantic*! [explicit instruction] It's a good thing dinosaurs didn't have to brush their teeth! [feedback]

Note that later when the child encounters the word "tyrant" in listening or reading, the basic part of the word "tyrannosaurus" will supply some help.

Parents and teachers often assume they need to be feeding the desired words into the child. This works when the words are useful and meaningful from the child's point of view, but just as with other learning, vocabulary growth occurs when the child is active in the process. The meaning the child creates in the presence of the words, rather than sheer memorization, is the memory-building ingredient that helps the child understand and use concepts and the words that represent them. Direct teaching can involve giving children a key word that links to the new word (tyrannosaurus/ tyrant), presenting images or models (a picture or 3-D model of the *T. rex*), making explanations (as in the *T. rex* exchange), and helping children act out word meanings (How big would that toothbrush have to be? As big as you? Bigger?). Direct teaching is most effective when it involves presenting definitions in an active way that requires students to do something with the words. Students can be prompted to add context and to talk and write using the words. They need to be brought into contact with the words multiple times and be expected to use them in various settings and ways in order to situate the words into schemata with related words and concepts. For the teacher, this can be very exciting, as it demands thinking about how to make connections from known parts of a child's environment to new experiences and things that make sense to the child because of that connection. Of course, dinosaurs didn't use toothbrushes, but children do, and the child can imagine the dinosaur using a *gigantic* toothbrush to learn about that word.

Children can also choose the words they want to learn. Blachowicz (2000) describes studies done in which children in school choose their own vocabulary lists. This has been shown to result in students choosing harder words than their teacher would choose for them and in remembering the words better than teacher-chosen words. Giving students instruction on how to choose important words yields even better results (p. 507). Reciprocal teaching in which students help each other in figuring out parts of a text they do not understand aids students in building comprehension, and this may be associated with helping them enlarge their vocabularies, possibly because it puts the process within their control (p. 507). Building language together through conversation goes a long way in extending students' vocabulary.

Analogies, similes, and metaphors provide many ways of understanding new words in relation to known words because they contain within them the meanings shared across the words (Lakoff & Johnson, 1980). Considering a window in a house in comparison with the eyes in a face provides many new ideas to think about. The analogy is "window is to house, as eyes are to face," the simile is "the eyes are like a window," and the metaphor is "the eyes are a window." It is not so much that the student learns to label these word images, but that the student becomes actively involved in thinking about the similarities of meaning embedded in the suggested relationships. This is language learning at its most delicious!

Parents and teachers must think intentionally about setting up experiences in which children can become involved actively in order to learn what makes sense to them; they must also teach directly about words and concepts.

> These realizations imply that teachers need to be knowledgeable about what they want students to know with respect to both the depth and breadth of learning and the kinds of connections to be made. Also, they must take into account the students' starting points. What do they already know that can help make the connections to new learning? What might conflict or confuse them? Teaching vocabulary becomes not a simple process of teaching words, but one of teaching particular words to particular students for a particular purpose. (Blachowicz, 2000, p. 517)

In order to prevent a fourth-grade reading level from becoming the achievement ceiling for the child with hearing loss, both formal and informal vocabulary learning must take place daily and in every way possible, both intentional and through serendipitous discovery. Children who learn to love and appreciate words continue to seek new ones to add to their repertoires, gaining much in background knowledge, phonology, and word function in the process.

Comprehension Growth

In general, comprehension in listening and comprehension in reading parallel one another, as both involve language, including vocabulary, and active thought. For some individuals, with or without hearing loss, the aural route is easier, and for others, the easier path is the visual. The child who learns to use both and who continues to strengthen both is likely to become a strong student. It may be tempting to "go with a child's strength," but that can result in the child not building both capacities. Comprehension involves learning, of course, and knowing how to learn is the desired outcome of schooling. At least one observer, R. Allington (2006), is concerned that school curricula too often put assessment of comprehension in the place of helping students develop strategies for comprehending. Worksheets, word searches, and the ubiquitous end-of-chapter questions may supply evidence of whether a child has remembered, but they do not instruct the child. Teachers need to demonstrate to children how to take specific steps in coming to understand something, and they need to give children repeated opportunities to practice the steps with both familiar and new materials. Such steps include thinking about what one already knows (activating prior knowledge), summarizing (selecting the most important information and reciting or writing it for one's own use or for someone else), use of elements in a story such as setting, characters, and plot (story grammar elements), imagery (of a character or of a concept or word), creating one's own questions, and thinking aloud during the reading process (p. 122).

It is useful to think about Bloom's taxonomy when thinking about comprehension (Bloom et al., 1956). This familiar taxonomy lays out cognitive processes from the simplest to the most complex. The task for the teacher is to help children gain facility with all its levels, as each level is supported by the simpler processes beneath it.

From simplest to most complex, the levels are as follows:

1. **Knowledge** involves demonstrating facility with the literal words used to express an idea, and it is usually accomplished by memorizing.
2. **Comprehension** involves demonstrating an understanding of an idea by explaining it in other words and being able to use it in some way. Interpretation, inferring, and predicting may be involved.
3. **Application** involves using the knowledge and comprehension of an idea to solve a practical problem.
4. **Analysis** involves identifying the component parts of an idea and understanding their relationship to each other.

5. **Synthesis** involves formulating something new using one or more ideas.
6. **Evaluation** involves judging one idea in comparison to another.

Helping students contemplate ideas using all these levels is critical in their becoming literate adults who can think for themselves. For this to happen, instruction must be about more than literal knowledge, and students need to be instructed about the steps involved in any of the simpler processes that comprise the more complex ones. The genius of Bloom's taxonomy is its applicability in all disciplines and its succinct description of what it means to think and comprehend. It is useful in thinking about instruction throughout the grade levels, for it tells us that memorizing is a low-level activity, and that if we want students to be able to do even a simple analysis, that student will need to know, understand, and be able to apply a particular idea. The teacher who makes use of this powerful hierarchy will not leave out the necessary steps in using an idea and will be more likely to be able to demonstrate strategies for using an idea in a highly developed way. That is the goal of moving children with and without hearing loss through the school years.

Academically Successful Young Adults with Hearing Loss

Recently, I have had the privilege of corresponding with four young women with hearing loss about their educational and work experiences. One of them is my own daughter, whom I describe in Chapter 12. These women are in their 20s and early 30s and all have advanced degrees spanning the fields of audiology, psychology, social work, and deaf education. Two have finished doctorates. They represent the coming of age that is available to the younger children addressed in this book.

Two of these women grew up with severe-to-profound hearing loss and two with profound loss, and all wore hearing aids from the time they were toddlers. Three obtained a cochlear implant after the age of 18, one of these is considering implanting the other ear, and the fourth is thinking seriously about getting an implant. All would identify themselves as individuals who use their listening skills to good effect and who participate in all that life has to offer. They enjoy hearing and remember assigning great value to their hearing aids, even as toddlers. The women with CIs express great joy about them: "I absolutely love my implant and cannot imagine not having it!" They all go on about how lovely it is to hear birds and crickets, whispers and music, and the words of professors and friends. They learned spoken language with hearing aids and, as adults, are learning even more about hearing and listening with their cochlear implants.

All began with intensive listening, speech, and language therapy. For some, this was called auditory-verbal; for others, the program had the word "oral" in it. They do not tend to use formal labels for what they experienced. In any case, they had intensive work from at least one therapist, and their parents, particularly their mothers, were highly involved with them from infancy through high school and college. Their fondest memories of therapy include listening and speech production games. Two were in mainstream classes from preschool on, one went to a special class one hour each day in second through fourth grade and was mainstreamed the rest of the time, and the fourth was in a program for children with hearing impairment until grade two.

Today they use cell phones, FM systems, and microphones that augment their implants in certain instances. They listen to the radio and to television with closed captioning filling in what they miss. They use flashing fire alarms and alarm clocks that shake their beds. In classes, some just listen, and a few use Computer Assisted Real-Time Captioning (CART) and sound-field systems. Before CART, they used note-takers, got notes from friends in the class, and talked with others about what had happened in class.

As children, they encountered teachers who understood and were accommodating and a few who either babied them or conveyed very low expectations. One woman's mother took her out of her special classes when she decided, against the advice of the professionals, that not enough was being expected of her daughter. She reports thriving in her new school alongside children with typical hearing.

In elementary school, some had support from tutors, itinerant teachers and teachers of the deaf periodically, but mainly all four blended in with and found acceptance from their peers with typical hearing. Several mention their experiences with FM systems, with two relating funny stories about their teachers forgetting to turn off their systems when they were reprimanding other students out in the hall. Apparently, they were able to tell all the other students in the classroom what the teacher was saying! One tells about a child with typical hearing who accepted her need for the FM system without question. They did not like their FM systems, however, because in their youth, FM systems only allowed them to hear the teacher and not themselves or other students. Another complaint was of being afraid at that age to remind their teachers to wear the microphone. In general, these young women report childhoods filled with activity, much like those of children with typical hearing.

Middle school brought more responsibility for their listening equipment, along with a new self-consciousness about their hearing aids and FM systems. During this time, they all gave up speech and language therapy and gave two reasons for doing so. First, their speech-language specialists at their schools seem to have lost interest in working actively with them, giving them mainly articulation drills and not expanding the work to include intricacies of language. Second, a few of them felt the typical teenage pressure of not wanting to be or even to appear to be different from other teens.

In high school, these women remember being part of the social network in their schools. They dated and enjoyed all kinds of activities, even though they did not feel a complete erasure of the difference their hearing loss made for them. Two of them told stories about forming close relationships with other students and having those students react with surprise, some time later, to learn of their hearing loss. Another became the "designated caller," the person who used the phone outside the noisy gym during school dances, because she could use the telephone switch on her hearing aid and hear the person on the other end; her friends with typical hearing could not hold a conversation in such noise. Perhaps this sort of advantage led to her saying that she became more comfortable with her hearing loss during her high school years. In the classroom, these women sat in front and used CART, closed captioning, and note-takers. Some of them had tutors and experienced advocacy and support from a school disability guidance counselor and/or speech-language teachers who visited periodically. They found good success as students.

Proceeding to college seems to have been a given for each of these women. One had to transfer to a different college when her first school would not provide CART services. She also found a support group for students with hearing loss to be very helpful at this time in her life. They all began to realize how much they depend on listening, yet at the same time, one learned sign language during this period of her life, and she enjoys being able to bridge from the hearing world to the Deaf culture. A leadership experience with other college students with hearing loss provided two of the women with the important information that they had rights, including the right to speak up, as individuals with hearing loss.

The decision to earn graduate degrees comes out of real interests each woman developed, and they report being well prepared for rigorous study.

In the world of work, they are making their way, drawing help from supervisors and coworkers when they need to solve listening problems. All are in fields that demand close attention to listening and using spoken language. The audiologist believes her patients relate better to her as a person with hearing loss and that she represents someone with whom they can identify and share their frustrations. Parents of young children with hearing loss see in her evidence that their children can become high functioning. Of the three women, only one reports experiencing discrimination on the job, and she has filed a complaint signifying her understanding of her rights and worthiness.

In musing about their lives, these women reveal high self-esteem, resilience, and real joy. One says that her hearing loss "helped me become the person I am today." "Another speaks of "appreciation for different things in life . . . a different way of listening." They share an attitude of not letting hearing loss prevent them from doing what they like and want to do. One remembers her mother saying when she began fifth grade, "you are starting a new school in our hometown. This is your chance to simply be yourself. Relax, be honest about yourself and with others, and be *you*. Strive to be your best and be kind to others. If you do this, you will not have a problem making friends." Then she says her mother was right. Another says:

> As I've gotten older, I have appreciated the ways my hearing
> loss has taught me about life. Since I use my vision often to

make up for my loss of hearing, I have enjoyed observing what's around me. While there are many times it's frustrating and that I wish I had normal hearing, it's a part of me that I don't know if I would want to get rid of!

Conclusion

Of course, these young women represent only themselves, but they signify that children with hearing loss can grow into adults who listen, speak, read, write, and think in highly complex ways. They can choose who and where they want to be in the world, and their achievements can be compared to the achievements of people with typical hearing, even to those of people operating at the highest levels of their professions. The advent of cochlear implantation in very young children, combined with appropriate listening and spoken language therapy, solid schooling, and attention to their social development makes this outcome even more feasible.

References

Allington, R. (2006). *What really matters for struggling readers; Designing research-based programs.* Boston, MA: Pearson.

Blachowicz, C. (2000). Vocabulary instruction. In M. Kamil, P. Mosenthal, P. D. Pearson, & R. Barr (Eds.), *Handbook of reading research: Volume III.* Mahwah, NJ: Lawrence Erlbaum.

Bloom, B., Englehart, M., Furst, E., Hill, W., & Krathwohl, O. (1956). *Taxonomy of educational objectives: The classification of educational goals. Handbook I: The cognitive domain.* New York, NY: Longman.

Daya, H., Ashley, A., Gysin, C., & Papsin, B. (2000). Changes in educational placement and speech perception ability after cochlear implantation in children. *Journal of Otolaryngology, 29*(4), 224–228.

Dornan, D., Hickson, H., Murdoch, B., & Houston, T. (2007). Outcomes of an auditory-verbal program for children with hearing loss: A comparative study with a matched group of children with normal hearing. *Volta Review, 107*(1), 37–54.

Elbow, P. (2004). Write first! Putting writing before reading is an effective approach to teaching and learning. *Educational Leadership, 62*(2), 8–13.

Farber, P. (1999). Johnny *still* can't read. *Harvard Education Letter, 15*(4), 1–3.

Gallaudet. Retrieved July 18, 2008, from http://gri.gallaudet.edu/~catraxle/sat10-faq.html

Geers, A. (2003). Predictors of reading skill development in children with early cochlear implantation. *Ear and Hearing, 24*(Suppl. 1), 59S–68S.

Goswami, U. (2002). Early phonological development and the acquisition of literacy. In S. Neuman & D. Dickinson (Eds.), *Handbook of early literacy research* (pp. 111–125). New York, NY: Guilford Press.

Lakoff, G., & Johnson, M. (1980). *Metaphors we live by.* Chicago, IL: University of Chicago Press.

Leach, J., Scarborough, H., & Rescorla, L. (2003). Late-emerging reading disabilities. *Journal of Educational Psychology, 95*(2), 211–224.

Metsala, J., & Walley, A. (1998). Spoken vocabulary growth and the segmental restructuring of lexical representations: Precursors to phonemic awareness and early reading ability. In J. Metsala & L. Ehri (Eds.), *Word recognition in beginning literacy* (pp. 89–120). Mahwah, NJ: Lawrence Erlbaum.

Moog, J. (2002). Changing expectations for children with cochlear implants. *Annals of Otology, Rhinology, and Laryngology, 111,* 138–142.

Padden, C., & Hanson, V. (2000). Search for the missing link: The development of skilled reading in deaf children. In K. Emmorey & H. Lane (Eds.), *The signs of language revisited: An anthology to honor Ursula Bellugi and Edward Klima,* (pp. 435–447). Mahwah, NJ: Lawrence Erlbaum.

Snow, C., Burns, M., & Griffin, P. (1998). *Preventing reading difficulties in young children.* Washington, DC: National Academy Press.

Vacca, R., & Vacca, J. (2002). *Content area reading: Literacy and learning across the curriculum.* Boston, MA: Allyn and Bacon.

Chapter 12

PARENT, THERAPISTS, AND TEACHERS WORKING TOGETHER

Don't stop the person from telling you everything that
they had planned to tell you. A person in distress
wants to pour out his or her heart, even more than
they want their case to be won. If you are the one who
stops a person who is pleading, that person will say,
"Why does he reject my plea?" Of course not all that
one pleads for can be granted, but a good hearing
soothes the heart. The means for getting a true and
clear explanation is to listen with kindness.

Ptahhotep, (ca. 2400 BCE) in Hord and Lee, 1995

Introduction

In this chapter, I write as the parent of a child with severe-to-profound hearing loss. At this time, my daughter, Annie, is 35 years old, and a successful user of spoken language learned though listening. She has earned a doctorate in clinical psychology and will soon complete a post doc year in a university counseling center. She lives comfortably and effectively in the world of those with typical hearing and has many friends with hearing loss who do the same. She accepts and understands the challenges her deafness brings her and values the quiet that deafness can offer. Together, our family has followed a path that began with two hearing aids and the auditory-verbal approach taught to us by Helen Beebe, and then proceeded through the sort of childhood and young adulthood enjoyed by the average child in the United States. Annie always attended schools for children with typical hearing and was never in a special class for children with hearing loss. Her teachers encouraged her, and we exhorted them to set high expectations for her. Throughout her schooling, she has sat up front, conferred one-on-one with teachers and professors, and gotten notes from other students. She took Suzuki piano lessons, was a Brownie and then a Girl Scout, played on soccer and basketball teams, swam on the summer swim team, was co-captain of the girls' tennis team, babysat, held a job at the local library, and learned to make friends easily. After high school, Annie went 300 miles away to Kalamazoo College, where she majored in Sociology with concentrations in writing and Women's Studies and served as reporter and then editor of the college newspaper. During her junior year, she lost the little hearing she had and chose to have a cochlear implant in one ear. In her first job as an adult, she was an admission counselor at Kalamazoo College; she traveled widely for the college and routinely met with and had phone conversations with prospective students and their parents. Her next stop was the University of Wisconsin at Madison for a master's degree in rehabilitative psychology, after which she stayed for two years to work with students with disabilities who needed accommodations in their classes. She has now earned a doctorate in clinical psychology, a PsyD, from the Massachusetts School of Professional Psychology and is nearing the completion of a post doc year in the counseling center at Salem State University; she plans to spend her career in a college counseling center, working with college students.

Annie and her husband, a physician with a similar hearing history who uses bilateral cochlear implants, have recently become parents. They have numerous friends with similar hearing losses who have completed graduate, business, law, and medical school degrees and are currently working as professionals in their chosen fields. They also have many friends with typical hearing who work in a wide variety of settings.

I write about this to underscore that it is becoming more frequent that children with hearing loss grow into adults who embrace and participate in the whole world. These individuals have developed high-level skills that take them wherever they want to go. They do not forget they are deaf, and, in fact, they value their deafness, but they do not restrict themselves to communications only with other people who are deaf, and they do not need elaborate accommodations or interpreters in order to get along in school and in work.

How does this happen? Can we be intentional about helping our children become whole, well-rounded adults? The answer, of course, is "yes" to both questions. From the earliest time in the child's life, parents, therapists, and teachers must work together to support all the hard work the child must learn to do and continue to do. It is the working together that is critical. Too often, I hear about parents who must take a school district to court to get a high-level program for a child, or about a teacher who has a student whose parents are uninvolved. In this chapter, I reflect on what worked for us in terms of schooling, why it worked, and how parents, therapists, and teachers can work together for the benefit of the child.

Emotional Connectedness and a Team Approach

My experience tells me that each child needs a "team" of people on his or her side, and this team should at minimum be comprised of the child's parent(s), the child's therapist(s), the child's classroom teacher(s), and the child's tutor(s). Other team members can include the child's audiologist, a school psychologist, the school principal, the guidance counselor, a special education teacher, and the child. Depending on circumstances, some teams also recruit the director of special education, a social worker, a child advocate, or a representative from the Bureau of Vocational Rehabilitation. Getting along is the first step, and doing so demands emotional connectedness. Too often, one or more of the players in the parent-therapist-teacher triad or on the team becomes overly defensive and demanding, and everyone loses sight of the reality that they are adults with particular responsibility for the life of the child in question. Instead of turning to their legal rights as a last resort, they begin by asserting them in aggressive ways, alienating the very people they need on the child's "team." When adults fail at connectedness, there is less chance they will be able to give the child high-quality attention. We have good evidence that emotional connection makes a difference. Beginning in infancy, emotional connectedness (attunement) with an adult is shown to boost listening, learning, feelings of self-efficacy, and a sense of self (Stern, 1977, 1985). We want all this for our children and need to keep in mind that these are precisely the qualities we want and need in our adult-to-adult relationships. People in charge of a child's social and academic education must listen to and learn from each other, and all the participants in the team have a right to good feelings about who they are and what they can accomplish. When these are in place, it is more likely that the parent's description of a problem is taken in by the therapist or teacher and that the therapist's or teacher's guidelines for a particular course of action are understood and followed. It is more likely that the parent's expert knowledge about the child and the therapist's and teacher's professional knowledge will be incorporated into the process. Everyone on the team needs to take seriously that all the others have particular and useful knowledge that is necessary in making decisions that help the child. Too much can get lost in the shuffle as adults compete for power in such situations, and the child is the one who suffers while the adults are busy arguing.

It is clear that teacher-to-student attunement is related in a positive way to academic outcomes such as performance, motivation, interest, and attention (Poulsen, 2001). Children benefit from attunement with all the people involved in their lives, and so this should be the goal as the triad/team makes decisions about the child's social and academic education. The child with hearing loss has enough to make up in terms of learning spoken language without having to suffer from hostilities among the adults in his or her life. These are difficulties the child is not equipped to understand, and they get in the way of the child's learning because the adults' attention is on their disagreement and not on the child.

IDEA and IEPs

The Individuals with Disabilities Education Improvement Act (IDEA) of 2004 spells out the responsibilities of the schools relative to children with special needs. Depending on how well development is progressing, a child with hearing loss may or may not qualify for particular services. Certain accommodations in the classroom, such as note-taking service, audio recordings and transcripts of them, preferential seating, and use of an FM system generally are thought to be necessary and will be written into the Individualized Education Program (IEP) when requested. In some circumstances, Computer Assisted Real Time Captioning (CART) is made part of an IEP. It is to everyone's advantage to make sure the parents are fully informed about their rights and responsibilities under IDEA and that they are full members of the team. Parents need to know they can request an evaluation, participate in the IEP and its annual review, see the results of reevaluations, and request an Independent Educational Evaluation (IEE) by a professional who is independent of the school district (Ohio Department of Education, 2008, p. 2).

An IEP is designed by the team, with input from everyone, for each child determined to be eligible for special services. Each IEP is a plan for a unique child and includes:

- [the] child's strengths and needs;
- measurable annual goals and short-term objectives or benchmarks;
- appropriate special education and related services for [the] child to be involved and progress in the general curriculum;
- other considerations based on [the] child's needs.
  (Ohio Department of Education, 2008, p. 6)

The IEP is shared with all members of the team so that parents and teachers know what to expect and have a guide for goals for the child. For ethical reasons, information about the child and his or her needs is not shared beyond the team. Before each IEP meeting, parents and teachers are obligated to write their "concerns, questions, and suggestions" so they are available for discussion during the meeting (Ohio Department of Education, 2008, p. 7). Teachers need to keep in mind that these procedures that come to seem ordinary to them are usually quite new to the parents, who may feel intimidated. Some parents did not like school themselves and/or do not feel well educated, and so they are uncomfortable about going to the school for any purpose. Therefore, the teacher needs to communicate carefully with the parent(s) so as to welcome them and avoid creating hard feelings. The following people should be present at each IEP meeting: the parent, the child, one of the child's mainstream classroom teachers, one of the child's special education teachers (if applicable), a special education supervisor from the school district, a person "who can explain how the evaluation results will affect teaching," persons who have particular expert knowledge about the child's needs, and, when and if the need arises, a representative of an agency that will help the student transition from school to another setting at age 18 (Ohio Department of Education, 2008, p. 21). The meeting agenda will include planning for the future, discussing current academic achievement, setting annual goals and short-term objectives, deciding upon appropriate services, designating the least restrictive environment (LRE), and discussion of when and how the IEP will be reviewed and revised (Ohio Department of Education, 2008, p. 22). When disagreements arise, IDEA includes multiple venues for parents to make complaints and recommends mediation and/or facilitation by a neutral special educator who will help the team come to agreement and develop a solution.

Using Mediation and Mediation Skills

Mediation is a commonly used procedure that can be very useful in resolving difficulties involving any combination of parents, therapists, teachers, and others concerned with the child. Its basis is that everyone has a point of view that feels reasonable to him or her and that conflict is normal. It holds that attempting to understand the other's point of view can lead to agreements acceptable to all involved in a conflict. Anyone in the team can use the principles of mediation in daily interactions with the others. Johnson and Johnson (1995) observe that conflicts usually revolve around concern for oneself in combination with the extent of one's desire to maintain a relationship with another. Depending on the relative importance of these to a person in the conflict, the person seeks different paths, moving from greater to lesser interest in preserving the relationship; this continuum encompasses problem-solving negotiations, smoothing, compromising, forcing or win-lose negotiations, and withdrawing (pp. 34–35). For problem-solving to work, the relationship must feel very important. Smoothing involves giving up one's goal in order to preserve the relationship. Compromising can result when both parties regard their own goals to be about as important as preserving the relationship. In a win-lose negotiation, at least one side sees his or her goals as far more important than the relationship. One person—especially if that person has more power than the other—may make threats, attempt to impose penalties, and/or take preemptive actions that ignore the other person's needs. Or, the person may employ persuasion, impose a deadline, commit to a rigid position, or make unreasonable demands. When neither one's own goal or the relationship seem important enough to do anything about, or a person wants to avoid conflict altogether, a person may simply withdraw from the situation (p. 35). Johnson and Johnson were writing about conflicts between and among students, but I have seen adults use all of these tactics and, most likely, you have, also.

For our purposes, because a child is involved, problem-solving negotiations are the preferred approach for conflict resolution. Teachers and therapists forcing decisions or practices onto parents, or parents forcing decisions or practices onto teachers simply alienates the "other side." Withdrawing by either side allows the problem to fester, and it certainly ends essential communication. Smoothing and compromising are often the socially-approved approaches, but they may result in a lesser education for the child; one side may see the decision made as involving some kind of loss for the side, and little losses add up over time. Because the relationship between and among those responsible for the child is critical, it must be nurtured with care so as to maintain it.

Problem-Solving Negotiations

Active listening is the core of problem-solving negotiations, whether in day-to-day interactions with others or in a formal mediation. In training I received from Community Mediation Services of Central

Ohio, I learned that active listening requires concentrating one's efforts to encourage the speaker to express him- or herself and that one must be attentive both verbally and nonverbally. Especially when a conflict is brewing, each person should give full attention to the other (no looking around or answering of cell phones allowed!) and should try to imagine him- or herself in the other's place. Body language is important: presenting oneself as open to the other's ideas shows up when one faces the other squarely, opens one's arms and hands, leans forward slightly, makes eye contact, and relaxes face, body, and tone of voice. Some of this may take some practice, but intentionally trying to look open can have the effect of creating openness in oneself. Asking questions is critical to learning about the other's views; it is helpful to ask open-ended, rather than closed questions, so as to get the other person thinking and talking. When the person is finished speaking, check on what he or she said by paraphrasing the statement and asking whether it is accurate. This can uncover areas of simple misunderstanding. It can be very helpful to comment on the person's feelings: "It sounds like this is difficult for you" or "I now understand how hard this has been from your point of view."

Here is an example in which both sides were able to be open enough to the other that no real conflict arose because each side came to be understood by the other. When Annie was about three years old, we began talking with the local elementary school, wanting them to be ready for her when it was time for her to begin kindergarten. They had never had a child with a severe-to-profound hearing loss; they were not sure they wanted one; and, at that time, they had less legal obligation to admit her than they do now. We had a meeting with the school psychologist who was open to us, but she expressed doubt about whether the school could serve Annie well. After all, there were at least two schools for the deaf in our area, and they could offer a specialized approach. This, of course, made us uncomfortable, as we had become committed to an auditory-verbal approach and were feeling knowledgeable and successful with it, but we listened to her and understood she was entering new territory and felt similarly uncomfortable. She listened carefully to us, talked with Annie's speech and language therapist, and decided the least she could do would be to observe Annie in her preschool setting. We had the feeling she would be looking for the many reasons she had in mind to turn us down, but that is not how it turned out. In a lovely irony, when the school psychologist visited the preschool, she mistook several other little girls for the "deaf child" before actually locating Annie among her peers with typical hearing. After that, she was ready to help in all the ways available to her. Because everyone in the situation was willing to listen and learn, we did not have to think about any extreme actions such as bringing suit against the school district, although that had been suggested to us by some as a likelihood.

There are times, though, when a situation becomes so difficult that it could disintegrate into a legal battle. Before taking that step, anyone on the team can suggest a formal mediation procedure in an attempt to create a solution everyone can accept. Everyone should keep in mind that should the matter get into a court of law, even though someone "wins," it is hard to set aside the bad feelings created, and the child will be the ultimate loser. This should be powerful incentive for all sides to enter into mediation.

Steps in a Formal Mediation

Formal mediation can vary some from one practitioner to another, but the basic elements are the same. The goal is for the participants in the conflict to arrive at a solution that meets everyone's needs. This is done with the aid of a mediator who offers a structured procedure for each to tell his or her story or side and then gets both parties in the conflict to listen deeply enough that they can put themselves into the other's shoes. Mediation is also an opportunity to share information that may have been passed by in the compromised communication that led up to the conflict. It is critical to understand that the mediator will be helping the parties come to an agreement and will not be formulating an agreement to foist onto them.

The seven basic steps in mediation include:

- Introductions
- Each party tells his or her story and describes the conflict
- Summarizing by the mediator
- Issue and interest identification
- Generation and evaluation of alternatives
- Agreement
- Closure

Mediations usually take place with the people involved sitting at a table. Those in conflict sit across from each other with the mediator between them at the head or foot of the table. No one is seated higher or lower than the others. First, the mediator introduces him- or herself and makes some general comments thanking the parties for coming together to try to solve a problem. The mediator asks each person how he or she would like to be addressed and explains the ground rules for mediation: each party will speak to the mediator and not directly to each other, each will speak and behave with respect, and each will keep what is said confidential. For mediation to be attempted, both sides must come to the process wanting to find a solution short of seeking a legal determination through the courts. This desire usually allows people to be respectful of each other during the process.

The process begins with the mediator asking one of the parties to describe the conflict as he or she is experiencing it. This person "has the floor" for as long as it takes to describe the problem. Then, the mediator summarizes the person's statements for both sides to hear and asks the person whether the summary is accurate. There are no comments or rebuttals allowed from the other side during this process. Next, the other side has the same opportunity to describe the conflict, and the mediator summarizes that statement and asks whether the summary is accurate. Careful attention is paid to getting the statements to reflect what each party asserts and feels about the problem. This is a critical step, because the conflict may have been the result of a missed communication or a misunderstanding of the role each should be playing in the situation. It also allows each person a sense of being heard and gives each a chance to hear and begin evaluating what he or she has asserted. At times, we can see that we are being unreasonable when we hear our story coming from another.

In the issue and interest identification phase of mediation, the goal is that the parties come to view the conflict as a mutual problem to be solved rather than as a win-lose situation. This can be hard to achieve if there have been hard feelings, and so the mediator leads the parties in focusing on the issues and interests underlying the conflict. For example, the parent may want the child in a special class, whereas the principal wants the child in a regular class but with no support. The issue is not really the class placement, but the kind of support the child will receive and the accessibility of that support. Or, the regular classroom teacher may take the view that children with hearing loss will always be behind academically, while the parent wants to make sure the child is challenged sufficiently in school. The basis of the conflict may really involve the identification of this particular child's strengths and weaknesses as a student and as a communicator.

When the underlying issues are identified and agreed on, then the conflict is reframed. No longer do the parties accuse each other of not doing their jobs and of not caring about the child. Hurt feelings and angry thoughts about what someone is and is not entitled to can be set aside.

Now, the mediation can proceed to generating and evaluating several alternatives that could solve the problem. The mediator asks the parties involved to participate in brainstorming a list of suggestions without commenting on them or criticizing them. When the parties are satisfied the list is complete, then the ideas are examined and discussed. Alternatives should be specific (who, what, when, where, how), realistic, and shared. Applying these criteria can elevate a vague idea into a pragmatic plan. In the first example, the parent and principal arguing about class placement have come to reframe the issue as being the kind of support the child will receive and the accessibility of that support. Alternatives could include: (1) The child spends some time each week with a specialist away from the regular classroom, (2) The specialist comes to the regular classroom and observes each week, (3) The teacher and the specialist confer each week about the student's progress during the week, and (4) The parent, the teacher, and the specialist share their observations each week. In the second example, the conflict has been reframed as the necessity to identify the particular child's strengths and weaknesses. Alternatives could include: (1) The teacher will take steps to get to know the child better through having daily conversations with him or her, (2) The parent will agree to monitor homework completion, (3) The teacher will pair the child with children who communicate easily, and (4) The parent will follow all directions given by the speech-language pathologist. Depending on what has surfaced during each mediation, one or some combination of these alternatives could become the plan for each child in question.

The penultimate step in the mediation is for the parties to articulate the agreement formulated. The mediator asks each whether the agreement is acceptable. Then, the agreement is written down and both parties sign it. This provides a sense of formality and legitimacy to the process and its result, and it yields a tangible statement of what each party is now to do. Each can have confidence that the other understands and will proceed as promised.

In closing the mediation, the mediator thanks each party for working on the conflict and coming to an agreement. He or she observes once more that conflict is normal and that it can arise again. The mediator invites either party to return in the future to work further on resolving any problem that arises with the agreement just reached or on a new area of disagreement. Finally, the mediator reminds the parties that what has been said in the mediation is to be held in confidence.

Practical Ways for the Team to Communicate

Establishing and maintaining clear communication is essential. Parents appreciate it immensely when the teacher, therapist, school psychologist, principal—in short, any representative of the school—reaches out and gets such communication started. Parents have so much to learn and do in dealing with their child with hearing loss, and they usually do not have a background in education to use in doing so. This needs to be recognized by school personnel, and they should welcome the parent(s) onto the team.

Preschool and Early Elementary School

Most important is that the adults in the child's life develop a sense of working together on the child's behalf. At times, this will mean setting aside criticisms and perceived slights. Essential steps for all involved include:

1. Speak with each other about being on the same "team."
2. Use a notebook in which parents and teachers write notes to each other about what has happened during school and at home. Devise a way to pass the notebook back and forth

regularly. Keeping it in the child's backpack is one way of doing this.

3. Have regular e-mail and phone conversations.
4. Send encouraging notes and messages to each other.
5. Maintain access to developmental milestone charts, share information about the child's progress, and create ways that both parents and teachers will work with the child on these matters.
6. Make sure the child sees people on the team smiling and talking with one another.
7. Gradually increase the responsibility the child has for remembering the notebook, the backpack, homework materials; for positioning him- or herself in the best places to listen in class; for handing in schoolwork; and for monitoring the hearing technology.
8. Teach the child to speak for him- or herself in multiple settings and to make phone calls using whatever technology is necessary.
9. Provide sheltered opportunities at first and move toward the child accomplishing these moves on his or her own. Remember the team's goal is self-sufficiency in the child.

Middle and High School

By middle and high school, the student should be in control of his or her hearing technology and school assignments, with an attentive parent looking in periodically out of interest in the subject matter, not out of some sense of being in control of the student. The desirable outcome at this point is that the student has taken on these responsibilities and is feeling a powerful sense of self-efficacy. At this point, the student should have become part of the team and become an active participant in IEP meetings, so he or she is an integral part of the communication system. If this is not the case, the team should be discussing a plan that helps the student take on such responsibilities. It is tempting to be a "helicopter" parent, therapist, or teacher of a child with hearing loss, but doing so adds a handicap where there should not be one. There are so many hovering parents of children with typical hearing who keep their children from learning responsibility that the child who is deaf or hard of hearing who is also self-sufficient will stand out in a group of children with typical hearing as being unusually mature. This will aid him or her immeasurably in learning to read, write, and do academic work. As hard as it may be to visualize a little child as a competent adult, the time will come when that adult must be responsible for him- or herself. Parents and teachers will no longer need to monitor equipment, make appointments, and make sure work is done and deadlines are met. This is the reward for all the social and emotional work contributed by all the team members on behalf of the child.

Conclusion

Children benefit greatly from the adults in their lives working carefully together. Of course, this can be difficult to achieve; instead of accepting a bad situation, parent(s), therapists, and teachers should seek out help when they recognize a lack of communication between and among them. Children who get lost in the shuffle are far less likely to learn what they need to know. Some useful resources that all involved can share include:

> The Alexander Graham Bell Listening and Spoken Knowledge Center: http://www.agbell.org/Landing.aspx?id=549

> Ohio Department of Education Learning Supports: http://www.ode.state.oh.us/GD/Templates/Pages/ODE/ODEDetail.aspx?Page=3&TopicRelationID=981&Content=53503

References

Community Mediation Services of Central Ohio. 67 Jefferson Avenue, Columbus, OH 43215.

Hord, F. (Okpara, M.), & Lee, J. (1995). *I am because we are: Readings in black philosophy*. Amherst, MA: University of Massachusetts Press.

Johnson, D., & Johnson, R. (1995). *Reducing school violence through conflict resolution*. Alexandria, VA: Virginia Association for Supervision and Curriculum Development.

Ohio Department of Education. (2008). *Whose IDEA is this?* Retrieved from http://www.ode.state.oh.us/GD/Templates/Pages/ODE/ODEDetail .aspx? Page=3&TopicRelationID=981&Content=53503

Poulsen, J. (2001). Facilitating academic achievement through affect attunement in the classroom. *Journal of Educational Research, 94*(3), 185–190.

Stern, D. (1977). *The first relationship: Infant and mother.* Cambridge, MA: Harvard University Press.

Stern, D. (1985). *The interpersonal world of the infant.* New York, NY: Basic Books.

Chapter 13

ENGLISH LANGUAGE LEARNERS AND BILINGUALISM

Children [with cochlear implants] from a multilingual background were able to achieve similar educational placements and similar rates of progress of speech perception outcome as the only English-speaking children. Children from a multilingual background were able to achieve similar educational placements and similar rates of progress of speech perception outcome as the only English-speaking children.

Daya et al., 2000

Introduction

The progress in spoken language learning being made by a significant number of children with cochlear implants is, happily, cause for a question that has not been entertained widely: Can a child who is deaf learn to listen to and speak in more than one spoken language and then learn to read and write in those languages? Very little study has been done on this question, and so this is a short chapter.

In the United States, educating for bilingualism in children with typical hearing has been fraught with controversy, with arguments arranging themselves along a spectrum from immersion of children in two languages in the home from birth, to immersion in two languages as early as possible in school settings, to introducing a second language in special language classes in the elementary, middle, or high school years. Some decide there is need for only one language and that it is English. Often these points on the spectrum are argued on the basis of cultural power, creating a conflict between conserving the culture of the family when English is not the first language and staking a position that the United States should have one official language.

And then there are those whose reasoning is based on what they think may happen cognitively for the child. Some argue for one spoken language out of worry that the child will become confused in moving between two languages and will suffer in the end from not knowing either language at a high level. These fears are allayed by evidence that language development proceeds in comparable and predictable ways for children with typical hearing who are becoming either monolingual or bilingual (Waltzman, Robbins, Green, & Cohen, 2003). Many people in the United States have little or no experience with more than one language, and so it is not apparent to them that children can learn languages more easily than adults. In reality, children have a huge capacity for learning multiple languages and for differentiating among them (Snow, Burns, & Griffin, p. 157), and one need only travel a bit in Europe or Africa to find numerous people who are multilingual.

Problems with language can become evident in either a monolingual or bilingual child, of course, but from this frame of reference, the impairment in the bilingual child with typical hearing would not occur due to being immersed in two different languages; instead, problems with multiple language learning may be attributed to factors involving quantity of experience with the languages, extent of cultural knowledge, and attitudes toward the languages (Brisk & Harrington, 2000, p. 11). Of course, as has been made abundantly clear, diminished hearing can be a major factor in compromised spoken language learning. But what if the child learns to use hearing aids or a cochlear implant so well that he or she is not operating as a person with significant hearing loss? And what can this child's family do about the cultural issues that affect them just as they affect families with typical hearing?

In doing a search of academic papers regarding deafness and bilingualism, all but a few "hits," which I discuss below, turned up studies and essays about the bilingual-bicultural approach to teaching children in the Deaf culture sign language first and then presenting English or another spoken language when the child is of school age and ready to become literate. As I have written elsewhere in these chapters, I wish the proponents of this approach well and hope they find ways to make it successful at increasingly higher levels, but I am interested in developing spoken languages in children with deafness, particularly because of the well-established link between knowledge of spoken language and literacy achievement. This chapter, then, deals with bilingualism and literacy in two populations: children with typical hearing and children who use cochlear implants or sophisticated hearing aids and thereby live as individuals with nearly typical hearing.

Can Children with Hearing Loss Learn More Than One Spoken Language?

I turn, first, to the question of whether more than one spoken language is possible for children with hearing loss, because if it is not, then parents, therapists, and teachers should aim their work with the child at the acquisition of one spoken language. In spite of all that technology is making possible, some maintain it is close to impossible, or at least very difficult, for children with hearing loss to learn even one spoken language, and they recommend concentrating on the learning of just one. But, that is not necessary, as the following investigations demonstrate.

Viewing linguistic diversity as a strength, not a deficit, Guiberson describes Julia, whose parents spoke both Spanish and English to her at home and whose therapist focused on her learning to listen to English (2005, pp. 30, 36). By age eight, three years after receiving a cochlear implant, Julia knew both Spanish and English and could differentiate between them (p. 34). In her situation, literacy in Spanish was not going to be supported at school, so her teachers and therapist used literacy activities focused on English. Guiberson concluded in his report that learning Spanish as well as the English needed for her schooling has "been a critical piece in helping Julia feel like a part of her family and culture" (p. 37), thus supporting a cultural argument for fostering two spoken languages in this child.

Children of families that do not speak the dominant language of the place in which they live are often at odds with the school they attend if that school uses only the dominant language. They feel out of place, and they *are* out of place, if they cannot communicate effectively. Julia is a good example of the child with or without hearing loss learning to navigate two linguistic settings.

Waltzman, Robbins, Green, and Cohen (2003) looked at the backgrounds of 18 children with prelingual profound hearing loss, implanted by age 5. The average age of implantation was 2.5 years, with a range of 1.2 to 5.4 years; at the time of the study, the children had had their implants for an average of 4.5 years, with a range of 10 months to 12 years. These researchers found that some of these children were learning two spoken languages and had an age-appropriate first language that they used both receptively and expressively. These children demonstrated success with recognizing words in both languages in open-set presentations. Waltzman et al. assert that high levels of language learning are possible with early implants: "The majority of the children showed age-appropriate receptive and/or expressive language abilities in their primary language commensurate with normal-hearing children," (p. 761). They hold that some children can simultaneously learn a second language, although they found in most cases that the second languages "were in the early stage" (p. 762). These authors theorize that as the individual becomes older and more experienced with language, the capacity to remember both languages grows, and thereby facility with both languages is established. Some of the parents in the group reported they had been advised originally to use only English with their children and so had stopped using their home language with their children. When they realized that English was becoming well established, they began trying out the second language in spite of that advice. Because of this, their children had not had consistent exposure to the second language, and so it is not surprising that their acquisition of the second language was lagging behind their acquisition of English. Waltzman et al. conclude that bilingual development is dependent on "speech perception postimplantation, the linguistic environment, type of intervention, and educational placement" and urge further work in this area (2003, p. 757).

Robbins, Green, and Waltzman (2004) studied 12 children who received cochlear implants by age 3 and found their average scores in their first language to be age-appropriate. Learning in the second language grew in the two years post-implant according to how much exposure to the second language they received and how long they had had the implant.

Thomas, El-Kashlan, and Zwolan (2008) investigated the cases of 12 pairs of children who received cochlear implants before age 6. Each pair had a monolingual and a bilingual child matched as closely as possible for "age of implantation, cochlear anatomy, educational setting, and device type" (p. 230). The object of the study was to determine whether the presence of a second language would be detrimental to learning English by comparing the acquisition of spoken English in these children from monolingual and bilingual homes (English and Arabic, Spanish, French, Marathi, Gujarati, and Cantonese). Using a variety of tests (the Infant-Toddler Meaningful Integration scale, IT-MAIS; the MacArthur-Bates Communicative Development Inventory; Words and Gestures; the Peabody Picture Vocabulary Test, PPVT; the Listening Comprehension and Oral Expression portions of the Oral and Written language Scales; and the Student Oral Language Observation Matrix, SOLOM), the researchers rated each child's capabilities in "comprehension, fluency, vocabulary, pronunciation, and grammar," and placed each child's proficiency in one of the following categories: "preproduction/early production, speech, emergence, intermediate fluency, and advanced fluency" (p. 231). Their finding was: "Matched-pairs t tests and matched-pairs mixed-model analysis revealed no significant difference between groups on any measure at any interval tested" (p. 233). The researchers conclude that children with cochlear implants can learn more than one language without the second interfering with learning the first. They suggest that in homes where the first language is not English, the parents use their own first language with the child in order to present good, well-formed language models to the child.

In instances where parents speak a language other than English better than they speak the language to be used at school, it is preferable to speak that first language with the child (Kohnert, Yim, Nett, Kan, & Duran, 2005). It is important that the child learn the spoken language of the parents, because the parents know it well and can present good models of its use. "When non-native English-speaking parents speak English with their children, they use less vocabulary and engage their children in less language discourse"

(Guiberson, 2005, p. 30), thus impeding their children's learning of English. Being in a rich listening environment, whatever the language, is the most important factor in promoting good spoken language achievement in children. The second spoken language can be learned along with the first spoken language; in fact, English was the dominant language for the bilingual children in the Thomas, El-Kashlan, and Zwolan study, probably because much of their education in school and in therapy was conducted in English (p. 233).

Learning to Read in the First Language First

Now that we have established that learning more than one spoken language through listening to and interacting with others by using it is possible for children with hearing loss, we can move to thinking about developing literacy in the languages. Let us begin with what is known concerning children with typical hearing who speak a language other than English at home while learning to speak English at school. It has been demonstrated in such children that " . . . learning to read in one's native language—thus offsetting the obstacle presented by limited proficiency in English—can lead to superior achievement" (Legarreta, 1979 and Ramirez et al., 1991, as cited in Snow, Burns, & Griffin, 1998, pp. 28–29). This makes perfect sense in light of the arguments I have described earlier. One must know the language to be read, so learning to read in, for example, Spanish or German or Arabic, will offer the best chance for literacy for children for whom those are first languages. Expecting a child with typical hearing or a child with hearing loss to come to school and begin reading instruction in a language he or she does not know will produce less than optimal results. For the purposes of reading instruction, the first language needs to be secure so that literacy can be built on it. In commenting on this, Snow et al. write, " . . . learning a second language cannot take the place of learning with one's own first language" (1998, p. 157), by which they mean that the school should not suddenly start teaching reading in a language the child does not know well. This argument applies also when thinking about sign language as the first language, and it provides insight into why making learning to read simultaneous with learning a new mode of communication, a spoken language, is so difficult that it leaves most adults who are deaf and use sign language at the fourth grade level in reading. The obvious problematic factor is that sign language does not have a written form; if it did, then reading instruction in the language could proceed as easily as it would for any other language known by the child.

It is the case, though, that a well-established first language spoken by the child facilitates good achievement at school in the second language (Cummins, 1979; Lanauze & Snow, 1989, as cited in Snow et al., p. 157). Children with typical hearing who are given time to learn two spoken languages can fare well in both, with each helping the other. Cummins (1984) holds that in developing two spoken languages, children build a common foundation that supports both (pp. 142–143). The academic and social advantage is that children become able to apply more numerous words and grammatical constructions in both languages to concepts they come to know through their lived experience. The more meaningfully the children use both languages, the better it is for language acquisition. This is borne out by Snow et al. who report that children who stay for a lengthy period of time in true bilingual programs in which the focus is on developing both spoken languages achieve more academically than children for whom the approach is to switch them to English as soon as possible. Literacy in the first spoken language influences literacy in the second as knowledge in one is mapped onto knowledge being acquired in the other (1998, p. 236).

These researchers caution against pushing children who come to school not knowing English to begin their reading instruction in English without first preparing them with good background in speaking English. The importance of fluency in the language in which one is instructed about reading is that it allows for matches to be discovered between what is heard and what is seen. This involves discovering the alphabetic principle, as well as learning to hear and see the structure of the language itself (word order and grammatical markers that designate words as having specific functions as nouns, verbs, adjectives, adverbs, articles, conjunctions, prepositions, and interjections). Being able to assign meaning to the language in its spoken form is a prerequisite to deciding about its meaning in written form (Snow et al., 1998, p. 324). Therefore, they recommend teaching reading in the language known first, as long as there are materials and a teacher who knows the language, while the child learns the second language, which in the United States is usually English (p. 325).

To support this argument, Cummins (1984) describes the findings of a study done by Malherbe in 1938 in South Africa:

1. Learning the second language was easier when it was used as one of the languages of instruction;
2. Instruction in the second language did not interfere with proficiency in the first language;
3. In the early years of schooling, there was a lag in learning subjects taught in the second language, but it disappeared by the end of elementary school; and
4. Children with all levels of intelligence did better school work in the bilingual school than in the monolingual school.

In reviewing this study, Cummins concludes that helping children learn language for actual communication purposes works better than teaching language in a traditional way (pp. 145–146).

Cummins also describes two studies done in California. The first was done in a San Diego immersion program in 1975. Students were instructed mainly in Spanish through third grade, with increasingly more English instruction each year, and then they spent half of their school time with instruction taking place in each language. By grade six, children were performing above grade norms in both languages. In the second study, done in 1982, Carpinteria School District found that children from economically disadvantaged Spanish-speaking homes were more ready for both Spanish and English literacy learning when their preschool experience was entirely in Spanish. One goal of the program was to help parents understand their roles as first teachers of language to their children. The researchers concluded that achieving fluency in their first language, Spanish, enabled the children also to learn the English they found in their environment, reasoning that it takes knowing a language to learn a new language (Cummins, 1984, pp. 146–149).

Multilingual Mastery Is Possible

Recently, I had the opportunity to interview a multilingual teen named Sunny and his mother. Born in India and diagnosed at 10 months with a 90 dB loss, Sunny was fitted with hearing aids at

14 months, and when he was 16 months old, his parents took him to the AURED auditory-verbal program in Mumbai directed by Aziza Tyabji Hydari. His family embraced AV therapy and sent Sunny as soon as possible to a "regular" school, because they valued a hearing environment. He started at age three in the local preschool for children with typical hearing while also having regular speech and language therapy at AURED. His mother reports that she always wanted her son to be in a harder, better school and that she worked hard to help him learn to listen and speak, so at age four, he went to kindergarten, then therapy, and finally home to sleep, four days a week. The school needed to be convinced to let him and another boy of the same age come, and they worked out an arrangement in which the teachers gave his mother the schedule ahead of time for the next week, and she prepared him for his lessons, so that he knew what was coming. In this way, Sunny learned the new words before they came to him at school. The school never treated him as different, which he said helped him a lot.

At one point, the teachers made him a compere, the host for the plays the children gave; his mother was very proud of him, and, of course, this gave her confidence that he was talking well enough to be understood. He progressed so well that he stopped daily therapy at age seven and began to go only twice a week, continuing on in a school for children with typical hearing. Throughout his elementary education, his mother continued to work with him at home on a daily basis.

At age seven, Sunny got his first implant, and then the second one at 11 years old, making him the first child to receive bilateral implants in India; they followed a protocol in which they removed the first implant and worked with only the newly implanted ear for the next year and a half. It is now clear that his hearing loss was progressive. His AV therapy stopped at age 14, his mainstream school placement continued, and he is on track to graduate from high school in 2013. He plans after that to study engineering at a major research university.

Sunny's mother reports that when they put the hearing aids on him, people told her that he should learn the language in which they planned for him to study. She is the only one in her family educated in English. At that time, Sunny's family lived with their extended family, some of whom wanted him to learn Gujarthi, but she wanted him to know a language used at the university. So she spoke with him in English, and worked toward improving her own speaking of English by reading extensively. Even so, she tried talking with him in Gujarthi and Hindi, but he wanted only English from her. Sunny's three drivers spoke in Hindi, and he learned to converse with them, starting around 5½. He learned Gujarthi from his grandmother beginning at 8 years old and then learned French at 14. Sunny told me he doesn't get the languages confused and doesn't mix them together and that, although he prefers talking in English, he talks with his dad mainly in Gujarthi.

It is important to note that the sentence order in Gujarthi and Hindi are the opposite of English, which was hard for Sunny to begin with, but he has mastered the structures of these languages.

Sunny's experience in learning multiple languages is not unusual in India where more than 1000 languages are spoken; Sunny's mother knows and uses seven languages. It may be that it is the expectations that people have about learning more than one language that either help or hinder the child in learning multiple languages.

Hearing or Deaf, Language Learning Is Possible

It is clear that the child with hearing loss can learn more than one spoken language through listening to it and interacting with people using it, just as children with typical hearing do, and that doing so is desirable because it increases the child's knowledge. Parents who find themselves living in a culture where their own first spoken language is not used do not have to choose to make their child with hearing loss an outsider in their family, and they do not need to give up their family's spoken cultural identity. In terms of seeking education for their children that prepares them for literacy and for academic success, they can feel confident in using their favored spoken language with the child, knowing that such a foundation will equip the child to learn other languages. If the child does not know the spoken language of the school when he or she begins, then time should be provided for that learning to take place before formal reading instruction begins. If at all possible, formal reading instruction should begin in the first language, if it is the stronger language for the child. Of course, it is to the child's advantage to become fluent in the dominant language of the society in which he or she lives, and so the parent should help that to happen, even if it means learning the language along with the child.

Learning language is easiest for very young children, after which a decline in capacity for learning both first and subsequent spoken languages sets in. Although learning a second language as a teen or as an adult is not impossible, it is much harder, and there is much variation in such ability among adults. Children are more like each other in their ability to learn spoken language and tend to do it well when presented with it (Johnson & Newport, 1989). For these reasons, it is a good idea to begin as early as possible to present a child, with or without any degree of hearing loss, with opportunities for learning spoken language(s).

Conclusion

With good hearing technology, used consistently and well, children with hearing loss can learn many spoken languages, and doing so builds a good foundation for literacy in all of them. Global conditions give the advantage to those who communicate across many languages, and children who are deaf or hard of hearing can be part of this phenomenon.

References

Brisk, M., & Harrington, M. (2000). *Literacy and bilingualism: A handbook for ALL teachers*. Mahwah, NJ: Lawrence Erlbaum Associates.

Cummins, J. (1984). *Bilingualism and special education: Issues in assessment and pedagogy*. San Diego, CA: College-Hill Press.

Daya, H., Ashley, A., Gysin, C., & Papsin, B. (2000). Changes in educational placement and speech perception ability after cochlear implantation in children. *Journal of Otolaryngology, 29*(4), 224–228.

Guiberson, M. (2005). Children with cochlear implants from bilingual families: Considerations for intervention and a case study. *Volta Review, 105*(1), 29–39.

Johnson, J., & Newport, E. (1989). Critical period effects in second language learning: The influence of maturational state on the acquisition of English as a second language. *Cognitive Psychology, 21*, 60–99.

Kohnert, K., Yim, D., Nett, K., Kan, P., & Duran, L. (2005). Intervention with linguistically diverse preschool children: A focus on developing home language(s). *Language, Speech, and Hearing Services in Schools, 36,* 251–263.

Robbins, A., Green, J., & Waltzman, S. (2004). Bilingual oral language proficiency in children with cochlear implants. *Archives of Otolaryngology-Head and Neck Surgery, 130*(5), 644–647.

Snow, C., Burns, M., & Griffin, P. (Eds.). (1998). *Preventing reading difficulties in young children.* Washington, DC: National Academy Press.

Thomas, E., El-Kashlan, H., & Zwolan, T. (2008). Children with cochlear implants who live in monolingual and bilingual homes. *Otology and Neurology, 29*(2), 230–234.

Waltzman, S. Robbins, A., Green, J., & Cohen, N. (2003). Second oral language capabilities in children with cochlear implants. *Otology and Neurology, 24*(5), 757–763.

Chapter 14

MUSIC LEARNING AND SPOKEN LANGUAGE DEVELOPMENT

The ability to focus the mind, or concentrate, is a great asset in any and all activity. Using music as a vehicle for its development from an early age is ingenious. Almost without our realizing it Suzuki [music] training fosters this growth.

Stark and Starr, 1983, p. 228

. . . children taking music lessons improved more over the year on general memory skills that are correlated with nonmusical abilities such as literacy, verbal memory, visiospatial processing, mathematics and IQ than did the children not taking lessons.

Laurel Trainor, in Vedantam, 2006

Introduction

New emphasis on establishing listening for children with hearing loss is leading to changes in thinking about the role of music in the lives and learning of such children, and the purpose of this chapter is to explore those changes and to give particular attention to the possibility that experiencing, learning about, and even learning to produce music may have some impact on the literacy development of children with hearing loss.

In thinking about music for children with hearing loss, we need to differentiate between developing musicality in children, that is, making musicians of them, and fostering participation in music-making for other reasons such as promoting cultural knowledge, providing listening pleasure, and establishing a foundation for literacy development. For example, regarding music appreciation and the cochlear implant, one source concludes, " . . . children who are, in general, more successful with communicating via listening and speaking can use these skills to enjoy the musical experience" (Gfeller et al., 1998). In the realm of academic success related to music, I have located reports of children with typical hearing whose language learning and reading achievement have been enhanced by their participation in music instruction, but, I have not found a study concerning the influence of music training on the language acquisition and reading development of children with hearing loss. For that reason, I begin this chapter by saying that such studies need to be done, but that, nevertheless, it is my hunch that children with hearing loss can benefit from intentional exposure to music and music-making and that such benefits include enjoyment, performance with voice or instrument, and an increased understanding of certain properties of language foundational to reading and writing.

Issues Involved in Learning About Music

Music is a frequently chosen activity for children in school and after-school programs, but it is apparently not offered frequently to children with hearing loss. Some have assumed that children with hearing loss cannot listen to, appreciate, and learn to make music. Furthermore, adults who have become deafened and then receive one or two cochlear implants (CIs) often report disappointment when they try to listen to music; they say that music with the CI doesn't sound as they remember music as sounding, or that it sounds harsh and discordant to them (Trehab, Vongpaisal, & Nakata, 2009). Some professionals observe that implant technology precludes the processing and enjoyment of music because of frequency limitations that make impossible the perception of at least some portions of music, particularly information about pitch, (Hopyan et al., 2012; Yennari, 2010; Trehab, Vongpaisal, & Nakata, 2009). At least one study has suggested that children who have had even a little low frequency hearing and some time to use it for listening before receiving one or two cochlear implants perform better on musical discrimination tasks than children who receive CIs very early in life (Hopyan et al., 2012). This finding, in theory, puts the spoken language learning made possible with early implantation at odds with the possibility of learning music. Understandably, some generalize this information about CIs in ways that may cause parents and teachers to think it unproductive to present music to children with hearing loss, especially children who use CIs exclusively.

On a more hopeful note, a recent study involving twenty-seven children ages 5 to 14 reports that duration of musical training correlated positively with pitch perception (Chen et al., 2010). The children in the study all have congenital prelingual profound hearing loss and use one cochlear implant; all but five of the children also use a hearing aid in the other ear. Prior to the study, thirteen of the children had participated in structured music lessons at YAMAHA Music School for between two months and three years. This instruction included listening, singing, score reading, and instrument playing. In the study, the children were asked to indicate whether piano tones presented were the same or different; for tones judged correctly by a child as different, the child was then asked the follow-up question of whether the pitch of the second tone was higher or lower than the first. The researchers speculate that, over time, auditory plasticity may be involved in the increase in the children's ability to discriminate between pitches. Children in the study who were age six or younger performed better on the presented task, prompting the researchers to recommend starting musical training early in a child's life and to include such training as part of rehabilitation beginning soon after cochlear implant surgery. The presence of a hearing aid in the second ear is not discussed in the report of this research, so questions that arise about its contribution to information about pitch are not addressed. The issues involved in learning to listen to and produce music include the age when hearing loss occurs, the age at which a child or adult begins using hearing technology, the contribution of hearing aids, and the capacity of the cochlear implant to deliver sufficient information about pitch.

Music Learning in Children with Hearing Loss

Much can be learned from music and music lessons, and for children with hearing loss the gains are thought, generally, to be apart from musicianship. A recent study that focused on seven cochlear implant users under 4 years of age found these children with prelingual profound deafness to be developing musically (Yennari, 2010). They sing often and enjoy music, particularly in the presence of others with whom to sing. The emotional value of music provides motivation for learning more songs, and the children were observed to respond well to content, humor, surprise, movement elements, and props used to make a song come alive. In Yennari's words,

> I would therefore like to argue that although hearing loss imposes limitations on how an individual develops musically, it does not obstruct the presence of an innate need to sing in the company of others or alone . . . I suggest that the environment of the child (technological advances like the CI, significant others, musical stimuli in children's everyday life, variety of opportunity in "musics," maturation and learning) can compensate for the losses of perceptual information and incidental learning. (Yennari, 2010, p. 294)

In another study, Trehub, Vongpaisal, and Nakata (2009) report that "child implant users who were born deaf or became deaf as infants or toddlers typically find music interesting and enjoyable," they are motivated to listen to music before they come to understand language, and "they prefer singing to silence" (p. 534). In this study, children with CIs were observed to have difficulty with pitch, but relative strength in dealing with rhythm. Hopyan et al. (2012) also report the ability of children to identify changes in rhythm and that children in their study could remember musical pieces.

Music performs many functions in a person's life, and fidelity to an ideal of production need not get in the way of a person with hearing loss gaining access to many, even most, of those functions.

Music Learning in Children with Typical Hearing and Its Association with Literacy

Just as it is helpful to know about the development of children with typical hearing in other realms as we think about the development of children with hearing loss, it is helpful to know about the benefits of learning music for children with typical hearing.

For children with typical hearing, the learning of music has been associated in some studies with learning to decode from print to sound. "Most basic skills used in text reading or decoding (i.e., the breaking of the visual code of symbols into sounds) find parallels in music reading" (Hansen & Bernstorf, 2002, p. 2). These writers relate learning music to learning about syllables, phonemes, sight identification, orthography, and patterns, and they connect knowledge of all of these to reading fluency. In a year-long study of 12 four- to six-year-olds with typical hearing, half of whom received Suzuki music lessons, the children participating actively in listening to and learning to produce music according to the Suzuki method scored higher on tests of digit span memory, suggesting that music training can enhance nonmusical abilities, specifically working memory, verbal memory, and visiospatial processing. Additionally, the children who received such music training scored better than the control group on tests requiring a same–different discrimination task involving harmony, rhythm, and melody (Fujioka et al., 2006).

Another study equates music and spoken language learning (Anvari et al. 2002). Beginning with the understanding that pitch discrimination correlates with phonemic awareness and that phonological and phonemic awareness are associated with learning to read, the study investigated 4- and 5-year-olds' perceptions of music in relation to their early reading development.

> Music, like language, is based in the auditory modality and the primary mode of music production, singing, uses the same vocal apparatus as speech. Both speech and music involve combining small numbers of elements (phonemes, notes) according to rules (referred to as grammars in music theory) that allow the generation of unlimited numbers of phrases or utterances that are meaningful. . . . Learning a language requires learning the basic building blocks of words, syllables, and

phonemes. The elements of music are different from those of language, but the basic learning processes may be similar. (Anvari et al., 2002, p. 112)

These researchers tested 100 children on rhyming, rhythm, blending, chord analysis, reading melody, digit span, mathematics, and vocabulary; they interpret the results as suggesting that skill in the perception of music is related to both auditory processes and auditory memory which are, in turn, related to early reading development.

The relation between phonological awareness and music perception suggests that they may share some of the same auditory mechanisms. Phonological awareness requires the listener to be able to segment speech into its component sounds, and to recognize those sound categories across variations in the pitch, tempo, speaker, and context. The perception of music also requires the listener to be able to segment the stream of tones into relevant units, and to be able to recognize compositions across variations in pitch (key), tempo, performer, and context. (Anvari et al., 2002, p. 127)

Marin (2009) found in her study of 31 children around the age of five that those with early musical training produced higher scores on a test of language development and, more specifically, on morphologic rule formation, memory for words, phonological processing, and sentence memory. She observes that skills in these areas are associated with syntactic development (p. 190).

The identification of the relationship between early music learning and reading development is important to our thinking about how to make better readers of our children, with and without hearing loss. Perception of music and perception of language have much in common.

Music Lessons for Children with Hearing Loss Who Are Learning to Listen

A study by Abdi et al. (2001) used music presented through the Standard Orff Method and Se-tar, for children older than eight, as ways to habilitate children with cochlear implants, and they report that "all children showed appreciable progress in playing a musical instrument" (p. 105). For the reader unfamiliar with the Orff method:

> Orff Schulwerk is a way to teach and learn music. It is based on things children like to do: sing, chant rhymes, clap, dance, and keep a beat on anything near at hand. These instincts are directed into learning music by hearing and making music first, then reading and writing it later. This is the same way we all learned our language. (American Orff-Schulwerk Association, 2013)

Abdi et al. recommend that children with cochlear implants receive music training between the ages of four and five, after they have had at least four months CI experience, to help them learn new concepts of sound as a part of their habilitation. These researchers see such auditory training experience as having a beneficial effect on children's speech, particularly in the areas of "understanding of rhythm and higher frequency differentiating skill" (p. 106).

The literature by music teachers includes studies suggesting an openness to helping children with cochlear implants and hearing aids, with an emphasis on developing musicality and capability with voice and instruments. Music teachers suggest focusing on detection, discrimination, identification, and comprehension:

1. Detection is demonstrated by a response to the presence or absence of music (for example, moving when the music starts and being still when the music stops).
2. Discrimination is demonstrated by differentiating between two or more rhythms and melodies.
3. Identification is demonstrated by the identification of rhythm and melody patterns and the use of music terminology in talking about musical patterns.
4. Comprehension is demonstrated by connecting rhythm and pitch to elements such as characterization in a story being told in the music.
(Schraer-Joiner & Prause-Weber, 2009, p. 51)

Creating a musical audiogram is another way to come to an understanding of how to meet an individual child's needs. One way of doing this involves these steps:

1. Select one melodic phrase from a children's songbook, specifically one the child is familiar with.

2. The teacher should inform the child that the tune will be performed in three different ways, each in a different register and at a different dynamic level.

3. The child should indicate which example sounded the best or was the most comfortable to listen to.
(Schraer-Joiner & Prause-Weber, 2009, p. 51)

Using this information, a music teacher can select and present music experiences that are more likely to be accessible to the individual child.

Despite the fact that CIs do not, as yet, offer access to every musical sound, the young CI and/or hearing aid user who is learning to listen can at least have access to rhythm, intonation, emphasis, words in songs, and certain kinds of pitch information, all of which are involved in becoming able to identify and use these musical nuances in learning to read and write. Both children with typical hearing and children with hearing loss can draw knowledge from music and apply it to their emerging literacy, and this usually happens unconsciously and without direct teaching. Whether or not a child can become a proficient musician does not matter when one realizes the important effects music can have on the child's developing literacy. Coming to understand that aspects of music such as rhythm, syllabication, rhyme/voice, intonation, pitch, and memory are foundations for language learning and reading comprehension is a powerful argument for providing all children with music instruction.

The Work of Two Talented Therapists

Christine Barton, a board certified music therapist, and Amy McConkey Robbins, a speech language pathologist, have developed the *TuneUps Music Program* to bring music to children with hearing loss. The premise of *TuneUps* is that music enhances communication development, and communication enhances music in a reciprocal relationship. *TuneUps* focuses on the appreciation and performance of music for music's sake, simultaneously recognizing the links between music perception and spoken language that support literacy. *TuneUps* is composed of 19 songs and activities, a music listening game, and information for teachers, therapists, and parents (Barton & Robbins, 2007).

Barton (SpeechPathology.com, 2007) observes that "children with hearing loss respond pretty well to steady beats or the pulse of a piece of music," just as children with typical hearing do, by vocalizing and moving arms, legs, bodies, and heads, all of which indicate strong physical involvement with music. The next step for the child is participating in the music by clapping, patting, and moving to the music. Gradually, Barton sees "little bits and pieces of familiar songs start entering their world like, 'Twinkle, Twinkle,' and 'Mary Had a Little Lamb' and maybe some lullabies." She asks the parents to tell her when their children with hearing loss begin to sing as they play, as that is part of the development of children with typical hearing between the ages of two and four. The next steps for children will be to pick up words and phrases from nursery rhymes and then to sing a song from beginning to end. Whether the tune is accurate, or not, singing an entire song signifies the developing ability to remember a sequence of sounds. "Then, if they can conserve it in their minds, they can actually hear it in their minds; and they can think it. Then we can start doing rounds like 'Row, row, row your boat.'" (SpeechPathology.com, 2007). It is this holding of sound in memory, rehearsing it, and "thinking it" that contribute to children's becoming ready for literacy. Barton has also come to understand that both reading and music are discovered and developed by the child through repeated exposure, rather than being taught directly (Barton, 2011a).

In pursuing these connections, Barton and Robbins have laid out important considerations for using music with children with hearing loss:

1. Your voice is the most important instrument you can own!
2. Don't reserve singing for "music time."
3. Use music purposefully and not as "background."
4. Always introduce the CD player and any other electronic device before using it.
5. Experiment with using different voices.
6. Turn-taking is essential.
7. Turn any important phrase into a song.
8. Rhythm is a powerful cue for spoken language.
   (Barton, 2010; Robbins & Barton, 2008)

Barton includes a collection of Song Books on her website (Barton, 2011b) as aids in bringing children's attention to words, pictures, pitch, timbre, intensity, and rhythm. This is a series of delightful electronic picture books accompanied by singing and instrumentation that can be used in ways similar to language experience books. Barton is continuing to publish in this area, and I encourage the reader to pursue her work as it emerges (Barton, in press).

The Suzuki Approach and Literacy

Before the advent of excellent hearing aids, cochlear implants, and approaches such as Barton's and Robbins', my husband and I wanted our daughter with hearing loss to have music in her life. We turned to the Suzuki method for instruction on the piano, choosing this method because of its use of the aural as the foundation for learning how to play the piano. Suzuki is a "mother tongue" musical approach that treats learning music and the playing of an instrument in ways that make one think of descriptions and theories of spoken language acquisition, as well as the auditory-verbal approach to teaching children with hearing loss to listen (Suzuki, 1983).

> . . . an underlying principle is that the child's musical education, insofar as the development of his ear is concerned, should parallel the manner in which he acquired his mother tongue. Young children have an uncanny aptitude for recognizing and later reproducing delicate nuances of spoken languages. Suzuki believes and has demonstrated through his teaching that a young child can develop, in the same manner, a highly discriminating musical ear. Much repetitive listening is necessary, just as it is in the acquisition of the mother tongue. (Starr & Starr, 1983, p. 125)

Accordingly, the Suzuki approach offers much to us as we think about bolstering language and literacy learning in children with hearing loss. Suzuki music lessons are designed to accentuate the child's focus on aural components of music long from the earliest age possible: pitch, tempo, rhythm, and intensity. Consistent listening and practice result in the development of musical memory in the child, and just as with the auditory-verbal approach, the role of the parent is to support listening and practice in a continuous manner at home.

Elements of the Suzuki approach include:

- Begin early with listening from birth and playing from 2½ or 3 years of age.
- Postpone reading [music] until the child's playing is well established in technicalities of fingering, positioning hands on the keys or strings.
- Involve parents in home teaching and practice.
- Create a favorable learning environment with parent-child-teacher cooperation.
- Use carefully graded, musically excellent pieces and play their recordings frequently to provide repeated listening.
- Use private lessons to provide careful, thorough, technical foundations and nurture the abilities of each child; provide group lessons for motivation and support.
- Use repetition and reinforcement effectively through constant review of previously learned music.
- Minimize competition and maximize self-development as a goal.
(Kendall, 1996, p. 43)

As can be seen in the list above, the Suzuki approach to acquiring the language of music is in many ways similar to the auditory-verbal approach to learning spoken language. Both emphasize learning through listening. Rather than teaching the reading of music right away, for the first year or more, Suzuki piano lessons involve intense repetition of each song to be learned. The teacher will play the song repeatedly and provide a CD of the song to be listened to over and over at home and in the car. Only after extensive listening does the child begin learning to play the song. Technique is emphasized, and nuances of rhythm and intensity are polished through repeated listening to the model and then playing and listening to one's own playing in order to discover its similarities to and deviations from the model.

> . . . due to Suzuki's emphasis on listening to recordings, the Suzuki student does have a built-in error recognition system

in that he notices when something he plays doesn't sound like the recording. A wrong note should leap out at him if he has listened enough. This, however, is not sufficient feedback. Parents need to provide additional information. (Starr & Starr, 1983, p. 19)

As we worked with the Suzuki approach, we observed our daughter learning music as though it were a spoken language during the same time we were working with the auditory-verbal approach to help her learn spoken language. We observed memory for intonation, phrasing, pitch, and rhythm being built bit by bit, just as memory for these and other attributes of spoken language were being developed in the auditory-verbal approach. As our daughter progressed, it became clear to us that the listening required in Suzuki music training was helping her make connections and to remember longer and longer sequences of both music and language. In retrospect, I realize that the experiences she had in learning to clap to the music probably taught her how to isolate syllables in words which aids the isolation of phonemes and builds the careful listening that helps with word identification and memory for words. Although I can only report this anecdotally, I can say that she has not had difficulty with working memory, verbal memory, and visio-spatial processing, and she learned to read easily, all of which align with the findings of Fujioka et al. (2006). Learning to read music was easy when the time came to do it, because knowledge of the aspects of music contained in its written form was so well established. This is the same approach to learning to use and read spoken language I have been discussing in this book. Interestingly, for our daughter, the ability to play some pieces from memory has persisted well into adulthood.

Conclusion

I recommend music training for all children and suggest that using the Suzuki approach with children who use hearing aids and cochlear implants be investigated in formal studies. Further, I recommend that parents, teachers, and therapists provide music in the child's environment in intentional ways; *TuneUps* is a good place to start. If music lessons enhance working memory, verbal memory, visio-spatial processing, harmony, rhythm, melody, and phonemic awareness in children with typical hearing, then such experience should do at least something of the same for children with hearing loss who are learning to listen. It is clear that further investigation concerning the relationship between the learning of music, spoken language, and literacy in the development of the child with hearing loss is needed. I look forward to seeing this unfold.

References

Abdi, S., Khalessi, M., Khorsandi, & Gholami, B. (2001). Introducing music as a means of habilitation for children with cochlear implants. *International Journal of Pediatric Otorhinolaryngology, 59*, 105–113.

American Orff-Schulwerk Association. (2013). *What is Orff Schulwerk?* Retrieved from http://www.aosa.org/orff.html

Anvari, S., Trainor, L., Woodside, J., & Levy, B. (2002). Relations among musical skills, phonological processing, and early reading ability in preschool children. *Journal of Experimental Child Psychology, 83*, 111–130.

Barton, C. (2010). *Music, spoken language, and children with hearing loss: Using music to develop spoken language.* Retrieved from http://www .christinebarton.net/PDF/SpeechPathologyBarton5-25-10.pdf

Barton, C. (2011a). *Music and literacy development in young children with hearing loss: A duet?* Imagine 2(1). Retrieved from http://www .christinebarton.net/PDF/Barton_imagine2_1_2011.pdf

Barton, C. (2011b). *Song books. Central canal creative arts therapies.* Retrieved from http://www.christinebarton.net/

Barton, C. (in press). Children with hearing loss. In M. Hintz (Ed.), *Guidelines for music therapy practice in developmental health.* Gilsum NH: Barcelona Publishers.

Barton, C., & Robbins, A. M. (2007). *TuneUps: A music program designed to foster communication development.* Valencia, CA: Advanced Bionics.

Chen, J., Chuang, A., McMahon, C., Hsieh, Tung, T, & Li, L. (2010). Music training improves pitch perception in prelingually deafened children with cochlear implants. *Pediatrics, 125*(4), 793–800.

Fujioka, R., Ross, B., Kakigi, R., Panter P., & Trainor, L. (2006). One year of musical training affects development of auditory cortical-evoked fields in young children. *Brain, 129*, 2593–2608.

Gfeller, K., Witt, S., Spencer, L., Stordahl, J., & Tomblin, B. (1998). Musical involvement and enjoyment of children who use cochlear implants. *Volta Review, 100*(4), 213. Retrieved from Academic Search Complete database.

Hansen, D., & Bernstorf, E. (2002). Linking music learning to reading instruction. *Music Educators Journal, 88*(5). Retrieved from Academic Search Premier.

Hopyan, T., Peretz, I., Chan, L., Papsin, B., & Gordon, K. (2012). Children using cochlear implants capitalize on acoustical hearing for music perception. *Frontiers in Psychology: Auditory Cognitive Neuroscience, 3*(425), 1–9.

Kendall, J. (1996). Suzuki's mother tongue method. *Music Educator's Journal, 85*, 43–46. Retrieved from Academic Search Premier.

Marin, M. (2009). Effects of early musical training on musical and linguistic syntactic abilities. *Annals of the New York Academy of Sciences, 1169*, 187–190.

Robbins, A. (2012). *TuneUps music program*. Retrieved from http://www .amymcconkeyrobbins.com/tuneups.html

Robbins, A., & Barton, C. (2008). *Music and pediatric cochlear implants: Bringing science to intervention*. American Speech and Hearing Association Conference, Chicago, IL. Retrieved from http://www.amymccon keyrobbins.com/PDF/MusicPedsCochlearImplants11-08sm.pdf

Schraer-Joiner, L., & Prause-Weber, M. (2009). Strategies for working with children with cochlear implants. *Music Educators Journal, 96*(1), 48–55.

SpeechPathology.com. (2007). Interview with Christine Barton, MM, MT-BC, Music Therapist. Retrieved from http://www.speechpathology .com/interviews/interview-with-christine-barton-mm-1334

Starr, W., & Starr, C. (1983). *To learn with love: A companion for Suzuki parents*. Los Angeles, CA: Alfred Publishing.

Suzuki, S. (1983). *Nurtured by Love* (2nd ed.). Mattituck, NY: Amereon.

Trehub, S., Vongpaisal, T., & Nakata, N. (2009). Music in the lives of deaf children with cochlear implants. *The Neurosciences and Music III—Disorders and Plasticity: Annals of the New York Academy of Sciences, 1169*, 534–542.

Vedantam, S. (2006). Musical training benefits kids' brains. *The Washington Post*. (Source of opening quote by Laurel Trainor).

Yennari, M. (2010). Beginnings of song in young deaf children using cochlear implants: The song they move, the song they feel, the song they share. *Music Education Research, 12*(3), 281–297.

Chapter 15

ASSESSMENT ISSUES AND APPROACHES

. . . tests are generally very small samples of behavior that we use to make estimates of students' mastery of very large domains of knowledge and skill.

Koretz, 2008, p. 9

Introduction

When I typed in "assessment," in .22 seconds, Google reported 246,000,000 hits (up from165,000,000 hits four years ago), demonstrating clearly how increasingly enamored people are with the concept of finding out how well someone is doing or how much someone knows. Usually, this is expressed as finding out about a person's knowledge, skills, attitudes, and beliefs/values. Compared to whom? Compared to what? For what purposes? We tend to think about assessment as testing in some formal way so as to rank people on some set of criteria, and so it often is. Assessment can also be done informally. This chapter discusses both approaches.

The first matter in thinking about assessing an individual child's achievement is to determine the questions one has about the child's learning and what kinds of feedback could help one in making instructional decisions on the child's behalf.

Norm-Referenced Standardized Tests

The way we have come to think about achievement is heavily
influenced by the way norm-referenced standardized tests are set
up. First, the content of such a test is selected based on expert
opinion about what should be known by a given population, but
the test will contain questions that very few can answer and that
very few cannot, and such tests are not linked to particular curricula delivered to students. The lowest score sits at the far left side
of the normal distribution, known as the bell-shaped curve, and
the highest score sits at the far right side, with all the other scores
stacking up in a predictable and symmetric hump in between. By
testing and then manipulating the questions asked, standardized
norm-referenced tests are created to produce such results, and then
much is made of finding the mean or average score or the median
score and then gauging whether a particular child has scored above
or below average. Scores on a standardized reading test are usually
expressed as percentile scores, with any particular score signifying
that it is higher than that percentage of the scores resulting from
giving the test for norming purposes. A score at the 50th percentile
means that it is better than 50% of the scores obtained when the test
was administered to a representative sample of children in order to
"test" or "norm" the test. A 73rd percentile score is better than 73%
of the norming group, a 32nd percentile score is better than 32% of
the scores, and so on. All percentile scores then, are comparisons
between any test-taker's score and the achievement of the original
representative group of students who took the test. For tests that
will be marketed for widespread use, representative groups are
chosen, usually from across urban, rural, suburban, and small town
schools, and they usually include children from all socioeconomic
backgrounds and major racial groups. In examining and thinking
about a child's score on any test, it is useful to examine the test's
technical manual to learn about the norming group(s) used in setting the standards for the test.

Percentile ranks are often expressed as grade-level scores. An
exactly average score translates as being exactly at grade level at the
start of the school year. A fifth grader who scores at the 50th percentile at the beginning of the school year is said to be at the fifth grade
level. If he or she scores a bit higher than the 50th percentile, then

the score might be expressed, for example, as 5.2 or 5.3, depending on how the numbers work out statistically. (See Koretz, 2008, for an extended discussion of standardized testing.) An important point to make is that, by definition, half the children taking any test will produce scores above the 50th percentile and half will produce scores below that mark. Bemoaning the fact that half our children are below average misses the point of how standardized tests work.

Although it does not appear to be widespread, there has been some effort to produce norms for children who are deaf or hard of hearing in order that an individual's scores be compared with those of a representative group of children with deafness, rather than with children and older students with typical hearing. One example is the Stanford Achievement Test, 10th Edition, for which special norms were developed during the 2003 to 2004 academic year for use with children who are deaf and hard of hearing (Gallaudet Research Institute). The Carolina Picture Vocabulary Test is a test of receptive sign vocabulary developed for children who are deaf or hearing impaired. It is norm-referenced, based on a norming sample of 767 children who signed as their main mode of communicating (Pro-Ed). The Test of Early Reading Ability: Deaf or Hard of Hearing (TERA-D/HH), developed specifically to assess the child's "ability to construct meaning, knowledge of the alphabet and its functions, and awareness of print conventions," was normed using a sample, drawn from 20 states, of more than 1,000 students who were deaf or hard of hearing (Pro-Ed), and is used to compare the achievement and progress of that population.

These kinds of test norms take children with deafness out of comparisons with children with typical hearing, in an effort to minimize the great differences so often seen between children with and without hearing loss. The greater achievement being recorded for children who use cochlear implants is making this approach to normative assessment unnecessary; it is now entirely informative to compare the achievement levels of children who are deaf or hard of hearing with those of their peers with typical hearing. If tests that offer D/HH norms are administered to the child with hearing loss, measures using norms derived from children with typical hearing should be requested, as well. In this situation, comparing the results of norms drawn from the two populations should be useful in making educational decisions concerning the child. No longer must parents and teachers accept that a child with hearing loss reads "pretty well for a child with hearing loss." Expectations can be set in terms that compare the child's achievement with all other children of his or her assigned grade level in school.

Criterion-Referenced Tests

Often, instead of wanting to compare one student with many others, one wants to know how much an individual has learned of what has been presented or experienced. In this case, a body of knowledge is designated, a test of some sort is created and administered, a cut score that designates the difference between passing and failing is established, and a score may be reported that represents the percentage of correct answers. This sort of testing is done regularly by teachers in schools when they want to measure the results of recent instruction, and some of the high stakes proficiency tests being administered by states to the children in their schools are of this sort. In the first case, it is the teacher who decides the content of the test, guided both by his or her own knowledge of the subject being taught and by manuals in which state-adopted standards for the subject area are set out by experts in the field. This is termed informal testing because the teacher prepares and gives the test for specific instructional purposes on a day-to-day basis and does not test the questions in a comprehensive way before the students get the test. In the second case, experts determine what should be known by students at a particular grade level, and tests go through a formal vetting process in an attempt to make all the questions clear and to decide the position of cutoff points signifying proficiency or lack of it on the part of the child. (See Koretz, 2008, for further discussion of criterion-referenced testing.)

The Relative Value of Norm-Referenced and Criterion-Referenced Tests

Both norm-referenced and criterion-referenced test results are useful, though how they are used can become controversial. When scores of groups of students on such tests are used to say something about how well our educational system is doing, they become highly politicized, and educators and citizens need to understand that phenomenon. But my purpose here is to explain them in neutral fashion to give a basic idea of what such scores represent. The important distinction between these two kinds of tests is that a norm-referenced test yields information about how the individual test taker's responses on the test stack up when compared to the responses of a specific set of test takers selected to represent a particular range of people in the overall population, and a criterion-referenced test yields information about the test taker's responses to questions selected to represent mastery of a given subject. So, the percentile rank score on a norm-referenced test suggests some sense of how a student is performing compared, usually, to students across the nation, and a numerical or categorical designation is designed to signify some measure of how well students are doing in mastering the subject matter as it is defined within the classroom or in some larger district, state, or national arena. For example, the National Assessment of Educational Progress (NAEP) categories are: "advanced," "proficient," "basic," and "below basic" (Public Schools of North Carolina).

Scores are always going to be relative to something, and in looking at them, one must ask what that something is. If I am told that my fourth grader is at the 95th percentile in reading, I need to ask with whom she is being compared. If the comparison is with children with typical hearing, then I can be pleased, because her score is high in the ranking; if it is with children who are deaf, then she is likely way behind children with typical hearing, even though she is at the top of the heap in her comparison group. If my son comes home with a 95% on a school test, I must ask about the rigor of the curriculum. Has it been made easier for children for whom not much is expected? Or, is it demanding in its presentation and in its assessment? A child who is doing well in a particular classroom may not be seen as doing well when that classroom's achievement is compared to the achievement of multiple classrooms in a state, region, or country. All such testing must be put into perspective, especially if the results are to be used in making instructional decisions.

Practical Reading Assessments for Teachers to Use

A major problem with standardized tests, whether norm- or criterion-referenced, even those labeled "diagnostic," is that they are not a source of specific information about what an individual child needs instructionally. In looking at a standardized test score or scores, one might find that the child scored at an average level in comprehension, but below average in vocabulary knowledge; that the child is good at letter identification, but not as good at identifying three-syllable words; that he or she remembered 75% of the literal information presented, but does less well in making inferences. This information may be helpful in general, but it does not give the teacher information about how the student processes the marks on the page and what sense he or she makes of them, and so it does not help the teacher decide exactly what to do next in instruction. One aspect of norm-referenced or criterion-referenced standardized testing I have not mentioned is that sometimes all a low score means is that the test taker did not want to take the test or did not know what to do and just filled in answers at random, or that the test taker may have been hungry or anxious, or just had a "bad day." Such tests do not provide that sort of information. Fortunately, teachers have some particular observational strategies they can put to good use in conjunction with their critical review of standardized test scores.

Observation Strategies

Reading Recovery is a program that uses extensive observation in working over many weeks with children identified early in the first grade as being at high risk for having difficulty in learning to read. Children so identified are placed in daily one-on-one contact for 12 to 15 weeks with a Reading Recovery-trained teacher who identifies and works on the child's particular difficulties in learning to read. Although Reading Recovery is designed for children of all capabilities and backgrounds, it is important to note that it has been shown in one study to work well with children with hearing loss (Charlesworth, A., Charlesworth, R., Raban, & Rickards, 2006). Marie Clay, the teacher/researcher from New Zealand who developed Reading Recovery, has brought together numerous observation strategies for teachers to use in gathering knowledge about individual learners. Clay recommends that teachers observe, record, and analyze the following aspects of a particular child's reading behaviors:

1. Oral language, and a child's control over sentence structures and inflections

2. The reading of continuous text (running records)
3. Letter knowledge
4. Reading vocabulary (words known in reading)
5. Writing vocabulary (words known in writing)
6. Concepts about print (how print encodes information)
7. Hearing sounds in words (dictation)
8. Making links between those sounds and letters.
   (Clay, 1993, p. 1)

These approaches can be used by any teacher to gather information about a child's reading without applying the entirety of Reading
Recovery. Their use is based on the theory that children are continuously hypothesizing about how language, reading, and writing work
and that their functioning in these areas at any given time reflects
their understanding of these language processes (Clay, 1993, p. 2).

Listening to the Child's Language

Careful listening to a child's language helps the teacher understand
the child's understanding of the spoken language. Does the child
leave out words ("I from Ohio")? Does the child leave out important endings on words (such as the "-ed" that signifies past tense)?
Does the child use words in the conventional order ("I went home,"
instead of "I home went")? Does the child use the conventional
forms of irregular verbs ("went," instead of "goed")? These categories from Clay (1991, p. 72) are some suggestions of what a teacher
can listen for. A teacher can record these uses by a child and concentrate on using well-formed conventional constructions of this
language in conversing meaningfully with the child; in addition, the
teacher can design experiences that cause the child to produce language in the company of people who use language conventionally
(Clay, 1991, p. 72). *The Record of Oral Language* (Clay, Gill, Glynn,
McNaughton, & Salmon, 2007) offers an assessment designed for
the 5- and 6-year-old in which he or she is asked to repeat a series
of sentences. It is the differences between what the sentence is and
what the child says in trying to repeat it that offer insight into the
child's command of a language's structure. The assessor proceeds
by reading a test sentence aloud, asking the child to repeat it, and
making a record of what the child says. Of particular interest are
omissions, substitutions, expansions by adding a word or words,

and transpositions (moving parts of the sentence to other positions in the sentence). Examples from the assessment include: "Sally is riding her bike," "For his birthday Mary gave him a truck," "My mother usually puts the cat out of the house at night," and "All the children talked loudly to each other at the table" (Clay et al., 2007, pp. 19–21). Other sentence forms include imperatives, questions, negatives, phrases, and clauses (pp. 25–29).

The score on the test suggests the approach the teacher, therapist, and parent should use with the child linguistically so that assessment leads directly into instruction. The adult should be a good language model for the child, while being careful to address the child using language that is just a bit more complex than the language the child uses. In studying the pattern of mistakes the child made in repeating the sentences, the adult should look for patterns that recur. One way to discover whether the child has a grip on particular sentence structures is to create sentences with those structures using words the adult knows are familiar to the child. "This is the chocolate that was in my bag," (p. 29) could turn into, "This is the dog that was in my house." When the adult determines the forms the child has not yet mastered, these can be used in meaningful ways with the child. Conversations should start with words and structures the child knows and add new structures as they fit conventionally, and practice sentences can be generated by changing the words while preserving the structures of the assessment models (pp. 32–33). Clay also makes recommendations for children for whom English is not the first language and says that children need to keep their home language, learn the new structures in English at school, and progress to knowing both; she points out that it takes several years to learn the rules of the new language (p. 35).

The Language Experience Approach to Observation

Another source for observation of a child's language is in the stories he or she tells during language experience book writing. This language should be progressing over time toward conventional usage; if it is not, the child should be having more extended conversations with someone who uses the language well so as to be presented regularly with good form. The importance of this cannot be overstated because at least part of the progress the child will make in reading is dependent on knowing the conventionally used structures of words and sentences. The child who usually says, "He goed" will not be able to predict and then identify the written "He went" as easily as the child who already knows the irregular verb form and says, "I went." The task for the child becomes larger as the language becomes more complex, and having knowledge of the language makes it easier to learn how the letters and the sounds match up, as well as the exceptions when they do not.

Observing While Reading Aloud with a Child

Children who listen to books read aloud learn that what is often called "the language of text" is different in subtle ways from the language people speak in day-to-day conversations. They go through predictable stages of holding a book and trying to "read" it by telling a story based on the pictures, by incorporating story language such as, "Daddy said . . . " by memorizing what they hear and repeating as much as they can, and by making up sentences that sound to them like book language (Clay, 1991, pp. 77–81). The teacher can learn much from noting the child's spoken language during shared reading.

Running Records, Miscue Analysis, and Informal Reading Inventories

In order to gauge what the child has come to understand about reading, a teacher can make what Clay (1991) calls a "running record" or what Goodman calls a "miscue analysis" (Goodman & Burke, 1973; Weaver, 2002). The object of each of these observations is to record exactly what the child says in response to a written text. The running record system uses a blank sheet of paper on which the teacher places a check mark for each conventional reading of a word and inserts words that do not correspond to the text. Miscue analysis begins with a copy of the text to be read by the child, and the teacher annotates it according to the child's reading of the text, for example, crossing out a word that isn't read and writing above it the word that is pronounced instead, circling a word that is skipped, and inserting words that are added by the child. These approaches begin with the premise that the reader is constructing a sense of the text based on the range of cues he or she knows at that point: reading left to right and from top to bottom, turning pages, letters and their sounds, whole words, vocabulary and other background knowledge, word order, word structure, and the ways texts are written. It is useful to see whether and when a child relies on syntax, semantics, and graphophonemic knowledge, and the teacher can make instructional decisions based on the patterns revealed in the analysis. Rather than calling changes of the text "mistakes," they are called "miscues" to signal departures from the text. When the text is, "The bear family lived in the house in the tree," and the child reads, "The bear family lived in the horse in the tree," it would appear that the child is not thinking enough about creating sensible meaning and may just be calling words, as "house" and "horse" do look a lot alike. On the other hand, if the child's reading of the text is "The bear family lived in the house in the woods," the child is creating meaning that makes sense to him or her and is not mistaking a "t" for a "w."

An Informal Reading Inventory (IRI) relies on the same approach. These validated and published assessments provide a series of word lists and a series of reading passages that grow increasingly harder. The teacher listens to the child read and marks the words and paragraphs in much the same way as with running records and miscue analysis. One intent of such inventories is to determine what the child reads with ease and then can read independently and what the child can read with teacher assistance, at an instructional level; another is to zero in on language, vocabulary, decoding, and reading rate issues that are assisting the reader or getting in the way of constructing suitable meaning from text. It should be noted that these inventories may also be used to learn about a child's listening capacities; for this use, the teacher reads the passages to the child and records his or her answers to a set of comprehension questions. Manzo, Manzo, and McKenna (1995) lay out ways of assessing reading as well as thinking in an Informal Reading-Thinking Inventory by adding the following to the traditional Informal Reading Inventory:

- reconstructive comprehension (literal plus inferential comprehension)

- constructive comprehension (critical and creative comprehension)
- degree of "engagement" (attention) in listening and responding to questions
- observations of self-monitoring
- language development
- cognitive style.
  (modified from Manzo, Manzo, & McKenna, 1995, pp. 10–11)

In this inventory, the teacher asks questions designed to learn about the child's background knowledge for each passage, asks the child how well he or she thinks he or she has answered the comprehension and inference questions, and prompts the child to think beyond the passage, perhaps by applying it to his or her own experience. These approaches are all described in great detail in the sources I have listed for them, and I urge teachers and therapists to take the time to learn to perform them so as to have additional information about each child's reading achievement levels as he or she proceeds through school. Seeing children demonstrate specifically what they do and do not know is immensely helpful in deciding about their instruction.

Informal Discussions with the Child About a Book

Although there are many good reasons and many good ways to record, quantify, and classify a child's reading progress, I want also to suggest that assessment and instruction can take place simultaneously and fruitfully when an adult (teacher, therapist, parent, friend) sits down and reads with a child. The adult can and should interact with the child about all the aforementioned aspects of reading: how a book works, letter and word identification, word meaning, word structure, word order, and constructing an overall understanding of the story or explanation. The adult can see what the child doesn't know and then make an explanation on the spot. The adult can offer strategies for figuring out what the child gets stumped on (for example, "Let's look at the glossary and see what that word means," "Let's read again from the beginning and see if we can figure out where this story is happening," and "Do you know the word 'can' and the word 'not'? What would you get if you put them together?")

Conclusion

The development of productive reading demands interactive feedback concerning a text, and this can take place at all points in reading development, from the beginning pre-reading stages through to the achievement of mature reading. All that is required is for someone to take the time to engage with the reader in formal and informal ways in order to think about what he or she is doing while reading.

References

Charlesworth, A., Charlesworth, R., Raban. B., & Rickards, F. (2006). Reading recovery for children with hearing loss. *Volta Review, 106*(1), 29–51.

Clay, M. (1991). *Becoming literate: The construction of inner control.* Portsmouth, NH: Heinemann.

Clay, M. (1993). *An observation survey of early literacy achievement.* Portsmouth, NH: Heinemann.

Clay, M., Gill, M., Glynn, T., McNaughton, T., & Salmon, K. (2007). *The record of oral language.* Portsmouth, NH: Heinemann.

Gallaudet Research Institute. *Norming of new Stanford for Deaf students.* Retrieved from http://research.gallaudet.edu/SAT/SAT-10.html

Goodman, K., & Burke, C. (1973). *Theoretically based studies of patterns of miscues in oral reading performance.* Detroit, MI: Wayne State University. ERIC: ED 079 708.

Koretz, D. (2008). *Measuring up: What educational testing really tells us.* Cambridge, MA: Harvard University Press.

Manzo, A., Manzo, U., & McKenna, M., (1995). *Informal Reading-Thinking Inventory.* Belmont, CA: Wadsworth/Thomson.

Pro-Ed. Retrieved from http://www.proedinc.com/customer/productView .aspx?ID=667 and http://www.proedinc.com/customer/productView .aspx?ID=557&SearchWord=Carolina%20Picture%20Vocabulary%20Test

Public Schools of North Carolina. Retrieved from http://www.ncpublic schools.org/newsroom/news/2007-08/20070925-01

Weaver, C. (2002). *Reading process and practice.* Portsmouth, NH: Heinemann.

Chapter 16

PROMISING LITERACY PRACTICES

. . . time spent reading for pleasure has a stronger impact on increasing reading test scores than time spent on traditional "skill-building" activities, such as vocabulary drill and reading comprehension exercises . . .

Cambourne, 2005, p. 1

Introduction

It is increasingly common for people in the current national scene in the United States to say that our teachers do not know what they are doing. The media portrayal of U.S. education is highly critical, which spreads the impression that our children are not doing well compared to children from our own past or compared to children in other countries. Anyone who takes a close look at the history of education, though, will discover there has never been a "golden age" of U.S. education when achievement levels were higher than they are now. In fact, we have expanded our schools' reach continuously over the years since our country's founding and have established a rich foundation of knowledge about teaching and learning.

Richard Allington reports, " . . . at all grade levels children today outperform children from earlier eras of U.S schooling," and ". . . in general, the best readers are reading better and the worst readers are reading about the same or slightly worse than was the case a decade ago" (2006, pp. 7–8). Our best schools are excellent, but, paradoxically, our worst are terrible. Despite our failures, which are probably due to all sorts of social forces, our successes make it evident that teachers know a great deal about how to teach reading as well as all the subjects opened to students by literacy.

In an effort to bring together what is known scientifically about the teaching of reading, the National Reading Panel (NRP), tasked by Congress to identify scientific studies that program developers could rely on in deciding about reading instruction, developed and issued a report: the *Report of the National Reading Panel: Teaching Children to Read* (NICHD, 2000). It is important to note that, as with many studies, this one is not without controversy: the NRP focused exclusively on experimental studies that fit with certain parameters, and not all researchers in reading agree with their conclusions. The NRP findings designate five areas as important to beginning reading: phonemic awareness, phonics, fluency, vocabulary, and comprehension. In some people's minds, this has translated into putting the greatest emphasis on phonics, and we have seen a proliferation of phonics-based programs as a result. I prefer to think about how the five aspects of reading interrelate, with an ultimate emphasis on comprehension, for without comprehension, reading gets one nowhere.

Word identification is necessary, but it is not enough because word identification could be simply word pronunciation. Especially as the foundation for reading is being built, one simply must know the meanings of the words and how they are used, as well as how to think about them in flexible ways. This involves having extensive experiences both first-hand and through listening to and learning from others. Many children learn basic word identification and to remember literal information from text, but then fall back in terms of mastering higher levels of thinking, reading, and writing. Some of these students lag behind because they have not become fluent, some have not developed vocabulary and pertinent background knowledge, and some have not learned to synthesize, summarize, draw conclusions, generalize, or relate text information to what they already know. Even worse, some students think they are reading for meaning when they are not (Farber, 1999, p. 1). Many students simply do not read often enough and long enough to discover the rich complexities of the system; practice does indeed contribute to making perfect.

Rather than prescribe particular "canned" programs for reading, this chapter offers suggestions about what to incorporate into a school's offerings for a child with or without hearing loss. Keep in mind that reading is a spoken language-based act and that at the beginning one must make sure the child's language is sufficient for the words and ideas offered through reading. As language and reading mature, the child learns how to expand his or her language through the act of reading. Good reading instruction shows children how to interact with a text in order to identify main ideas and details, how to articulate the purpose and general meaning of a text, and how to relate the text to previous knowledge and decide whether it fits or not. Good reading depends on monitoring one's understanding and using "thinking strategies," such as creating one's own questions about the text, predicting what will come next in the text, summarizing what one has read, and stopping to figure out what the text means when it seems confusing (Farber, 1999, p. 2). These thinking strategies can be used when reading with a small child who does not yet know how to read, and they should be fostered throughout school. (In fact, whether you are a student or not, I hope you are employing these strategies as you read this text.) Beyond these capabilities are the aspects of critical reading that involve deciding about the validity of an author's assertions, the strength of the evidence offered to support them, and the worth of the argument and the way it is expressed. When reading and writing are not regarded and taught as thinking in response to marks on a page, the point of learning to read and write is lost.

Four General Suggestions

Richard Allington (2006) makes four suggestions about reading instruction that I would urge folding into reading instruction at all levels and in multiple settings, including the classroom, speech and language therapy, and the home. Note that these suggestions suggest a broadening of the length of reading instruction. They argue, in effect, that reading should receive attention in all instruction throughout a person's school years. This means that one does not learn to read once and for all; we continue to learn more about reading and writing as long as we continue to read and write. When I teach a college course, for example, I consider myself to be teaching my students how to read works written about some aspect of teaching and learning. When I read something in an unfamiliar area, I recognize that I have some learning to do about reading in that subject in order to make the subject cohere in my thinking. Different disciplines use language, words, and content in different ways; sentences, paragraphs, chapters and arguments are structured differently from one discipline to another. It takes some work to get used to making sense of these differences.

The first suggestion is that to become a good reader, the child needs a lot of practice. This concept is often overlooked when adults think about children and reading. The child must read extensively and often; according to Allington's conclusion based upon numerous studies on the amount that children read, " . . . there exists a potent relationship between volume of reading and reading achievement" (2006, p. 44). Better comprehension, higher achievement scores, faster mastery of reading, and positive thoughts about oneself all result from reading frequently and actively (McPherson, 2007, p. 71). The *Harry Potter* phenomenon in which we find children bemoaning the fact that the longest book in the series has "only" 734 pages is surprising in an environment in which people are always looking for the quickest way to get through their reading and on to something else. Instead of giving children that message, we should be encouraging them and applauding them when they spend days reading their favorite books.

Not only should children read often, they should read "real" texts, not just school-related texts, including both stories and informational works. Over the course of their reading, children should encounter increasingly complex language that draws them into higher levels of thought. Over time, picture books and books with simple words should give way to ever-longer chapter books and descriptive works. J. K. Rowling, author of the *Harry Potter* series, increased the difficulty and length of her books from the first through the last several and thereby maintains the interest of the millions of children reading them as they grow older. By following their growing interest, children also increase their vocabularies and their ability to comprehend extended text.

In a description of how an effective teacher uses an hour of instructional time, Allington envisions the teacher doing a 5- to 10-minute preparation for reading, the children reading for 40 or 45 minutes, and then the teacher doing a 5- to 10-minute activity with them. He found that the more effective teachers he observed had their children reading two or three times more than the less effective teachers. The less effective teachers spent more time within such an hour on having children respond to questions, do workbook pages, review stories, and check on vocabulary (2006, p. 45). It may not be that such activities are useless, but that if they routinely take the place of actual reading, they deprive the child of valuable reading practice. Another way to increase the amount of reading children do is to use Sustained Silent Reading (SSR), a practice in which everyone in the room or even in the school, including the teachers, principal, and janitor, reads something he or she chooses for an extended period of time. SSR has been associated with greater achievement in children who participate in it regularly (Krashen, 2006) and with children developing more favorable attitudes about reading (Yoon, 2002). A vital component of SSR is that children have access to enough reading material that they can find texts they are passionately interested in reading (Hartley, 2008).

Allington's second suggestion is to make sure that children have access to many books they are capable of reading. Using a practical point of view, he points out that adults choose easier (but not easy) texts for their own pleasure reading and then argues that children should be able to do the same. He writes, "The evidence available has convinced me that lots of high-success reading is absolutely critical to reading development and the development of positive stances toward reading. So why is assigning such reading so often ignored in schools?" (2006, p. 57). As evidence, Allington cites work by Berliner (1981) that demonstrated that students give up and often act up when a task is too hard, but engage more fully, develop positive attitudes, and learn more when they feel successful in doing a task (p. 58). Such tasks should not be overly easy, but of moderate to high challenge for the child (Ormrod, J., 2008, pp. 390–391). This observation applies both to books to be read for schoolwork and for fun, both of which should supply good practice in reading. Allington concludes that classrooms in which children experience the conditions in the following list are more likely to foster good reading achievement (p. 62). I have modified his list to make it apply to actions the parent(s) and therapist can perform, as well. Children need:

- access to books that range from being easy to challenging for each individual child to read;
- a teacher, therapist, or parent who regularly brings in new books;
- a role model for trying hard;
- choices in what to read;
- engagement in reading and writing tasks that accomplish something;
- activities that foster inference-making, application, analysis, synthesis, and evaluation;
- quality time interacting with adults and children; and
- frequent reading sessions with an adult or older child who reads in an interesting way.

Helping children explore the library at school and the local public library is critical in helping them find what they like and want to read, as that flows into what they actually do read. The teacher and parent must be part of the search. It is not enough to just point the way and say, "go find a book!" Adults who show delight in books, reading, and writing become role models whose behavior encourages the child to read and write. Teachers and parents must build this interest in the child over a period of years by reading and writing not only with the child, but also by reading and writing for their own needs in the child's presence.

The third suggestion is to help children read fluently. Children who read word by word, rather than phrasing words together in the ways they are usually uttered when speaking, do less well in reading (Allington, 2006, p. 91). At the very least, it is hard for anyone to understand a message that comes in one word at a time. What goes with what? Where do the intonations go? When reading is a laborious sounding out of words, by the time the end of the sentence is reached, the beginning is forgotten. A child who reads in word-by-word fashion may think that is the point of reading and probably needs to be read aloud with more frequently. The speech-language therapist should evaluate the child's expressive language development and decide whether the child needs help in speaking more fluently. Reading words in isolation can happen when the text being read is too hard for the child, not just in terms of word identification, but for ready comprehension of it. Developing fluency in reading demands practice with texts that make sense to the child and, especially for children with hearing loss, constant practice in making sense while listening and speaking.

The fourth suggestion involves helping children think about what they read. Allington calls this "thoughtful literacy" (2006, p. 109), by which he means developing in children the capacity for thinking and talking about what they read. If the end result of reading is always a test or a request to recite the information from the text, then a child's approach to reading is apt to be less than thoughtful. He or she could easily adopt the attitude that reading is just an unpleasant task to endure. Allington points out that adults who have read the same text often talk about the text. This happens, for example, in book groups about a selected book, in chats in the hallway about the latest newspaper story, and even in party conversations. These interactions enhance comprehension of a text, not because its readers have asked each other literal questions about the content of the text, but because they have constructed an understanding of the text and its nuances by bringing up various parts of it for analysis and/or debate. When they ask questions of each other, the questions are usually designed to find out what the other person thinks about some aspect of the content. Such talk yields better comprehension of the content of the text, as well as better memory for the elements of the text, even if those elements are not recited by the people involved, because it takes the interaction to a higher level. We want our children to learn the excitement of reading something, to think about the reading for themselves, and to enjoy finding out what someone else makes of it. This is not to say that reading for details is not important, but that details are usually remembered as a result of inference-making, application, analysis, synthesis, and/or evaluation. People remember best what they comprehend. The easiest way to get children engaged in and thinking about their reading is to talk with them about it in ways that require they think about it.

Before, During, and After Reading

Regardless of the age of the person doing the reading, doing something with the content of a text before, during, and after reading it helps the person build good understanding and facility with it, and so I recommend looking for that feature if one is looking for a program for teaching reading.

The prereading phase of reading can be as simple as looking at the title and asking, "What do I know about that?" or, in the case of a young child, asking something like, "Do you remember when we saw the *T. Rex* at the museum? What did *T. Rex* eat?" Having a discussion with someone else can be helpful at this point, and so can examining the pictures or diagrams, looking up some information, or being introduced to some new vocabulary. The idea is to activate prior knowledge and have it available for use in working memory during reading, so as to make connections between old and new knowledge.

During reading, the reader should be actively involved in thinking about the ideas, events, and emotions the writer has tried to create. Doing something active may be as simple as being aware and monitoring what the text seems to mean by continuously asking questions of the text, but it can also involve making a chart or web that shows the connections in and beyond the text or stopping at specified places to talk about the text with someone.

Postreading should involve extending one's thinking about the text, perhaps in a discussion with others. Planned activities in response to the reading could include building on a diagram begun during reading or creating something tangible, such as a homemade book or a journal entry. Again, the goal is to make and use connections between the reading and pre-existing knowledge in order to turn the new input into tomorrow's pre-existing knowledge, complete with as much inference-making, application, analysis, synthesis, and evaluation as possible.

Basic Elements of a Lesson Plan

A good lesson, whether done at school, at home, or somewhere else, needs to be built on a strong foundation. Of course, the sequence of activities and approximate time schedule (element #6 in the list below) are central to a plan; this is the part that comes to mind first as the parent, teacher, or therapist thinks about how to help a child learn. But, without the support of the other elements, the activities and schedule may not be sufficient. At first, attending to eight parts of a plan seems daunting, but with practice, planning a lesson becomes second nature.

1. *Goals for student learning for this lesson:*
   Think about what you want the child to know and be able to do as a result of the experience you are planning. For example, goals for a lesson might include:
   a. Demonstrating ability in handling a book and turning the pages.
   b. Identifying the characters and learning their names.
   c. Identifying and pointing to a character feeling sad and a character feeling happy.

2. *How the content of this lesson builds on what students learned previously:*
   Learning built on solid prior knowledge is more durable than learning that has little or no connection to a previous experience. For example, suppose you are working with a child who has had some experience with books, but you've usually been the one to turn the pages. Suppose the child understands that everybody has a name, and suppose you've been working on applying names for emotions. All of this would be the content on which you are planning to build.

3. *How the content of this lesson relates to what students will be learning in the future:*
   Practice doing something with the help of a person who knows how to do it is helpful in being able to move toward doing it independently. In this case, you would be preparing the child for being able to go back and forth within a book, by giving the child practice in turning the pages in a mostly independent way. By doing something about naming the characters, you would be preparing the child to expect that storybooks usually have main characters. By naming sadness and happiness in the pictures of the characters, you would be adding examples of sadness and happiness to the child's repertoire so they can be identified in other situations.

4. *How literacy is addressed in this lesson:*

   Every lesson can address literacy. Remember that literacy isn't just about identifying words and handling books. Using language in a conversation, practicing listening for a rhyme or for certain sounds or words, having a new experience that builds background knowledge, finding things that are alike and different, using new words, and remembering a sequence are just a few ways to address literacy, and each of them could be done with or without involving a book! Given the goals set forth in this example, literacy will be addressed by reading a book together and taking the time to check with the child about turning pages, identifying the main characters' names, and looking at the pictures to see when a character looks sad and happy.

5. *How you will make sure your students can listen during the lesson:*

   Whatever you are doing with a child, you need to make sure he or she can listen to you easily. This should involve checking on the hearing technology in some way, perhaps with the Ling 6–Sound Test and resolving any gap in hearing in some way. It also involves thinking beforehand about the listening conditions you will likely encounter during the lesson. For this example, you might think about which chair you will sit in with the child in your lap so you can speak into his or her ear and the fact that you'll need to mute your cell phone.

6. *Sequence of activities and approximate time schedule:*

   Pacing a lesson is important so that you can accomplish your goals. For this reason, you need to think ahead about how long each part might take; of course, it's fine to depart from your scheduled plan if the child seems to be learning something different from what you planned. But without prior planning, you might find that the lesson feels aimless. For this example, you might do the following:

   > Prereading (10 minutes): Make sure that the child has some experience with at least one of the activities depicted in *A Weekend with Wendell*, the story by Kevin Henkes that you are going to read with the child. These include: having an overnight guest, children playing "house," eating vegetables, playing with the hose outside in the yard pretending to put out a fire, and writing a note to someone. For example, you could

say, "We're going to read a book about a boy named Wendell who visits a girl named Sophie for the weekend while his parents go out of town. We're going to see how they played together. Do you remember when Charlie came over and you played house? Tell me about who was the mommy and who was the daddy and who was the dog." "At first, I'm going to turn the pages, and then I want you to turn the pages."

Reading (20 minutes): Start with the cover and read each page, giving the child the job of turning the pages and helping where necessary. Stop and talk about the parts that seem interesting to the child. Show the child who Sophie is and who Wendell is and ask him or her to point to them throughout the book. When you get to pages where Sophie has reason to be sad (because Wendell isn't a very nice guest at first), ask the child to find pictures where Sophie looks sad. Do the same with the places where Sophie has reasons to be happy and where she looks happy. Complete the book.

Postreading (10 minutes): After you've completed reading the book together, ask the child to tell you the story and help fill in the details. Pay attention, particularly, to the goals you set at the beginning. In this instance, the retelling might involve asking the child to turn the pages, look at the pictures, and talk about them. Prompt the child to point out Sophie and Wendell and the sad and happy images. You might want to make pictures of happy and sad faces.

7. *Instructional materials:*
   It's always a good idea to make a list of what you will need. In this example, you need a copy of *A Weekend with Wendell*, by Keven Henkes, and you may need paper and crayons.

8. *Evaluation Plan (how you will know whether the students have learned what you intended them to learn)*
   After the lesson is over, reflect on what the child was able to do in terms of your goals. Did he or she achieve all of them? How? Are there any gaps? Where is more practice needed? What can you use to build on during a future lesson? Use this information to plan what you will do next with this child. In this example, you may discover the child doesn't have a concept of a fire chief and a burning building, so you might decide to create an experience so the child will understand this.

Specific Steps for Meeting Literacy Goals

Many books are available that describe specific steps to take in meeting the gamut of literacy goals, and any of them can be worked into a lesson plan. A few I have found useful are listed below. (Please see the references at the end of this chapter for full citations.)

- Beaty, *50 Early Childhood Literacy Strategies* (2nd edition)
- Miller, *Strategies for Developing Emergent Literacy*
- Fisher et al., *50 Content Area Strategies for Adolescent Literacy*
- Yopp and Yopp, *Literature-Based Reading Activities* (3rd edition)
- Vacca and Vacca, *Content Area Reading: Literacy and Learning Across the Curriculum*

Some of my favorite approaches are:

- the anticipation guide (Fisher et al., 2007, pp. 7–9); Vacca & Vacca, pp. 203–206; Yopp & Yopp, 2006, pp. 20–23);
- the K-W-L chart (Fisher et al., 2007, pp. 47–49); (Vacca & Vacca, pp. 220–226; Yopp & Yopp, 2006, pp. 38–41);
- the semantic map (Vacca & Vacca, pp. 297–299; Yopp & Yopp, 2006, pp. 41–44), concept map (Fisher et al., 2007, pp. 10–13), pattern guide (Fisher et al., 2007, pp. 63–65), and web (Beaty, 2009, pp. 159–161);
- the contrast chart (Yopp & Yopp, 2006, pp. 36–38); and
- the quotation share (Yopp & Yopp, 2001, pp. 91–92) and popcorn review (Fisher et al., 2007, pp. 69–70).

I use these with my college students to help them in their thinking and reading, and they are used in elementary and secondary schools. To demonstrate they can be used with even very young readers who cannot read yet or who are just beginning to read, I offer examples below using the story, "Goldilocks and the Three Bears." One version of this childhood story can be found in Scarry (1975, pp. 31–38). Note that the story content focused upon in any of these approaches is determined by the teacher or parent according to what he or she wants the child to learn. My selections are arbitrary and meant only as examples. I am also conscious that these approaches could degenerate into some kind of "skill and drill" that sucks the meaning right out of the story for the child and urge caution while using these approaches.

Anticipation Guide

Teacher: I'm going to read you a story called "Goldilocks and the Three Bears." Before we start, I want you to think about what you know about some things. I'm going to ask you some questions, and I want you to tell me "yes" or "no."

1. Is porridge a cereal like oatmeal?   Yes   No
2. Is hot the opposite of cold?   Yes   No
3. Is little the opposite of big?   Yes   No
4. Is hard the opposite of harder?   Yes   No
5. Is it okay to walk into someone else's house   Yes   No
   without being invited?

After reading the story, the teacher or parent asks the questions again and talks with the child about the answers, clarifying where the child had the wrong idea before hearing the story. For example, items 1 to 4 of this anticipation guide focus on vocabulary. It is important to learn what porridge is, and it is necessary to learn what "opposite" means if that concept is not already known. The final question relates to the story's content and helps a child apply the story to daily life in a particular culture.

K-W-L Chart

To prepare for this approach, the teacher writes "Know," "Want to Know," and "Learned" on the board or on a large sheet of paper. Then the teacher gives a topic and asks the children what they know about it; the responses are written in the "Know" column. Next, the teacher asks what the children want to know about the topic and records the responses. The next step is to read the story aloud to the children or to have them read it silently. The final step is to ask the children what they have learned from the reading. For "Goldilocks," depending on what the child paid attention to, the chart could look like Table 16–1. Note that the content of the columns is not exhaustive; there is only so much that can be learned in one reading of a story.

> **Topic**—This is a story about a girl who went into the bear family's house without being invited. She ate their food, she sat in their chairs, and she went to sleep in their bed. What do you think could happen?

Table 16–1. K-W-L Chart

Know (This column is filled in before reading.)	**Want to Know** (This column is filled in before reading.)	**Learned** (This column is filled in after reading.)
The bears could be surprised.	What was the girl's name? What were the bears' names?	Goldilocks, Papa, Mama, and Baby Bear. The bears were very surprised when they came home and found Goldilocks asleep.
The bears could get angry.	Did the bears get mad?	The bears were both surprised and angry when they found Goldilocks. They wanted Goldilocks to get out of their house.
The bears could be happy to have a new friend.	Did the bears chase her away?	Goldilocks ran away fast when she saw the bears.
	What did the girl do inside the house?	Goldilocks ate the porridge that was not too hot, not too cold, but just right. Papa Bear had a big chair, Mama Bear had a medium chair, and Baby Bear had a tiny chair, and Goldilocks tried them all.
	Did the girl feel sorry?	Yes. Goldilocks was sorry and scared.

Semantic Map/Concept Map/Pattern Guide

A diagram can help a child master relationships and the words that represent them. Table 16–2 offers a brief example.

Contrast Chart

The teacher can ask the child after reading the story about things that were "not right" and "just right" for Goldilocks in the story. A diagram can help a child master relationships and the words that represent them. Table 16–3 offers a brief example.

Table 16-2. Semantic Map/Concept Map/Pattern Guide

A semantic map shows relationships in graphic form. Perhaps a teacher would want to focus on adjectives and their comparative and superlative forms, either before or after reading. A semantic map could look like this:

| Hard | Harder | Hardest |
| Soft | Softer | Softer |

Or, perhaps the teacher wants to focus on relative magnitude of an object or a sound:

| Tiny chair | Medium-sized chair | Great big chair |
| Tiny voice | Medium voice | Big gruff voice |

A focus on comfort changes the dimension, with the extremes on either end and "just right" in the middle:

| Too hard | Just right | Too soft |

Table 16–3. Contrast Chart

Not Right	Just Right
Mama Bear's cold porridge	Baby Bear's warm porridge
Papa Bear's big chair	Baby Bear's tiny chair
Mama Bear's medium-sized bed	Baby Bear's tiny bed

Quotation Share/Popcorn Review

This technique works with children who can read a story or article. After reading, each is asked to choose a passage to share aloud to everyone. Children take turns reading aloud the parts of the story or article that feel important to them, and they describe why they find their choices to be important. There is no necessity for the story to unfold in order, as the emphasis is on what is meaningful to each child. For the Goldilocks story, it could go like this:

> Child 1: "'Someone has been sleeping in *my* bed,' said Baby Bear in his wee tiny voice, 'and *here* she is!'" (Scarry, 1975, p. 37). Child's comment: "I like this part because it's the most exciting part."

> Child 2: "'Someone has been sitting in my chair,' he roared in his deep gruff voice'" (Scarry, 1975, p. 36). Child's comment: "Papa Bear has a big voice because he's big."

> Child 3: "But the tiny chair was not strong enough and it broke all to pieces" (Scarry, 1975, p. 33). Child's comment: "Goldilocks shouldn't break things."

Writing

Writing can grow out of any of the approaches above. As the child gains more control over writing, he or she can write about "what I thought before I read the story and what I think now," and "here's what I learned that changed my mind." A child can use a diagram, web, or contrast chart to organize his or her thoughts and then write about them systematically. Listening to other children read their favorite parts and tell why they chose them can help a child choose the most meaningful part to write about.

Reading and Writing as Thinking: The Basis of Good Programs in Reading

Teachers and therapists can help students get at the many ways people can organize thought, whether they are listening, speaking, reading, or writing. All of these language processes depend on thinking if they are to be at all meaningful. Using language receptively or expressively to create meaning is always the goal, and the intent of any literacy program must be that the child or older student is regularly creating meaning in the presence of symbols, not merely identifying someone else's description of meaning. Meaningful use of language results in better memory and greater capability to make connections between and among bits of information and larger ideas.

Conclusion

Children with hearing loss need even more emphasis on creating meaning than children with typical hearing, because they will always be more likely to be in the position of having to hypothesize about information or an idea that fits into the gaps that occur because of incomplete hearing. This capability proves to be very helpful as these children encounter reading material and create their own written texts, and it will hold them in good stead throughout their lives.

References

Allington, R. (2006). *What really matters for struggling readers: Designing research-based programs* (2nd ed.). Boston, MA: Pearson.

Beaty, J. (2009). *50 Early childhood literacy strategies* (2nd ed.). Upper Saddle River, NJ: Merrill/Pearson.

Cambourne, B. (2005). J. K. Rowling, Harry Potter, the Dolores Umbridge syndrome, and teaching reading. *New England Reading Association Journal, 41*(2), 1–6.

Farber, P. (1999). Johnny *still* can't read? *Harvard Education Letter, 15*(4), 1–3.

Fisher, D., Brozo, W. G., Frey, N., & Ivey, G. (2007). *50 Content area strategies for adolescent literacy.* Upper Saddle River, NJ: Pearson.

Hartley, J. (2008). "You should read this book!" *Educational Leadership, 65*(6), 73–75.

Henkes, K. (1986). *A Weekend with Wendell.* New York, NY: Greenwillow Books.

Krashen, S. (2006). Free reading. *School Library Journal, 52*(9), 42–45.

McPherson, K. (2007). Harry Potter and the goblet of motivation. *Teacher Librarian, 34*(4), 71–73.

Miller, W. (2000). *Strategies for developing emergent literacy.* Boston, MA: McGraw-Hill.

National Institute of Child Health and Human Development (NICHD). (2000). *Report of the National Reading Panel. Teaching children to read: An evidence-based assessment of the scientific research literature on reading and its implications for reading instruction: Reports of the subgroups* (NIH Publication No. 00-4754). Washington, DC: U.S. Government Printing Office. Also available online: http://www.nichd.hih.gov/publications/nrp/report.htm

Ormrod, J. (2008). *Educational psychology: Developing learners* (6th ed.). Upper Saddle River, NJ: Pearson Education.

Scarry, R. (1975). *Richard Scarry's animal nursery tales.* New York, NY: Golden Press.

Vacca, R., & Vacca, J. (2002). *Content area reading: Literacy and learning across the curriculum.* Boston, MA: Allyn and Bacon.

Yoon, J. (2002). Three decades of sustained silent reading: A meta-analytic review of the effects of SSR on attitude toward reading. *Reading Improvement, 39*(4), 186–195.

Yopp, R., & Yopp, H. (2001). *Literature-based reading activities* (3rd ed.). Boston, MA: Allyn and Bacon.

Yopp, R., & Yopp, H. (2006). *Literature-based reading activities* (4th ed.). Boston, MA: Pearson.

Chapter 17

EDUCATIONAL SETTINGS FOR CHILDREN WITH HEARING LOSS

I never thought of myself as being hearing impaired first—my hearing loss was always secondary to who I am as a person. . . . I also grew up with an attitude that my hearing loss wasn't going to stop me from doing things I like doing or wanted to do.

Young Adult, 2008

The kids were accepting of me and one time a boy that I had a crush on at the time asked why every morning I had to go to a corner of the room to put on my FM equipment. He thought that I should just put it on out in the open.

Young Adult, 2008

Introduction

Children's needs differ, and sometimes that recognition is used as an argument to keep children from being put where they can learn the most by rising to challenges presented to them in environments enjoyed by children with typical hearing. Parents need to adjust to the fact that their child who is deaf or hard of hearing is different from other children, but the adjustment should not be so complete that their main motivation is that their child will not ever be frustrated. Environments for children with typical attributes are populated by children who come with a wide variety of capabilities and weaknesses, and children with hearing loss can fit right in.

The Optimal Placement

The optimal placement for a child with hearing loss is with his or her typically hearing peers in a typical public, private, or parochial school designed for all children. At such a school, the child with hearing loss will have frequent opportunities to interact with children from a variety of backgrounds and will learn language, academic, and social skills in the process. Teachers in such schools can learn to make the individual accommodations each child needs while keeping the child on track academically. It does not matter that an individual child with hearing loss may be the only student with a hearing loss in the school; in fact, that possibility can be desirable, as the teachers involved with the child do not have a chance to adopt negative stereotypes that lead to low expectations or overly-helpful stances that create "learned helplessness" in the child. In the optimal situation I am describing, the child consistently uses the best technology available, fitted as early as possible, has had auditory-verbal therapy that has stimulated his or her parents to work on listening and language on a daily basis, and has been in preschool and playgroups with children with typical hearing. This child enters kindergarten having learned to listen and express himself or herself, how to pay attention when being instructed, and how to say what he or she needs in order to hear and get along in the environment. It does not matter whether this child is as fluent with spoken language as the children with typical hearing are; what matters is that the child is confident in interacting with others using whatever language capabilities he or she has at that point. Children with typical hearing adapt well to differences in other children, especially when they are present from the beginning of their own schooling. For them, having a child with hearing loss in their midst is how it has always been, and so it is "normal." In thinking about this optimally, waiting until third or fourth grade or beyond to put the child with hearing loss into the mainstream has numerous drawbacks. One, the child with hearing loss has large adjustments to make in meeting new children and new teachers. These social ties are very important, and yet adults often overlook them, thinking only about maximizing academic development. Such thinking is counterproductive because children aren't interchangeable parts of schools; it matters greatly to them to have continuity in their relationships. Academically, such continuity is part of the foundation for sustained academic progress. Two, children with typical hearing who have already established relationships with the other children in their classes can have difficulty making room for a new child, typically hearing or not, and may especially have little interest in trying to understand the new child in their midst who doesn't hear everything easily and who speaks differently. If they know the child from the start of their schooling, they accept and interact with him or her more easily, possibly not even noticing, but at least just accepting any differences between this child and their other classmates. Three, children can have a difficult time learning new routines at a new school, not because they have hearing loss, but just because they are young and inexperienced. Adding the hearing loss can make such adjustments even harder. The child with hearing loss is first a child, and then takes on all the other descriptors one might apply to the particular individual. Every child has many personality traits, interests, and academic strengths and weaknesses that have little or nothing to do with whether he or she can hear, see, or walk. The child in question may by inflexible or shy, quite apart from having a hearing loss, and such qualities could take their toll while he or she adjusts to a new environment. Fourth, the mainstream school may be more demanding than the school with only children with hearing loss, and by third or fourth grade, the child might be very far behind the other children. Closing this sort of gap is very difficult.

A parent can feel confident in sending the child who has learned to listen and who is learning to speak to school with children with typical hearing for all the reasons we send any child to school. Especially when such placements begin with preschool, the parent can depend on the child with hearing loss learning a lot from the children with typical hearing about language and social interaction. Everyone benefits as children with typical hearing learn patience and compassion for others who do not hear in the ways they do, and children with hearing loss learn they can get along and interact with everyone.

This optimal view depends on a teacher who monitors the child's progress in comparison to all the other children and expects comparable growth. This teacher understands and teaches self-reliance, interdependence, and responsibility to all the children, including the child with hearing loss. This teacher thinks about how best to present material to the child with hearing loss and often finds that such strategies benefit the class as a whole. This teacher welcomes the special educator (a Listening and Spoken Language Specialist/Auditory-Verbal Educator—LSLS AVEd—would be ideal), and the speech-language pathologist (ideally, a Listening and Spoken Language Specialist/Auditory-Verbal Therapist—LSLS AVT) into the classroom on a regular basis and discusses the child's needs with them. Rather than just sending the child to a special classroom for certain kinds of instruction, the specialists come into the classroom, to observe, participate, and help the teacher make necessary changes in the classroom and in instruction. Together, they decide on a course of action, always keeping in mind that it is in the best interest of the child to act upon high expectations that involve the child taking personal social and academic responsibility for her or himself. My daughter experienced this optimal setting from preschool through graduate school, and so have many children brought along with the auditory-verbal approach. It is not too ideal to contemplate.

What If the Optimum Is Not Possible?

Often, the optimum is not possible, and it is nobody's fault. Circumstances do not always line up in the ways we might like, and early learning of spoken language in an extensive way may not have been possible for some reason. Perhaps it took a while to diagnose the hearing loss, perhaps the parents tried sign language first, or perhaps there were equipment failures. This child probably presents more severe needs that can be addressed in a special classroom led by an auditory-verbal educator (LSLS AVEd). The child's peers in such a classroom will have similar needs in terms of their spoken communication, and they can all benefit from being put into regular contact with children who hear and speak and who are well on their way to mature spoken language use. This sort of classroom can be thought of as a safe haven where the child receives intensive instruction from a well-prepared teacher who understands language acquisition and socio-emotional phases of development, enforces the use of hearing technology with consistency, and works daily to draw the child's parents into enriching and expanding all aspects of the child's language development. The goal is mainstream education as soon as possible.

It may be that an individual child has a challenge beyond that of the hearing loss. For example, the child may also be diagnosed with Attention Deficit Disorder (ADD), Attention Deficit Hyperactivity Disorder (ADHD), learning disability, cognitive delay, or low vision. In these cases, the school's expert on the difficulty exhibited should be on the team with the child's other teachers and the parents and should assist in answering questions about what exacerbates the problem of the hearing loss and whether the hearing loss accentuates the other problem. For example, the child with hearing loss who also has ADD or ADHD needs help in paying attention and monitoring his or her own behavior in the classroom in addition to listening, speech, and language intervention. It would be unfair to the child just to treat one of the aspects of his or her being that get in the way of learning, and so all the people involved in the individual child's education need to work together to decide the best course of action for the child.

Schooling Is Not the Only Source of Education

Other opportunities besides school should be offered to every child with hearing loss, regardless of school placement. Once the parents stop thinking of the child in terms of the hearing loss, they can see that all the activities available to any child are available to their child, and they should feel free to seek out and enroll their child in activities they think their child will enjoy. This means learning music, sports, art, dance, crafts, and so on, alongside children with typical hearing. For some families, this will include religious education. There is great advantage for the child with hearing loss of being in small groups of children, guided by an adult, in which natural immersion in meaningful talking and listening takes place.

A Letter to a Mainstream Classroom Teacher

Therapists, speech-language pathologists, and parents need to communicate the principles of LSLS AVTs and AVEds (see Chapter 5 for these) to the mainstream classroom teacher. Here is a letter I would like to send at the beginning of the school year to the classroom teacher of children with hearing loss, in this case a generic "Ms. Smith" about a boy named Jamie. Feel free to use it, altering it to apply to each particular child's age, grade placement, and other circumstances. It lays out what I have come to consider essential for the child's academic and social growth the teacher will foster in the mainstream classroom:

Dear Ms. Smith,

You are about to experience something you may have been told is not possible. You are going to have a child in your classroom who listens by using hearing aids or a cochlear implant. I want to assure you that many people have spent many hours helping Jamie learn to listen and to speak, and Jamie is ready to learn in your classroom alongside all the other students you will have. You may be thinking that Jamie will claim too much of your time and attention, so I want to assure you that once you understand what Jamie can do, you will come to forget that Jamie cannot hear without the technology he uses.

You should talk with Jamie as you talk with any other child. This will require him to use what he knows and to learn what he doesn't know about communicating. Set yourself the goal of coming to know Jamie and his life experiences as well as possible, so you'll be able to fill in communication gaps when they happen.

Please resist the impulse to baby Jamie. Shielding him from responsibilities you give your other students will get in the way of building the self-reliance and responsibility he needs to develop. He is going to need to become even more self-reliant and responsible than your students with typical hearing, because there will be times when he doesn't hear you or the other students, and he needs to learn to speak up for himself. You need to develop high expectations for Jamie and to believe that he will learn to read, write, do mathematics, and learn other content just as your other students will.

Especially at the beginning of the school year, you should communicate with Jamie's parents and speech/language therapists and teachers daily in order to make sure everyone understands what to do. After you get this established, you will need to reach out to this group regularly and expect that you'll confer with them to set up goals for Jamie. Call Jamie's parents when something goes well and share the event. His parents have worked hard so he can listen and speak with you, and they deserve positive feedback from you. Also call Jamie's parents when a problem arises. They will want to work with you and Jamie to overcome it.

When you don't know something about Jamie, ask his parents and speech-language therapists and teachers. Ask Jamie, himself! Keep your biases at bay, and do not just assume that Jamie will be behind the other children in learning. Remember that children are not alike, and welcome the processes that help Jamie get along. Try first those approaches you use with other children, and then fall back to other ideas as necessary. Be willing to figure out new ways to help Jamie work with concepts, and expect Jamie to master them. You may discover that what you develop to do with Jamie helps all the other students learn better, too.

There will be times when you think Jamie is lazy, not interested, or even disobedient. The first thing to do is to check out the hearing aids or cochlear implant (CI). Some of what looks like problematic behavior is the result of not being able to listen well. Learn how to troubleshoot hearing aids and CIs so you can help Jamie get back on track by changing a battery or alerting Jamie's parents to some other problem with the equipment. Let Jamie know that you expect him to tell you when his hearing aids/CIs aren't working right.

Be willing to wear the microphone for an FM system when Jamie is in your room, so that he can always have the best possible sound delivered right into his ears, and check it every day to make sure it is working correctly. When it breaks down, which it will, make sure that it is replaced or repaired as soon as possible. It is not a frill; *even one day* without appropriate access to sound is detrimental to Jamie.

Help Jamie integrate into social groups with the other students. Help him explain his hearing aids, CIs, and FM system to them. Talk with your students about how different doesn't mean better or worse, but just different. Explain to them how to value the differences they see among themselves and in other people beyond their classroom.

Trust that you can communicate with Jamie just as you can with your other students, and expect Jamie to work hard and learn well. Imagine that in 20 years, Jamie will come back to see you because he wants to tell you he's finished college and working in his first job as a writer. Do everything you can to build the foundation that fulfills that vision, and one day you'll meet that future Jamie, and he'll be doing something important in the world.

Sincerely,
Lyn Robertson

Conclusion

Children with hearing loss present us with many challenges. The important message of this book is that we can meet them, whether they are cognitive, social, or emotional. I have seen the lives of many children with hearing loss and the lives of their families enriched beyond measure in the process of helping the children learn to use listening and spoken language. Developing literacy is just one aspect of their lives, yet it is central and powerful for them in making their way in the world. Perfection is not the goal; instead, I urge you to help each child explore his or her potential. The possibilities are without limit.

Chapter 18

PARENTING A CHILD WITH HEARING LOSS

Introduction

In preparing to write this chapter, I sat down with my husband to talk about how we have been parents of two children, one a child with hearing loss and the other a child with typical hearing. Neither of our families had any history of deafness in childhood, so we had no expectation that one of our children might have even a slight hearing loss and thus no preparation for having such a child. We have now lived with hearing loss for 34 years and are pleased to report that our experiences have enriched and improved our own lives and our family life.

Our children are happy adults, both married to well-adjusted, interesting people. One couple has profound hearing loss and uses hearing technology to listen, and the other has typical hearing. We made a conscious decision not to treat our children very differently, with two exceptions: we followed the advice of our auditory-verbal therapists, and we were scrupulous about making sure our child with hearing loss had access to the best hearing technology possible. Our children and their spouses enjoy their lives, pursue many interests, contribute to society, find fulfillment and success in their chosen professions, and spend time with each other. What follows are our thoughts about how all this has come about.

Some Precepts to Consider

Focus on the Child as an Individual

A child with hearing loss is, first and always, an individual. It can be easy to fall into the habit of letting a child's deafness define him or her—to think of the child as a "deaf child," rather than a "child who is deaf," and we were fortunate to learn early that much of what we might have attributed to our daughter's hearing loss included behaviors that any child might display. Inattentiveness, carelessness, stubbornness, too much or too little activity, and worrying about the smallest details, for example, can show up in any child, and it helped us immensely to hear complaints about such matters from parents of children with typical hearing.

When in the throes of adjusting to a life full of appointments with doctors, teachers, and therapists, it can be hard to think of one's child in terms of his or her personality and development apart from the presence or absence of the ability to hear, but it's best for the child if the parents strive for that. Who among us would want the people we love to define us by what we cannot yet do very well?

Refuse to Accept Low Expectations About the Child from Others

Perhaps because my husband and I are both teachers, we have always thought our daughter could learn what anyone else could learn, and we refused to believe anyone who intimated that our daughter's prospects were diminished because of her hearing loss. When we thought a person's low expectation was related to the increasingly antiquated assumption that deafness would prevent her from being part of the "hearing" world, we were motivated to prove that person wrong. As teachers, we had learned in educational psychology courses and from our own experience that high expectations are associated with better results. High expectations expressed in positive, encouraging ways create a hopeful atmosphere that spurs good behavior, curiosity, and successful learning. For example, there was a period of time during the upper elementary years when our daughter said she didn't like going out of her class to have speech therapy. We approached this by asking questions, making suggestions about what to do, and talking about how important intelligible speech is. We also told her to do her best, and to work to the point where she didn't need to go to that particular program anymore. At the same time, we invented little games at home that supported the speech targets. One game involved a special necklace that we dubbed the "s" necklace. We wrote little stories that had many "s" sounds in them and had her read them aloud while holding onto the "s" necklace to remind her to pronounce the sound carefully. The goal was to get as close to 100% of the "s" sounds correct as possible. We laughed and had a good time over the silly sentences, and her "s" production improved. In addressing another aspect of learning, we didn't encourage our daughter to drop a course in high school or college when the material seemed "too hard." We talked with her about what she needed to do in terms of talking with the teacher or professor, seeking outside assistance, and opening herself to whatever she could learn. We accepted that some of her grades would be average or low, but we didn't tell her that; we always emphasized that classes are places for learning, not for amassing grades. The point of these strategies is to help the child take ownership of his or her learning, to learn how to learn, and to believe that better performance is based on putting in more effort and finding new ways of understanding.

But, we also observe that high expectations imposed in a rigid way can damage a parent-child relationship and disrupt the child's love of learning. If we had insisted on high grades without supplying help in working toward them, or if we had equated grades with self-worth, our outcomes would have been unhappy. It is important to develop perspective about one's expectations and a situation's outcomes.

Learn About the Developmental Stages of Childhood

Knowing the typical trajectory of development in children is important in building an understanding of where a particular child is functioning socially, emotionally, physically, and cognitively. For example, four- to five-year-olds are usually becoming more independent, and five- to six-year-olds are increasingly able to follow directions that include many steps. Parents and teachers may "baby" a child with hearing loss and make him or her overly dependent, and they may assume their child will always lag behind children with typical hearing in memory tasks. Instead, they can pay attention to the overall development of a particular child compared to children with typical hearing and help everyone keep the child's development in perspective. Not expecting enough can get in the way of offering the opportunities for growth the child needs. Helpful descriptions of child development can be found on the PBS Parents website at http://www.pbs.org/parents/child-development/ and in *Yardsticks: Children in the Classroom Ages 4–14* (Wood, 2007).

Help the Child Develop a Sense of Responsibility

Helen Beebe counseled us to give our daughter responsibilities and to hold her accountable for completing them. We were surprised when she suggested that we show our two-and-a-half-year-old how to take plates and silverware from the table and put them in the dishwasher, but we followed this advice and found that she could do it, first with help, but soon on her own. Learning how to take care of a plant, to fill up the dog's water bowl, and to pick up one's toys are other examples of appropriate responsibilities for young children. Having jobs to do, along with the satisfaction of completing them and being thanked for doing them, helps a child know that she or he is capable and valuable and spurs on the desire to learn to do more. Children who feel responsible for contributing to their family, school, and community are seen as dependable and capable, rather than helpless and dependent, and this helps their parents and teachers know they can thrive.

Help the Child Learn Practical Skills

An extension of helping children become responsible involves teaching them how to deal with very practical matters. Because of what we had learned when our children were young, we made sure they learned practical skills as they grew older. Consequently, when our children went away to college, they found out quickly that they were among the few who knew how to do laundry, change a tire, cook a meal, and hammer a nail. Such skills aren't just "handy"; they create self-sufficiency and the ability to help others. Learning to do them can involve applying listening, thinking, and reading skills that are, in turn, strengthened through their application. Such skills carry over into adult day-to-day life and to the workplace where they represent maturity and promote the learning of additional skills. Accumulating skills and the sense of empowerment they insure contribute to success in personal life and promotions in the workplace.

Listen to the Child with Care and Respect

If we want our children to learn to listen, we must demonstrate good listening ourselves. Well beyond learning to interpret sounds and internalize language structures, listening is about understanding one another. Parents and teachers serve children best when we sit quietly while our children express themselves to us. We should take in our children's words, consider them, and ask questions that give us more information and support further thinking in our children. We should try to see what our children are seeing and to understand from their point of view. Only then can we see their insights, as well as their gaps in knowledge and experience. It is understandable that children with hearing loss might miss something said by a playmate and feel left out or disrespected. Parents and teachers can help the child come to see what may have happened and talk with him or her about how one's perceptions are not always reality. At the same time, we must understand that this applies to all children, not just to our children with hearing loss. Such talk helps build the self-knowledge, trust, empathy, and communication skills that create healthy relationships, and if such talk is maintained, parents and children will continue to communicate well throughout the highs and lows of adolescence and will weather disagreements without damage to their relationship.

Push for the Best Possible Listening Through Technology

Children can learn early to tell parents and teachers when their batteries are dead or something is wrong with their hearing aids or cochlear implants, and parents and teachers can learn to trouble-shoot the equipment. Equally important is that parents develop good relationships with providers of such technology and to stay abreast of new developments in technology. For example, the program in a cochlear implant is hugely important. If it's not helping enough, parents can push for a better program from the audiologist, recognizing that creating an optimal program for the individual child involves both art and science. I have seen instances in which someone has "settled" for less-than-helpful technology, only to discover later that more could be done. Parents are their children's best advocates in this regard.

Nurturing Healthy Sibling Relationships and Friendships

It is important not to make siblings feel an inordinate responsibility for the child with hearing loss. Siblings need to admire the child with hearing loss for everything the child is able to do. Parents can nurture sibling respect and friendship by being obvious about treating all the children fairly, by explaining the child's hearing loss to the children with typical hearing, and by encouraging healthy play and speaking with one another.

Similarly, parents should encourage healthy friendships with children who are respectful of the child with hearing loss. Parents can become friends with the parents of their child's friends and explain the hearing loss, what they are doing about it, and why it is important for their child to be in close contact with children with typical hearing who can carry on conversations and serve as good speech models. Making an effort to make one's house a place where classmates want to come play is a good move, as this fosters spoken language practice and allows the parents to monitor the child's relationships.

Encourage Public Speaking and Speaking for Oneself

People who speak easily in public have a great advantage. They can speak up anywhere and make themselves understood. As a young child of five or six, our daughter was asked to read something during a church service. She stood perched on a box at the podium and read as clearly as she could at that point. I could understand her, but most people probably could not, as her articulation had not matured yet. But, this was a starting point for her, she agreed to do it on other occasions, and she grew up confident in her right to speak and unafraid to talk in front of groups and with people she does not know. Her own memory is that we encouraged her to have many early experiences of public speaking and to practice beforehand in front of mirror and in front of us. Since learning to speak in public takes practice, it fosters a desire to make oneself understood. Another bit of advice we received and followed was to encourage her to give her own order at fast food places and restaurants. When there is a practical reason to work on making oneself understood, children will work hard to learn to do so.

Expect Children to Do Their Own Schoolwork

Some parents "hover" over their child when it comes to homework. They exhort the child to do the work and then interfere in unhealthy ways, sometimes even doing the work themselves, so that the child will get a good grade. Ironically, while trying to ensure their child's success in school, parents can deprive their children of the very learning they want their children to accomplish. It is better to communicate a love of learning and a sense of curiosity to the child and to make clear to the child that the homework is his or hers to do. I had several experiences of seeing another parent in the grocery store and being asked if we had completed our science report or some other project. I was happy to reply that I didn't know about whatever it was and that I hoped my child had done her work. There is much to be learned by getting feedback on one's own work. As a teacher, I can assure parents that teachers do not want to evaluate their work; teachers need to see what their students can do in order to make instructional decisions. What good is an "A" for a parent who has done a child's work? How will the child be able to do the next assignment without mastering the material or process that comes before it? This is not to say that parents should be uninvolved. A good balance involves the parent monitoring how the child is doing, asking questions that demonstrate genuine interest in what the child is doing in school, helping the child learn how to ask for help, and assisting in ways that help the child complete the work with independence.

Speak Respectfully About the Child's Teachers

However much a parent might be justified in criticizing a child's teacher, it is best not to convey this to the child. It is very difficult for a child to learn from a person his or her parents do not respect. Instead, the parent should speak with the teacher and try to work out an understanding; if that is not possible, the parent needs to find out if other educational arrangements can be made. Teachers become wary of the parent who is on the attack, and parents need to keep in mind that the best situation for their child is for the teacher to believe in the child's ability to learn, even when the child is still having difficulty expressing him or herself.

Expect the Child with Hearing Loss to Ask "Why Me?"

Very few children grow up completely happy with every facet of their lives. There is a point for most people when they ask, "why me?" about something. By listening carefully, parents can help a child with hearing loss come to terms with this question. Parents with typical hearing themselves have probably asked themselves the same question about their altered status as parents. Recognizing that different people come to different answers and that answers can change over time is helpful. Other children may tease the child because of the way he or she speaks or misses some of what others say, and it is important for the child to be able to come home and share this with parents and for them to validate hurt feelings, remind the child of his or her strengths, and reassure the child he or she is loved. In our daughter's case, she came after a time to the realization that "everyone has something," and she understood that many people have something far worse to deal with than hearing loss. Throughout the times when she felt sorry for herself, we just listened carefully, asked her genuine questions about her feelings, reassured her, loved her, and did not tell her how to feel, all the while monitoring unobtrusively what she was saying and doing.

Celebrate the Child!

The best approach parents can take is to concentrate on doing things as a family, even when the family is defined as one parent and one child. Involving the child with hearing loss in all kinds of experiences and activities enriches the child's life in social, cognitive, linguistic, and physical ways. Dinnertime can be a pleasurable time to talk and enjoy each other; so can grocery shopping and doing chores. Playing games, pretending and acting out stories, building things, and having fun together with puzzles and riddles builds capability, encourages imagination and learning, and creates bonds between the parent and child. As the child grows, activities will change, and the relationships will deepen. Parents who spend time with their children will be happy they did so.

Conclusion

The emphasis on communication that we gave to our daughter with hearing loss by necessity became the focus for everyone in the family, including us as parents. Developing openness to one kind of difficulty has fostered affirmation of other differences that exist between and among people. As a result, we, our children, and our children's spouses are close and communicative. We consider ourselves fortunate, indeed.

References

Public Broadcasting System. *PBS parents*. Retrieved from http://www.pbs
   .org/parents/child-development/
Wood, C. (2007). *Yardsticks: Children in the classroom ages 4–14*. Turners
   Falls, MA: Northeast Foundation for Children.

Chapter 19

Chapter 19

WHERE ARE THEY NOW? LISTENING AND SPOKEN LANGUAGE OUTCOMES

You have brains in your head.
You have feet in your shoes.
You can steer yourself
Any direction you choose.

Dr. Seuss, 1960, p. 2

Introduction

As you come to the end of this book, I'm guessing you're wondering what happens to the children with whom an oral or Auditory-Verbal/Listening and Spoken Language approach is used. In anticipating that, I sent inquiries to several of the young adults I have come to know, asking them to write about 500 words in response to a series of questions and to identify others to whom I might send the same questions. What follows is not the result of a study, and the respondents have not been selected at random. They are just interesting accounts of people with hearing loss making their way in the world. Not all children with hearing loss with whom this approach is used become as adept with spoken and written language as these respondents are. There is no approach available in all of education that can guarantee equal outcomes for all children, but I think that *just knowing* of the success of some using a particular approach is, indeed, inspiring.

The Questions

You have gone further educationally and professionally than most people with hearing loss. How have you done this?

1. Please describe:
   a. Your hearing loss
      i. (Prelingual? Later?)
      ii. technology used (HI, CI, FM systems, etc.)
   b. Your speech and language therapy/schooling
   c. Your school history (special programs, mainstreamed schooling, etc.)
   d. Your college, graduate school, professional school education
      i. Major, minor, concentrations
      ii. Activities (Resident Advisor? Newspaper editor? Athletic team?)
2. What do you do professionally as an adult?
3. What do you remember about learning to read and write?
4. How does your hearing status figure into your adult life?
   a. Does it ever help you? Hinder you?
   b. How do you talk about it to people with whom you live and work?
5. What else would you like to say?

The Respondents

Ari Sagiv

I was diagnosed with a medium hearing loss when I was 3 years old. It eventually progressed to a severe-to-profound hearing loss when I was 7. I started wearing hearing aids in both ears when I was 3, until just recently, when I got a cochlear implant on my right ear.

I started getting speech therapy at the age of 5, and I continued it until I graduated high school. One of my speech therapists for 13 years, Adele Markwitz, was one of the most prominent and influential figures in my life. I feel that I would not have been the person I am now if it was not for her, and I feel blessed for it.

Not long after I was diagnosed with my hearing loss, I went to a specialized preschool called The Little Room, which was a school for children with learning disabilities. My parents felt it was necessary to develop my language skills at The Little Room, which held me back an extra year academically. However, my parents say my language skills developed very quickly, as well as my reading and writing ability.

After graduating from The Little Room, I was mainstreamed at a Hebrew school, the Rabbi Harry Halpern Day School, from kindergarten to eighth grade. I relied mostly on my hearing aids and an FM system to follow along in class. Starting in eighth grade, I made use of CART (Computer Assisted Real-time Translation), which helped me immensely to get involved with class activities. I then went to the Leon M. Goldstein High School for the sciences, where I was involved with the bowling team and was the captain of the tennis team in my senior year.

I went to Drexel University for my bachelor's degree in Materials Science and Engineering, and Stony Brook University for my master's degree for the same major. I did my thesis on thermal spray engineering, a specialty I decided would be the focus of my career. Thermal spray technology is a key role player in the aeronautics and energy market.

I am currently working at Stony Brook University as a full-time employee, learning with some of the best minds in thermal spray technology to become a quality control specialist for thermally sprayed coatings. I hope this opportunity will lead me to a position in a well-known company in thermal spray technology.

My hearing loss has had a major impact on my social life. Because I still rely very heavily on lip-reading, I find it difficult to engage in group conversations or be involved at places with a lot of background noise. As I continue to adjust to my cochlear implant, I hope to rely less on lip-reading and start using my actual hearing.

I am very outgoing about my hearing loss. I take a lot of pride in what I've accomplished despite it, and I always make sure it's one of the first things people know about me when they meet me. I show that I have something to prove, and I believe that it is my strength and courage. I hope that this is an attitude that future children with a hearing loss can carry with them as they grow up.

David J. Rancourt Jr.

I have gone further educationally and professionally than most people with hearing loss because I seize opportunities when I see them and take advantage of them when they become available. People always ask me how I get all the cool jobs and projects and I tell them it's because people and my customers trust me enough to grab the bulls by the horns and get the job done right and for what it's supposed to be, no matter how difficult the challenges I face daily to achieve a successful end result.

I was born with severe profound deafness in both ears and was diagnosed at 6 months old. I received my first pair of hearing aids at the age of 1. I received my right side cochlear implant on May 26, 2005 and my left side cochlear implant on August 10, 2006. I am now on the latest processor Harmony which I received this past summer of 2012.

My speech and language therapy started at Millridge Center (MCHI) and went from preschool all the way to twelfth grade. I started school at Millridge Center (MCHI) and progressed through the entire Mayfield Schools organization graduating in 2006. I participated in 99% mainstreamed schooling with support from teachers within the special programs in classes such as captioning and notating services. I participated in the Alexander Graham Bell organization, which advocates for the rights and technology for deaf and hard of hearing individuals, and I am still an active member.

I attended Rochester Institute of Technology for university studies and majored in Networking and Systems Administration. I also completed two minors, one in Telecommunications Engineering and the other in Forensics.

At RIT, I was involved in Men's Hockey team, from 2007 to 2010, and industry groups such as IEEE Society in which I was part of a group to develop a new networking standards protocol to solve issues in video streaming technology in the format of h.264 which now helps the world view HD content in live streaming broadcasts. I am now an IT Systems Engineer specializing in servers, storage, and unified communications platforms.

Learning to read and write was a struggle in my early years because of the lack of phonetically understanding how words sounded against how you read them. My parents and teachers always had to correct me on how to phonetically read and say words. Nowadays I am often correcting a lot of people who are hearing because of my extensive vocabulary skills. When I got to high school and college, my writing skills took off because of an extremely tough writing teacher that I had for three years of high school who always knew I could do better work than what I had submitted. In college my writing skills increased in the form of very technical writing to ensure that technical documents are well written, thought out, and understandable by those who are not in a particular field that may need to understand technical interpretations for solutions to real world problems that many businesses face every day.

I don't consider my hearing status a problem in my life. I have always seen it as an advantage over many people. Because of my status, there are things that I can do better than my hearing counterparts can do. I do find myself at a disadvantage in some situations, because my lack of hearing can hinder my performance on the job because I do have a tendency to avoid using the telephone as a habit left over from my days of wearing hearing aids. I have enforced a policy at work where I communicate in person or via text formats that everyone can understand which has even helped my co-workers because they can backtrack and find something if they ever forget something in a conversation. I talk about it with people when I have difficulties understanding them or remind them to remove anything blocking their face so I can read their lips. I don't ask people to slow down too often. I do have to do that sometimes, but it doesn't bother me too much.

If you see an opportunity, no matter how challenging it is, it's always better to take on the challenge because you can always find ways to improve yourself, your skills, and have the satisfaction of success when completed successfully. In my job, having Google-fu skills is a tremendous asset because there is a wealth of information on the internet that can help you achieve successful results with a little bit of help and inspiration.

Evan Brunell

My hearing loss was discovered when I was a year old. I was outfitted with hearing aids and attended a local preschool before joining Clarke School for the Deaf (now Clarke Schools for Hearing and Speech) from kindergarten through grade six. At that point, I was mainstreamed into my public school system. I continued to utilize my hearing aids and also had an oral transliterator through high school. Although I did test out an FM, it did not benefit me, so I did not use it. I did so well in school, with advanced language and English skills for my age—never mind as a deaf child—that I was placed in a special program for children with advanced skills to further my education.

Through junior high school, I received speech therapy at the school to improve my speech, and this was discontinued in high school. At 16 years of age, I received a cochlear implant in my right ear. The internal piece failed, so I was re-implanted nine months later and underwent regular listening therapy to adapt to the implant. I successfully completed high school, playing on the junior varsity and varsity baseball program while also being involved with the school newspaper and literary magazine.

In my senior year of high school, I created a Red Sox blog titled Fire Brand of the American League (firebrandal.com), which quickly moved to being the most influential Red Sox blog on the Internet. I then spun this into the first online sports media network titled Most Valuable Network, which maintained operations for six years throughout college. While in college, I pursued a degree in journalism at Northeastern University in addition to a business administration minor. Most of my free time in college was spent helming MVN and writing at Fire Brand, although I did participate in intramural sports.

I graduated cum laude in 2009 and then began baseball journalism jobs for NBC Sports, NESN and CBS Sports before becoming Director of Marketing in the family business, a residential heating-oil provider in central Massachusetts. Three years after graduating, I returned to Northeastern for a master's degree in Public Administration.

In 2011, I began participating in volunteer work by taking over the Alexander Graham Bell Association chapter in Massachusetts, providing events and mentorship for children and teenagers with hearing loss. In early 2012, I was elected to the board of directors for the national A. G. Bell Association for the Deaf and Hard of Hearing by the membership base. I also volunteer for Clarke Schools, participating as a teen mentor as part of the *Making Connections!* program during their annual Mainstream Conference, and I have volunteered at other Clarke-related events.

In a way, I owe my journalism degree and career to Clarke School. When my parents decided to enroll me at Clarke School, the issue came up as to whether I would join the dorm or commute two hours round-trip every day to Clarke. The latter option was chosen, so I took the bus every day an hour west to Northampton, Massachusetts, and back. There were generally one or two other students on the ride as well. This was before the days of cell phones, portable DVD players or other modes of electronic stimulation, so I spent the vast majority of my time reading books and quickly grew into an avid bookworm. Due to my extensive reading, I developed strong reading, spelling, grammar and writing skills, which have sustained me well in my life.

Given my involvement in nonprofit organizations for the deaf, my hearing status is fairly significant in my adult life. I am proud of what I have been able to accomplish thus far. Hearing loss can be overcome, and although some hurdles may be harder to clear or some creative solutions need to be found to address issues, hearing loss does not end a life before it begins, nor should it be an excuse for not striving to reach your dreams.

Socially, my hearing loss is a struggle. Groups, dark areas and loud background noise are all struggles I deal with on a daily basis. I do best with a smaller group of people, as even going out to dinner with three other people is challenging enough to follow.

When I meet someone unfamiliar with deafness, I tend to just keep things simple and identify as hard of hearing, although I am really deaf. I wear two cochlear implants and speak well, so to the uninitiated, the concept of "hard of hearing" is easier to grasp than "deaf," as I have been subject to stereotypical, insensitive, or assumed responses from these people on how to best communicate or perform. "Hard of hearing" gives the impression of a hearing person who struggles to hear, but can still communicate fine. This way, I am able to establish a basic base of communication with the uninformed person, and then I can educate them on who I really am and how I differ from others.

Rachel Arfa

I was diagnosed at 18 months of age with a hearing loss. My hearing loss was a progressive, fluctuating hearing loss, so my hearing levels varied from severe to profound until I was three years old. After age three, my hearing levels continued to be profound until I eventually lost all my hearing. I was immediately fit with a body aid. I wore the body aid until I was five years old, and then upgraded to behind the ear hearing aids. I wore those until I was about 11 years old, when I realized I no longer had enough hearing for my hearing aids to function or be beneficial. I realized I could no longer hear when a fire drill caused everyone in my sixth grade class to exit unpredictably, a sound I previously was able to detect. I received my first cochlear implant when I was 15 years old, and re-entered a world of sound. The benefits were tremendous as I could hear myself again and hear environmental sounds and speech. It was the start of a journey of learning to listen all over again. I embarked on that journey again when I became a bilateral cochlear implant user at 31 years old. Being bilateral was life changing, as I could hear more than I had ever been able to, even eavesdropping on conversations at home without having to lipread.

I give credit to my parents, who sought out the spoken language option, eliminating other communication modes that they did not see as a fit for them or for us. Then they invested countless hours and dedication to teaching me to listen and to talk, and also to make sure that I had language. As I could not always rely on my hearing when I wore hearing aids due to my hearing fluctuations, I learned to communicate by relying on lipreading, and if my hearing was functional, by hearing speech and environmental sounds. My mom and dad took me to speech and language therapy four days a week to make sure I was on par with my peers, or in many cases, above my peers. I went to speech and auditory verbal therapy for a total duration of 18 years and was mainstreamed during my entire education. My parents used every opportunity possible to teach and expose me to language. For example, when my dad would take me with him grocery shopping, he would point out the names of many of the food items and, probably unintentionally, instilled in me a love of different food stores. I learned how to read at age three. My speech and language therapist wanted me to learn to read earlier, and I believe it helped me to be a better lipreader and acquire language faster. By third grade, I was reading at a high school grade level, challenging myself to read as many books as I could. The same therapist advised my parents to encourage me to speak and not to interrupt me when I was talking. To my brother's dismay, he did not get to finish a sentence until I left for college.

I started out at a Montessori school and then transferred to a private, progressive school in second grade where I remained until 8th grade. I then transferred to a large public high school for all of high school. I attended the University of Michigan where I earned a B.A. in American Culture. In college, I was involved in numerous student activities and student leadership, where I really blossomed after receiving hassle-free accommodations for the first time in my educational experience. Next, I attended law school at the University of Wisconsin School of Law and earned a J.D. I am now an attorney at Equip for Equality where I practice disability rights law, representing people with disabilities in employment discrimination and civil rights cases.

My parents set high expectations for me and I'm glad to say I've met their goals, and maybe even surpassed their wildest expectations. They also allowed me to make decisions for myself. When I was four and a half, my parents wanted to upgrade me from the body aid to the behind-the-ear hearing aids. I told them I wasn't ready until I turned five years old. My parents listened to me and allowed me to wait until I was five years old to upgrade, even though the behind-the-ear hearing aids were likely better technology and certainly much easier to wear. It was so important that they listened to what I wanted and gave me the choice to make my own decisions, a lesson that has helped me as an independent adult.

My hearing loss has shaped my life and who I am. Without a hearing loss, my life would have been simply ordinary. I have met many interesting people and made many friends due to my hearing loss, including others like myself who identify as speaking deaf. Growing up, I attended conventions held by the Alexander Graham Bell Association for the Deaf and Hard of Hearing. At AG Bell conventions, I experienced a level playing field where my world was accessible for those five days, and my friends with hearing loss were in the majority rather than the minority. Being among my friends, I thrived and built my confidence to continue to advocate for myself when I returned home. My AG Bell world showed me the potential of making the world accessible.

My daily experience living with a hearing loss nurtured a strong drive and passion to succeed and to create a career devoted to advocating for others. In my work as an attorney, I use my passion to help others and to remedy injustice.

Jeffrey Zuckerman

To me, it seems strange to think of deafness as a disability. It's more a communication disorder than anything. Certainly that's how my parents thought of it, and framing it in that way helped a great deal in making my life the best it could be. I was born deaf—the only one in my family—and my parents opted for me to speak rather than sign, so that I could communicate with as many people as possible. Similarly, they made the decision for me to get a cochlear implant at seven years old, just when most of my deaf classmates were also being implanted. And for the same reasons, they pushed for me to be mainstreamed in third grade from an oral school for the deaf to public school.

In the time since then, I've graduated from high school in the same public school system and majored in English at Yale University. I had always been passionate about books and writing— I ran my high school's literary magazine, and started up a literary publication in college—so after college I went into book publishing. Because I'd learned French and German, I found myself working with titles in translation. Being deaf is, professionally, both a liability and a nonissue: being unable to easily conduct a phone conversation makes it very hard for me to get hired, but once in the office, accommodating that single issue renders the issue of deafness nearly moot.

The path from getting my cochlear implant to working as an editor and a writer was not an easy one. I learned to speak inorganically, with flashcards and repeated practice of phonemes. To this day, I still often mispronounce my s's. But I learned to read and write at the same time I learned to speak, and so both modes are equally easy for me. When I got my implant, however, I had to actually learn how to hear. The first year was a horrible and frightening new world—an experience that, I imagine, explains somewhat why babies cry so much. But the difference my implant made was immeasurable. I was able to hear things I had never known made a sound and to talk to people whom I never could have understood by lipreading alone.

Because of my parents' perspective and their decisions, I find myself more comfortable around hearing people than around other deaf people. I've always been incredibly candid on a personal level about my deafness. It's as natural to me as having brown eyes or being right-handed, and so I'm accustomed to broaching the topic myself. I surprised myself by taking a class the very last semester of college on disability and culture. I had expected it to be easy; instead it raised questions I had hardly ever considered. "There is no disability," my professor declared, "only discrimination." I was shocked by the overt politics of her statement—and yet I could not disagree. And even as I faced the same discrimination I'd always experienced, I also chose to work with the written word—an arena in which my deafness means nothing, and in which my background and my talent means everything.

Reference

Dr. Seuss. (1960). *Oh, the places you'll go!* New York, NY: Random House Children's Books.

Chapter 20

THOUGHTS FROM TWO FOUNDERS OF THE AUDITORY-VERBAL APPROACH

What does seem to be clear is that the human brain is specially equipped to process spoken language.

Ling, 1978, p. 36

Introduction

This final chapter is comprised of two pieces about the auditory-verbal approach written by Daniel Ling and Helen Hulick Beebe. These were provided by Judith Marlowe, PhD, FAAA, who received them from Dr. Ling and Ms. Beebe in 1990 and 1989, respectively. She planned to include them in a work on auditory-verbal practice that she was editing, but that book did not come to fruition. The piece by Beebe, as she was known to many, is thought to be the last she wrote; with Beebe's permission, Dr. Marlowe edited and expanded it during Beebe's final illness, and Beebe approved the version as it is printed here. It was printed in *The Auricle*, a publication of Auditory Verbal International, an organization which merged several years ago with the Alexander Graham Bell Association for the Deaf and Hard of Hearing. I am grateful to Dr. Marlowe for providing these pieces, to Jane Ling for permission to include Daniel Ling's foreword, and to the Alexander Graham Bell Association for the Deaf and Hard of Hearing for permission to include Helen Beebe's chapter here.

Written many years ago, these pieces demonstrate the extraordinary vision of both Ling and Beebe. I hope as you read them you feel you have come full circle as you think back to other parts of this book and that you will appreciate the profound chain of connections between and among hearing and listening, listening and speaking, speaking and reading, and reading and writing, all of which support thinking and feeling. Literacy is a cognitive activity begun most easily by providing sounds and patterns for the brain to use in authentic language communication, thereby making spoken language meaningful in relation to its written forms. As you have read in these pages, this is a compelling argument for bringing listening and spoken language to children with hearing loss.

Foreword, 1990, by Daniel Ling, PhD

Hearing impairment can range from a transient mild deficit to a permanent and total loss of audition. When present from birth or early childhood it may jeopardize many aspects of development. The primary effect of severe, profound, or total hearing loss is to limit spoken language acquisition. As a consequence, it may also restrict opportunities for personal-social growth, educational achievement and, at a later stage, openings and satisfaction relating to employment.

Views on appropriate forms of treatment vary widely. At one end of the spectrum there are advocates for the exclusive use of American Sign Language (ASL). The attempt to circumvent the consequences of severe or profound hearing impairment through the simultaneous use of speech and sign language, however, is more widespread. Known as Total Communication (TC), the method was widely introduced over 20 years ago. Like ASL, it basically prepares hearing-impaired children for life as members of a deaf community. In contrast, those who advocate auditory-verbal communication attempt to meet the problem of hearing impairment head on, by minimizing its effects to the greatest possible extent. They do this through the use of carefully selected hearing aids and/or other technological devices such as cochlear implants, the adoption of teaching strategies that optimize the reception and production of spoken language, and through close collaboration with caregivers. As knowledge relating to speech, language, and hearing has emerged and as technology has improved, so too has the effectiveness of auditory-verbal training. Modern devices and strategies can reach even totally deaf children. Over the past few decades, many children treated in auditory-verbal programs from early infancy by competent teachers and clinicians have gone on to acquire excellent spoken language skills, to achieve high levels of education, and to compete and conform as fully independent and happy members of society. There is now a large and growing network of professionals who advocate auditory-verbal therapy, but the approach, though adopted in numerous countries throughout the world, is followed by too few, probably because it requires higher levels of professional awareness and competence than are generally available. In this volume, well-known and highly respected advocates of auditory-verbal therapy set out to make readers aware of the principles underlying this form of work, and in "how to" passages suggest ways of dealing with many of the problems associated with hearing impairment more competently. The authors were selected by Dr. Marlowe as diverse practitioners (not theorists) who were willing to describe how their particular type of involvement contributes to this form of habilitative treatment. Readers may be assured that the programs they have run are of the highest quality. In their diversity, they share high expectations of children who are hearing impaired and not one of them believes that there are inevitable limits to what such children can achieve.

Daniel Ling
Dean, Faculty of Applied Health Sciences
The University of Western Ontario
London, Canada

An Auditory-Verbal Retrospective: A Personal Account of Individual Effort and International Organization, 1989, by Helen Hulick Beebe, CCC/SP

Just before the turn of the century, Victor Urbantschitsch presented a practical demonstration of the so-called acoustic method to the Medical Society of Vienna (Urbantschitsch, 1982). (The acoustic method, acoupedic, and unisensory have in common the principle or philosophy now referred to as auditory-verbal.) The idea for the approach did not originate with Urbantschitsch. It had been known for centuries but he applied it systematically at the Cobling Institute for the Deaf in Vienna. Max Goldstein studied with Urbantschitsch and tried to introduce the method into institutes for the deaf in America. He published his book, *The Acoustic Method*, in 1939. Many other scientists and educators throughout the world studied and experimented with application of acoustic exercises. Goldstein had written in 1920 that " . . . the technique has not been applied with sufficient care, detail and persistency . . . and without sufficient regard for the fundamental principles on which the method depends for success" (Goldstein, 1939).

Interestingly, both Urbantschitsch and Goldstein, who suggested that the acoustic method be considered a separate form of pedagogy, applied the method in institutions for the deaf which in themselves carried the negative connotation that deaf children had to be separated from hearing peers in order to talk and to receive an education. In addition, the children in these institutions were beyond the age *critical* for development of speech/language skills (0 to 4 years).

Since Goldstein's writing there have been two major developments that contribute to the achievement of the Urbantschitsch goal: namely, the development of spontaneous speech and language via acoustic pathways. First, the electronic production of wearable hearing aids, and second, the growth of audiology as a science for the evaluation of hearing loss and appropriate prescription of hearing aids. As suggested by Pollack (1970), Goldstein was ahead of his time because without hearing aids, the child benefited only periodically from amplified hearing. (Hearing tubes, megaphones, etc. were used during therapy.) Since the advent of wearable hearing aids in the early 1940s, a child in a true auditory program is deaf *only when he takes off his aids.*

As to the early detection and measurement of hearing loss, the first experiments with the acoustic approach did not have to wait for the advent of audiometry. Medical men in the early centuries, specifically Ernaud in Paris (1767), claimed that total deafness did not exist. With my first case in 1944, the only encouraging signs of residual hearing were some positive responses to the Direct Tone Introduction Test of Froeschels, using the Urbantschitsch whistles (Froeschels, 1946). This case was presented in 1950 at the VIII Congress of the International Association of Logopedics and Phoniatrics (IALP) in Amsterdam. At the same Congress, Huizing, with Pollack, presented the acoupedic philosophy which stems from the Urbantschitsch teaching (Pollack, 1970).

As late as 1964, in a hospital clinic, a five-month-old baby's suspected deafness (due to maternal rubella) could not be confirmed by objective measurement. At my suggestion that there must be minimal residual hearing, the audiologist approved trial of a loaner aid under my supervision. That particular child, who has a profound hearing loss, is now a college graduate who speaks like a hearing person.

Of course, modern audiometric measurement provides a more sophisticated indication of the range of hearing deficit and, in turn, the opportunity to select appropriate amplification. Although there is ongoing research to find more efficient means of detection and measurement of hearing loss in neonates and infants, there are still too many reports of failure to recognize hearing deficits. Consequently, there is failure to give parents appropriate guidance to sources of help which can minimize the consequence of hearing impairment. Unfortunately, parents' suspicion of hearing deficit is too often not heeded by the professional to whom they turn for guidance.

My introduction to the Urbantschitsch philosophy was through my teacher, Emil Froeschels, M.D., who had studied with Urbantschitsch in Vienna. My first opportunity to apply the philosophy was in 1944 with a profoundly deaf 15-month-old girl whose mother had had rubella during pregnancy. My former experience as a teacher in oral schools for the deaf preceded the advent of wearable hearing aids. Consequently, in 1944 our goal to have this child achieve spontaneous speech through intensive auditory training, and to develop auditory oral communication adequate to matriculate in a normal school, seemed almost wishful thinking. But, it did happen and has continued to happen with most of the severe-to-profoundly deaf children we have treated in ensuing years.

During the last four decades, there has been parallel experience in many places around the world: Whetnall in England; Huizing in Holland (from whom Pollack took the term acoupedics); Wedenberg in Sweden; Ling in Canada; and more recently, Crawford, Simser, Estabrooks in Canada; Griffith and Grammatico in California; and many offspring. As therapists, all have been working to have children with hearing impairment in the mainstream of education and family life and have had these goals long before the advent of Public Law 94-142. There are now several universities where auditory-verbal practicums are included in the course of deaf education.

We can state specific requisites for our programs, some of which we have in common with other oral programs.

1. Early detection of hearing impairment.
2. Early fitting of adequate amplification binaural (with rare exceptions) *to be worn all waking hours.*
3. Full family involvement in carrying out therapy.

The above three might be shared with other programs in which a limited amount of auditory work is done. However, our goal of processing language via auditory channels emphasizes our priority of intensive auditory training, so we insist on:

4. One-to-one therapy with intensive auditory training eliminating visual cues to force *maximal* use of even minimal residual hearing.
5. Nursery school placement with hearing peers from the beginning.
6. Education placement with hearing peers.
7. *Firm* behavioral management.

In a unisensory program intensive auditory training means developing the use of amplified hearing to its maximum potential. Even *profoundly deaf children* can learn to hear. They can be brought to the point of handling conversational speech—repeating and discussing a story through hearing alone. They are not allowed to rely on lip-reading until they are *hearing oriented*. Eventually they become multisensory. These children just naturally develop the necessary lip-reading skill without special instruction.

In early training we know that the child with one sensory receiving modality (sight) intact and one impaired (hearing), will rely on the modality that is easier for him, and so we teach him to listen and to hear by preventing him from watching the speaker's mouth. If our goal is to provide maximal use of residual hearing and to develop spontaneous speech, he must be *forced* to hear enough to stimulate the motor speech center of the brain and to appreciate what hearing and discrimination can do for him. One does not just put a hearing aid on a child and expect him to hear. Pollack (1970) states that a child's hearing age dates from the time he is fitted with amplification. It sometimes takes months, or *even a year*, before there is objective evidence that the child *"knows" that he hears*. During that time we must "charge" the brain like a battery until sound perception and cognition are converted to motor speech response.

To those who say there is no one method of choice for children with hearing impairment, we would suggest that every parent be offered a choice and, as we suggested in Toronto in May 1979 (Learning to Listen—The First Option Conference sponsored by Voice, Toronto, May, 1979), that the auditory-verbal approach be considered the first option. Until the first two most critical requisites of such a program have been given a fair trial, that is intensive auditory training and full parental involvement, one cannot make a reliable prognosis. Efficient diagnostic therapy can determine whether the child should follow an alternate approach for speech/language acquisition. Children with profound losses *can* learn to hear and parents *can* learn to be effective.

In February 1978, a two-day conference hosted by the Helen Beebe Speech and Hearing Center was convened at Lafayette College in Easton, Pennsylvania. This was prompted by a suggestion of members of the staff returning from a Daniel Ling colloquium in Montreal. They felt that promotion of the auditory-verbal approach might be strengthened by combining the forces of Ling, Pollack, and Beebe, each of whom had demonstrated the viability of the approach for a number of years (Ling, 1976).

The thrust of the two-day discussion was how to provide all children with hearing impairments between the ages of 0 to 5 (including those with additional handicaps) the opportunity to develop communication through spoken language based on the optimal use of residual hearing.

To achieve our objective, we first discussed approaching universities with curricula which trained special education or communication disorders personnel. However, although this would be our ultimate goal, we decided that first we must demonstrate through workshops the viability of the approach, thus creating a demand from both parents and professionals that it be included in all programs related to educating the hearing-impaired child.

In ensuing months, as we sought support from both parents and professionals, a central (or executive) committee added members from Canada and Mexico who shared our involvement and our goals and thus we became The International Committee on Auditory-Verbal Communication (ICAVC). In 1980 we were invited to become a special committee of the Alexander Graham Bell Association. The general membership grew steadily and included members from Europe, Asia, India, and Australia.

Much as we appreciated the support of the Alexander Graham Bell Association, we decided in 1987 to incorporate as a separate entity in order to establish more clearly the difference between auditory-verbal programs and other oral approaches. At that time we changed our name to Auditory-Verbal International (AVI).

From the beginning, we have tried to state clearly the requisites of the system as well as the goals of our organization. Auditory-Verbal communication means "deaf" children learning to hear and speak naturally. This means:

- Early detection of hearing loss
- Immediate fitting of appropriate hearing aids
- Development of language and speech through listening with effective use of hearing aids
- A partnership of parent, child, and professionals working together
- Expecting the child to grow and live in the most normal learning and living environments possible.

As of this writing, we are beginning to compile a statistical report on the percentage of children following through in an auditory-verbal program to become fully integrated into a hearing society and to achieve their full potential to lead happy productive lives. Many of these children are absorbed in the mainstream and not recognized as "deaf." Consequently, they are not easily located. My own anecdotal account, however, would report that when we have had full collaboration of parents and a mentally intact child, we have achieved our goal. Degree of hearing loss has not yet been a critical factor, except in the few cases where there is no hearing to amplify. In these few cases, parents may expect to use classes that can be oral. In more recent years, the parents' role has been made easier in some cases by the availability of special resource faculty in school programs and, in some instances, infant-preschool parental guidance. I can recall a number of families who would have had better staying power had they been offered this kind of assistance, as well as some financial assistance for private therapy, when that was the only choice versus institutional care. Even in today's culture, too many hearing-impaired children are missing out on appropriate treatment because both parents have to work to support the household. As stated previously, in order to succeed, this program needs constant input from the mother or caretaker. Another must, of course, is appropriate amplification which involves sizable expense, in most cases not underwritten by any public agency. One might mention that in Canada, where auditory-verbal training and integration are very prevalent, both preschool therapy and hearing aids are subsidized by the government. In the United States, those in charge of public monies have not been persuaded that, in the long run, it would be better economics to get more children into the mainstream at an early age, thereby educating more productive citizens.

Parents usually receive the diagnosis, or at least suspected diagnosis of deafness, from their family physician, pediatrician, or otologist. Eventually, they depend on an audiologist for evaluation and guidance as to the possible educational road to follow in rearing their hearing-impaired child.

It is our contention that in addition to the need for competent audiologists, therapists, and teachers, the medical profession has a responsibility to be informed about the critical need for early diagnosis of hearing impairment. As suggested by Pappas (1985), intake histories, as reported by mother or caretaker, should receive careful attention. And as pointed out by Beebe (1982), the physician should be knowledgeable about the availability of reliable audiologic facilities to which he could refer families in need of such services.

Obviously, early detection of hearing loss is important for any program; however, it is critical for an auditory-verbal program because we are dependent on early, maximum, amplified input of speech and language as the first therapy option in a child's life. Beginning auditorily at age 8 to 9 is not reasonable. It is the auditory-verbal philosophy that hearing is the primary source of natural language development, and that this relationship of language to hearing can be maintained even with the profoundly hearing impaired. The hearing-impaired child should not be limited by the first therapy option. Initiating therapy without utilizing audition as the primary source of language acquisition is limiting a child's later opportunity to develop natural verbal language.

Auditory-verbal therapy is not the only option available in a hearing impaired child's life. This auditory approach is not indefinitely continued for years in the face of lack of auditory development. By definition it relies on constant, ongoing diagnosis and reevaluation during the course of therapy. Language development is a long-term developmental process and cannot be accomplished in a few months of auditory-verbal therapy within the profoundly hearing impaired. The therapist must be mindful of the child's development measured against time in therapy. One must be careful not to blindly continue auditory-verbal therapy because of commitment in the face of a total lack of development. Conversely, one should be careful not to sacrifice the future of normal adult communication on the altar of immediate, but limited, functional communication in an attempt to achieve feedback from the hearing impaired child.

References

Beebe, H. (1982). When parents suspect their child is deaf. *Hearing Rehabilitation Quarterly, 7*(4).

Froeschels, E. (1946). Testing the hearing of young children. *A.M.A. Archives of Otolaryngology, 43*, 93–98.

Goldstein, M. (1939). *The acoustic method.* St. Louis, MO: Laryngoscope Press.

Ling, D. (1976). *Speech and the hearing impaired child: Theory and practice.* Washington, DC: Alexander Graham Bell Association for the Deaf.

Ling, D., & Ling, A. (1978). *Aural habilitation: The foundations of verbal learning in hearing-impaired children.* Washington, DC: Alexander Graham Bell Association for the Deaf.

Pappas, D. (1985). *Diagnosis and treatment of the hearing-impaired child: A clinical manual.* San Diego, CA: College-Hill Press.

Pollack, D. (1970). *Educational audiology for the hearing-impaired child.* Springfield, IL: Charles C. Thomas.

Urbantschitsch, V. (1982). *Auditory training for deaf mutism and acquired deafness* (S. Silverman, translator). Washington, DC: Alexander Graham Bell Association for the Deaf.

Appendix A

KNOWLEDGE NEEDED BY LISTENING AND SPOKEN LANGUAGE SPECIALISTS

These domains and competencies are specified by the Alexander Graham Bell Academy International Certification Program for Listening and Spoken Language Specialists (LSLS). The LSLS examination is comprised of questions in these domains.

Domain 1. Hearing and Hearing Technology

A. Hearing Science/Audiology

1. Anatomy of the ear and neural pathways
2. Physiology of hearing
3. Physics of sound (e.g., decibel; frequency; sound waves)
4. Psychoacoustics (e.g., HL; SPL; SL)
5. Auditory perception (e.g., masking; localization; binaural hearing)

6. Speech acoustics
7. Environmental acoustics
   a. Signal-to-noise ratio
   b. Distance
   c. Noise
   d. Reverberation
8. Causes of hearing impairment
9. Types of hearing impairment and disorders (e.g., site of lesion; age of onset)
10. Early identification and high risk factors
11. Audiogram, audiogram interpretation and implications to speech perception
12. Audiologic assessments
    a. Behavioral
    b. Speech perception testing
    c. Electrophysiologic (e.g., OAE, ABR ASSR, acoustic immittance)
    d. Hearing aid evaluation (e.g., real-ear/probe microphone; electroacoustic analysis)
    e. Cochlear implant candidacy, surgery, activation, functional application of programs

B. Hearing Technology

1. Sensory devices (e.g., hearing aids; cochlear implants; vibro-tactile aids; transposition aids)
2. Assistive listening devices (e.g., personal FM/auditory trainers; sound-field FM and infrared (IR) systems)
3. Earmold acoustics (e.g., impact of the earmold characteristics on the transmission of sound)
4. Hearing technology troubleshooting strategies

Domain 2. Auditory Functioning

1. Auditory skill development
2. Infant auditory development (e.g., neural development; plasticity)
3. Functional listening skill assessments and evaluations, both formal and informal

4. Acoustic phonetics as related to speech perception and production
5. Functional use of audition

Domain 3. Spoken Language Communication

A. Speech

1. Anatomy of speech/voice mechanism
2. Physiology of speech/voice mechanism
3. Suprasegmental, segmental, coarticulation aspects of speech production
4. Sequences of typical speech development (e.g., preverbal; articulation; phonology; intelligibility)
5. Sequence of speech development in clients with various sensory devices (e.g., hearing aids; cochlear implants; vibrotactile aids; transposition aids)
6. Speech production assessment measures (both formal and informal)
7. Teaching techniques in speech production
   a. Prerequisite skills for phoneme production
   b. Developmental (habilitative) and remedial (rehabilitative) speech development
   c. Suprasegmental and segmental aspects of speech facilitation
   d. Auditory strategies for speech facilitation
   e. Visual and tactile strategies for speech facilitation
   f. Integration of speech targets into spoken language
8. Speech characteristics of children without auditory access to the full speech spectrum
9. International Phonetic Alphabet (IPA)
10. Impact of auditory access on speech production

B. Language

1. Impact of auditory access on language development
2. Aspects of language (e.g., phonology; pragmatics; morphology; syntax; semantics)

3. Sequence of typical language development (e.g., prelinguistic; communicative intent; linguistic)
4. Language assessment measures (both formal and informal)
5. Teaching techniques in receptive and expressive language
6. Impact of speech acoustics on choice of language targets (e.g., inside/beside; he/she)
7. Development of complex conversational competence
8. Development of divergent/convergent thinking
9. Figurative language and higher level semantic usage

Domain 4. Child Development

1. Sequence of typical child development
   a. Cognitive
   b. Gross and fine motor
   c. Self-help
   d. Play
2. Influence of associated factors on child development (e.g., cultural; community; family)
3. Conditions that are present in addition to hearing impairment (e.g., sensory integration deficits; visual challenges; Autism Spectrum Disorders; neurologic disorders; learning disabilities)

Domain 5. Parent Guidance, Education, and Support

1. Family systems (e.g., boundaries; roles; extended family; siblings)
2. Impact of hearing impairment on family (e.g., coping mechanisms, family functioning; stages of grief)
3. Family counseling techniques (e.g., active listening; reflective listening; questioning; open-ended statements)
4. Family coaching and guidance techniques (e.g., demonstration; modeling; turning over the task; providing feedback; co-teaching)
5. Impact of associated factors on parent guidance (e.g., cultural; language in the home; economic; lifestyle; community)
6. Behavior management techniques
7. Adult learning styles

Domain 6. Strategies for Listening and Spoken Language Development

1. Learning to listen strategies (e.g., creating optimal listening environment; positioning to maximize auditory input)
2. Pausing (wait time) appropriately
3. Language facilitation techniques (e.g., expansion and modeling)
4. Prompting techniques (e.g., linguistic; phonological; acoustic; physical; printed written prompts)
5. Responsive teaching (e.g., listening to the client and modifying according to the client's language and speech production)
6. Creating a need for the child to talk
7. Acoustic highlighting techniques
8. Auditory presentation prior to visual presentation (e.g., say before seeing)
9. Spoken language modeling
10. Meaningful, interactive conversation
11. Experience-based, naturalistic language activities
12. Experience and personalized books

Domain 7. History, Philosophy, and Professional Issues

A. History and Philosophy

1. History of education of individuals who are deaf or hard of hearing
2. Historical perspective of communication approaches
3. Current communication approaches and principles for individuals who are deaf or hard of hearing

B. Professional Issues

1. Ethical requirements and issues
2. Professional development requirements and opportunities
3. Evidence-based practice and research findings

Domain 8. Education

(The focus of this domain is on the development and expansion of the auditory and language skills that underlie and support the child's progress in the general education curriculum.)

1. Continuum of educational and community (e.g., child care; respite care) placements
2. Curricular objectives that meet local standards in areas of instruction
3. Strategies for preteaching and reteaching (postteaching) the academic curriculum
4. Strategies for preteaching and reteaching (postteaching) language needed for academics
5. Strategies to integrate auditory speech language goals with curriculum
6. Cognitive and academic assessments
7. Process for developing individualized educational plans
8. Collaborative strategies with school professionals

Domain 9. Emergent Literacy

(The focus of this domain is on the development of the auditory and language skills that underlie and support the acquisition and advancement of literacy.)

1. The learning sequence and pedagogy related to teaching the following skills in accordance with the child's level of language development:
   a. Reciting finger plays and nursery rhymes
   b. Telling and/or retelling stories
   c. Activity and story sequencing
   d. Singing songs and engaging in musical activities
   e. Creating experience stories/experience books
   f. Organization of books (e.g., cover; back; title; author page)
   g. Directionality and orientation of print

h. Distinguishing letters, words, sentences, spaces, and punctuation

i. Phonics (e.g., sound-symbol correspondences and letter-sound Correspondences)

j. Phonemic awareness (e.g., sound matching; isolating; substituting; adding; blending; segmenting; deleting)

k. Sight word recognition

l. Strategies for the development of listening, speaking, vocabulary, reading and writing

m. Contextual clues to decode meaning

n. Oral reading fluency development

o. Text comprehension strategies (e.g., direct explanation; modeling; guided practice; and application)

p. Abstract and figurative language (e.g., similes; metaphors)

q. Divergent question comprehension (e.g., inferential questions; predictions)

Source: Alexander Graham Bell Association for the Deaf and Hard of Hearing, the Academy for Listening and Spoken Language. Retrieved from http://www.agbellacademy.org/CoreCompetencies.pdf

Appendix B

LISTENING AND SPOKEN LANGUAGE SPECIALIST (LSLS) DOMAINS ADDRESSED IN THIS BOOK

Domain	Chapter	Competencies
1	3	A. 7 a, b, c; 12 b B. 1, 2
2	3	2, 3, 5
3	3 4 12	A. 4 B. 1 B. 1, 2, 3, 4, 7, 9 B. 4
4	3 6 17	1a 1, 2 3
5	3 4 7 10 13	1 5 6 3 5
6	3 4 7 8 9	1, 10, 11 3, 4, 6, 9, 10, 11 1, 2, 3, 4, 5, 6, 8, 9, 10, 11, 12 3, 6, 10, 11, 12 3, 4, 5, 6, 7, 9, 10, 11
7	1 5 10 15 Appendix A	A. 1, 2 B. 3 A. 3 B. 1 2, 3 B. 2
8	10 12 16 14	7, 8 6 3, 4 1
9	2 4 5 7 8 9 10 13 14 16 17	1. h, i, j, k, l 1. i, j 1. j, l 1. l 1. b, c, e, f, h, i, j, k, l, m, n, o, p, q 1. p 1. b, c, e, f, g, h, i, j, k, l, m, n, o, p, q 1. j 1. a, d, i, j, l 1. m, o, p, q 1. d

Appendix C

DESCRIPTION, APPROACHES, AND PRACTICE OF LISTENING AND SPOKEN LANGUAGE SPECIALISTS

Listening and Spoken Language Specialists

Listening and Spoken Language Specialists (LSLS) help children who are deaf or hard of hearing develop spoken language and literacy primarily through listening.

LSLS professionals focus on education, guidance, advocacy, family support, and the rigorous application of techniques, strategies, and procedures that promote optimal acquisition of spoken language through listening by newborns, infants, toddlers, and children who are deaf or hard of hearing.

LSLS professionals guide parents in helping their children develop intelligible spoken language through listening and coach them in advocating their children's inclusion in the mainstream school. Ultimately, parents gain confidence that their children will have access to the full range of educational, social and vocational choices in life.

Listening and Spoken Language Approaches

The two main Listening and Spoken Language approaches, historically, have been the Auditory-Verbal Approach (AV) and the Auditory-Oral Approach (A-O). Today, as a result of advances in newborn hearing screening, hearing technologies, early intervention programs, and the knowledge and skills of professionals, these two approaches have more similarities than differences and they lead to similar outcomes.

The A. G. Bell Academy for Listening and Spoken Language certifies Listening and Spoken Language Specialists (LSLS).

Currently, the designations of the LSLS certification program are:

> LSLS Cert. AVT (Certified Auditory-Verbal Therapist) and LSLS Cert. AVEd (Certified Auditory-Verbal Educator).

The LSLS must provide services in adherence to the A. G. Bell Academy Code of Ethics and the Principles of Auditory-Verbal Therapy or the Principles of Auditory-Verbal Education (available in the LSLS Candidate Handbooks and online at http://www.agbellacademy.org).

Listening and Spoken Language Practice

Listening and Spoken Language Specialists have similar knowledge and skills and work on behalf of the child and family.

The LSLS Cert. AVT works one-on-one with the child and family in all intervention sessions.

The LSLS Cert. AVEd involves the family and also works directly with the child in individual or group/classroom settings.

The LSLS Cert. AVT and the LSLS Cert. AVEd both follow developmental models of audition, speech, language, cognition, and communication.

The LSLS Cert. AVT and the LSLS Cert. AVEd both use evidence-based practices.

The LSLS Cert. AVT and the LSLS Cert. AVEd both strive for excellent outcomes in listening, spoken language, literacy, and independence for children who are deaf or hard of hearing.

Source: Permission to reprint granted by the Alexander Graham Bell Association for the Deaf and Hard of Hearing, the Academy for Listening and Spoken Language. Retrieved from http://www.agbellacademy.org/about-academy.htm

INDEX

Note: Page numbers in **bold** reference non-text material.

A

A. G. Bell Academy International Certification Program for LSLS
designations of, 92–98, 360–361
auditory-verbal education (LSLS Cert. AVEd), 92, 96–98, 360–361
auditory-verbal therapy (LSLS Cert. AVT), 92, 93–96, 360–361
principles on which work is based, 93–98
domains and competencies specified by, 349–355
addressed in book, 358
Domain 1. hearing and hearing technology
A. hearing science/audiology, 349–350
B. hearing technology, 350
Domain 2. auditory functioning, 350–351
Domain 3. spoken language communication
A. speech, 351
B. language, 351–352
Domain 4. child development, 352
Domain 5. parent guidance, education, and support, 352
Domain 6. strategies for listening and spoken language development, 353
Domain 7. history, philosophy, and professional issues
A. history and philosophy, 353
B. professional issues, 353
Domain 8. education, 354
Domain 9. emergent literacy, 354–355
A. G. Bell Association for the Deaf and Hard of Hearing
Academy Code of Ethics, 360
Auditory Verbal International merged with, 338
description of, 328–329, 331, 334, 338, 344
Listening and Spoken Language Knowledge Center, 92–93
Academic achievement, 75–79
description of, 215
Dickinson and Tabors study of, 75–77
Hart and Risely study of, 77–79

Acoupedics, 342

Acoustic method, 340–341

Acoustic Method, The (Goldstein), 340

Active listening, 239–240

Activities, for teaching writing, 183–185, **184**

Adams, M., 26

Adult-directed speech (ADS), 105

Advanced signal processing, 52

Allen, T. E., 9–10

Allington, Richard, 289–293

Alphabetic principle, 255

American Academy of Audiology

    Clinical Practice Guidelines for Remote Microphone Hearing Assistance Technologies for Children and Youth Birth–21 Years, 57–58

    HAT guidelines, 57–58

    Pediatric Amplification Guideline, 50, 51

    Pediatric Amplification Protocol, 51

    website, 51

American Annals of the Deaf, 6

American Sign Language (ASL), 71–73, 171, 338–339

Amplification technology

    auditory feedback loop, 59

    CADS, 56–57

    cochlear implants, 58–59

    computer analogy for understanding, 48–49

    HAT, 57–58

    hearing aids/instruments and, 50–55

    incidental learning through overhearing, 59–60

    literacy development and, 49–50

    overview of, 49–58

    personal-worn FM technology and, 55–56

Analogies, 225

Analysis level, in Bloom's taxonomy, 226

Anticipation guide, 298–299

Application level, in Bloom's taxonomy, 226

Application questions, 164

Arfa, Rachel, 332–334

Aronow, M., 8, 12

Assessments

    in cochlear implant children, 277

    criterion-referenced tests, 278–279

    norm-referenced standardized tests, 276–279

    reading. *See* Reading assessments

Attention, 165–166

Attention deficit disorder (ADD), 309

Attention deficit hyperactivity disorder (ADHD), 309

Attuned caregiving, 106, 112

Audiometric measurements, 341

Auditory/cognitive closure, 45

Auditory-verbal approach, 91–93, 173–178, 337–346

Auditory-verbal communication, 344

Auditory-verbal educator (LSLS Cert. AVEd), 92, 96–98, 360–361

Auditory-verbal practice, 96, 337

Auditory-verbal therapist (LSLS Cert. AVT), 92, 93–96, 360–361

Automated auditory brainstem response test (AABR), 108

B

Background knowledge, 138, 201–205
Background noise, 49, 53, 328, 331–332
Barton, Christine, 268–270
Basal reading program, 28
Beebe, Helen, 91, 140, 340–346
Beginning to Read (Adams), 26
Behaviorist psychology, 36
Behind the ear (BTE) hearing aids, 54
Bidirectional communication and IDS, 105
Bilingualism. *See also* Multiple languages; Second language
  in cochlear implant children, 252–254
  deafness and, 250–251
  educating for, 249–250
  factors that affect development of, 252
  fears regarding, 250
  in hearing-loss children, 251–254
  learning to read in first language, 254–256
  non-native English-speaking parents effect on, 253–254
Birth to age five (typical development), 113–116
  cognitive development and play, 113–114
  motor development, 114–115
  self-help skills, 115–116
Bloom's taxonomy, 226–227
Bluetooth (BT) technologies, 53–54
Body language, 240
Body-worn gateway device, 54

Book language, 176
Bootable, 54
Bottom-up processing, 27–29, 34
Breitkopf, Dara Ellen, 206
Brill, Richard, 7
Brunell, Evan, 330–332

C

Caregiver sensitivity, 104–105
Caregiving relationships, 104–105
Carolina Picture Vocabulary Test, 277
Celebrations, 323
Cephalocaudal development, 114, 115
Child development, 101–119
  caregiving relationships, 104–105
  developmental context, 116–117
  early identification of hearing loss, 106–112
  expectable events, 102–104
  experience-dependent development, 102–103, 104
  experience-expectant development, 102–104
  hearing impairment co-occurring with other conditions, 117–118
  nature-nurture question, 101–102
  optimal period, 102
  study of, 101–104
  typical development (birth to age five), 113–116
  useful links on, 118–119
Classroom audio distribution systems (CADS), 48, 56–57
Clay, Marie, 26–27

Clinical Practice Guidelines for Remote Microphone Hearing Assistance Technologies for Children and Youth Birth–21 Years (American Academy of Audiology), 57–58

Cochlear implants
  bilingualism in children with, 252–254
  case studies of, 227–228
  developmental outcomes and, 109–110, 111
  music listening affected by, 262–263
  music training in children with, 267–268
Cognitive development and play, 113–114
Cognitive psychology, 38–39
Communication
  with early elementary school children, 244–245
  with high school children, 245–246
  learning language for purposes of, 246
  with middle school children, 245–246
  with preschool children, 244–245
  team-based, 244–246
Competing noise, 53
Completely in the canal (CIC) hearing aids, 54
Comprehension
  in Bloom's taxonomy, 226
  growth of, 225–227
  guidelines for building, 138
  learning and, 226
  listening, 138
  of music, 267
  reading, 29–34, 137–138

Comprehension monitoring, 33
Comprehensive Assessment Program, 76
Compression component, 52
Compromising, 239
Computer assisted real time captioning (CART), 229–230, 237
Concept map, 301
Conflict resolution, 238–239
Congenital hearing impairments, 4, 107–108, 263
Conrad, R., 9
Contrast chart, 298, 301
Crawford, Louise, 91
Creativity, 196
Criterion-referenced tests, 278–279
Critical theory and pedagogy, 39–40
Croak, Tammy, 206–212
Crossmodal reorganization, 47
Cultural context, 117
Cumulative practice, 47

D

Deaf Children in America, 9
"Deaf," new context for word, 60
Deaf or hard of hearing (D/HH), 106
Dedicated wireless digital signal processing devices, 54
Detection, of music, 267
Developmental context, 116–117
  cultural context, 117
  family context as child 's immediate environment, 116
  social and economic context, 116–117
Developmental psychology, 111–112. *See also* Child development

Developmental stages of
     childhood, 317–318
Dialogic reading, 132–133
Dickinson, Emily, 28, 29, 30, 39
Differentiation, 114–115
Digital hearing aids, 52–54
     advanced signal processing and,
          52
     bootable and, 54
     compression component and,
          52
     dedicated wireless digital signal
          processing devices and,
          54
     frequency compression and, 53
     frequency response and, 52
     multichannel capability and, 52
     multimemory capability and,
          52–53
     multimicrophone capability and,
          53
     noise reduction capability and,
          53
     wireless connectivity and, 53–54
Digit-symbol testing, 3–4, 5
Discrimination, of music, 267
Distance hearing, reduction in,
     59–60
Down syndrome, 118
Drawing, 179, 191–192

E

Ear level hearing aids, 54
Early elementary school children,
     communication with,
          244–245
Early Hearing Detection and
     Intervention Programs
     (EHDI), 108, 112
Early identification of hearing loss,
     106–112
     before 2.5 years, 106–107

attunement and, 106
developmental outcomes and,
     109–110
intervention and, 106–107,
     108–109
recommendations, 111–112
screening for, 107–108
theory of mind and, 110–111
in U.S., 107–108
Early intervention, 215
Earshot, 50, 59–60
Economic context, 116–117
Educational settings. *See also*
     School(s)
     accommodations, 306
     mainstream classrooms,
          310–312
     optimal placement, 306–309
Elliott, A., 6–7
Emotion questions, 164
Emotional communication, 105
Emotional connectedness, 235–236
Environment
     least restrictive, 238
     for literacy, 136–137
Evaluation level, in Bloom's
     taxonomy, 227
Evaluation plan, 297
Expectable events, 102, 103, 104
Experience-dependent
     development, 102–103,
          104
Experience-expectant
     development, 102–104
Expressive One-Word Picture
     Vocabulary Test, 133

F

Family context as child's
     immediate environment,
          116
Fetuses, hearing of, 45, 46

FM technology, 229
"Fourth-grade slump," 216–218
Freire, Paulo, 39–40
Frequency compression, 53
Frequency response, 52
Friendships, 320
Frigate, 28–31, 39
Froeschels, Emil, 341
Functional speech perception
        measures, 55

G

Gates-MacGinitie Reading Test,
        173
Goldstein, Max, 340
Goodman, Kenneth, 35, 37
Greenough, William, 102

H

Harry Potter, 290
Hearing, in utero, 156
Hearing aids/instruments, 50–55
    digital. *See* digital hearing aids
    fitting issues in, 51
    functional speech perception
        measures and, 55
    multilingualism in child with,
        256–258
    new context for, 50–51
    styles of, 54–55
Hearing assistance technologies
        (HAT) guidelines
        (American Academy of
        Audiology), 57–58
Hearing impairment co-occurring
        with other conditions,
        117–118
Hearing loss
    academically successful young
        adults with, 227–231
    case studies of, 325–335

in children
    diagnosis of, 341
    early detection of, 346
    spoken word vocabulary in,
        220
    writing in, 198–201
Henkes, Kevin, 296
High expectations, 316–317
High school children,
        communication with,
        245–246
Higher academic achievement and
        spoken language, 12–18
Higher order comprehension, 217
High-frequency words, 219
Holt, J., 10
Home-School Study of
        Language and Literacy
        Development, 75–77

I

Identification, of music, 267
Illinois Test of Psycholinguistic
        Abilities, 133
Immediate talk, 70
Implicit questions, 164
In the canal (ITC) hearing aids, 54
In the ear (ITE) hearing aids, 54
Individualized Education Program
        (IEP), 237–238, 245
Individuals Educational Evaluation
        (IEE), 237
Individuals with Disabilities
        Education Improvement
        Act (IDEA), 237–238
Infants
    infant directed speech (IDS),
        105, 109–110, 112
    literacy development in, 45–46
Informal reading inventory (IRI),
        284–285
Intellectual disability, 117–118

Interactive theory of reading, 34–35
Interactive writing, 172
International Reading Association (IRA), 73
Intervention
  developmental outcomes and, 109–110
  early identification of hearing loss and, 106–107, 108–109
  screening, 108
  theory of mind and, 110–111
Invented spelling, 180, 182, 194

J

Joint roles for maturation and experience, 114, 115

K

Keys and Pedersen Visual Language Test, 7
Knowledge
  background, 138, 201–205
  in Bloom's taxonomy, 226
  phonological, 218
K-W-L chart, 298–300

L

Language(s)
  development of, in monolingual versus bilingual children, 250
  learning of, in children, 250, 258–259
  listening to, for reading assessment, 281–282
  multiple. See Bilingualism; Multiple languages
  spoken. See Spoken language
Language building, 224–225
Language experience approach
  to observation, 282–283
  to reading, 140–150
Language experience books
  adult's involvement in, 192
  background information and, 200–201
  background knowledge, 201–205
  content for, 193
  creating and using, 193–195, 213
  description of, 180, 182–183, 189–190
  developmental-based approach to use of, 191–192
  in early language development children, 194
  experiences of teachers who have been using, 205–212
  goals of, 195
  grammar and, 194–195
  language development stimulated by, 194
  language immersion, 194
  listening, 190
  mother's experience with, 212–214
  parental participation in, 140, 195
  reading learned by using, 140–150
  sample pages from, 142–150
  spelling and, 194–195
  spiral progression through, 190–192
  summary of, 214
  teacher and therapist comments about, 196–197
  tenses and, 195
Language impairments, 117

Learned helplessness, 306
Learning
asking questions as critical to, 240
comprehension and, 226
music. *See* Music learning
from shared book reading, 134
spoken language, 73–75
advantaged vs. disadvantaged parents and, 79–81
later academic achievement and, studies of, 75–79
social interaction and, 73–74
sounds of, 68–71
writing. *See* Writing, learning to write
Learning disabilities, 117–118
Learning to Listen, 91
Least restrictive environment, 238
Lesson plan, 294–297
Lexical restructuring, 218
Lexical restructuring theory, 69
Ling, Daniel, 91, 337–339
Ling 6 Sound Test, 55, 161, 296
Linguistic diversity, 251
Linguistic spillover, 135
Linguistics and psycholinguistics, 36–38
Listening
active, 239–240
care and respect during, 319
case studies of, 325–335
in hearing-loss children, 132
infants and, literacy development in, 45–46
to language, for reading assessment, 281–282
language experience books, 190
lesson plan provisions for ensuring, 296
neurological basis of, 44–48
outcomes of, 325–335
by parents, 319
in shared book reading, 132, 134
technology and. *See* amplification technology
Listening and Spoken Language Specialists (LSLS), 92–93, 359–360.
See also A. G. Bell Academy International Certification Program for LSLS
Listening comprehension, 138
Listening vocabulary, 219
Literacy
environment for, 136–137
goals, steps for meeting, 298–302
lesson plan used to promote, 294–297
practices for developing, 287–293
thoughtful, 293
Literacy development
amplification technology and, 49–50
author's study of, 173–176
differences in, 199
in infants, 45–46
Literal questions, 163–164
Literary criticism, 39
Logic, 156
Loop Systems, 58
Low expectations, 316–317
LSLS Cert. AVEd (auditory-verbal educator), 92, 96–98, 308, 360–361
LSLS Cert. AVT (auditory-verbal therapist), 92, 93–96, 308, 360–361

M

Mainstream classrooms, 310–312
Mediation
agreement reached in, 243–244

alternatives for problem solving, 243
case example of, 240–241
closure of, 244
description of, 238
information sharing during, 241
issue and interest identification phase of, 242–243
problem-solving negotiations, 239–241
setting for, 242
steps involved in, 241–244
Medical conditions, co-occurring, 118
Metaphors, 225
Middle school children, communication with, 245–246
Miscue analysis, 283–284
Moskowitz, S., 8, 12
Motor development, 114–115
Multichannel capability, 52
Multilingualism, 256–258
Multimemory capability, 52–53
Multimicrophone capability, 53
Multiple languages. *See also* Bilingualism
spoken
case example of, 257–258
in hearing-loss children, 251–254, 258–259
non-native English-speaking parents effect on learning of, 253–254
second language affected by achievement in first language, 255
written, learning to read in native language, 254–256
Music
cochlear implant effects on listening to, 262–263
functions of, 264

Orff method for teaching of, 266–267
Suzuki teaching approach for, 265, 270–272
Music learning
benefits of, 264
in cochlear implant children, 267–268
in hearing-loss children, 264, 266–268
issues involved in, 262–264
reading development and, 266
spoken language learning and, 265–266
studies of, 263–264
summary of, 272–273
in typical hearing children, 265–266
Musical audiogram, 267–268
Musicality, 262

N

National Assessment of Adult Literacy (NAAL), 2
National Assessment of Educational Progress (NAEP), 279
National Association for the Education of Young Children (NAEYC), 73
National Council of Teachers of English, 23
National Institute for Literacy, 2
National Reading Panel (NRP), 288
Native language
fluency in, 255
learning to read in, 254–256, 258
Nature-nurture question, 101–102
"Neighborhoods," 219
Neuroplasticity, 47
Noise reduction capability, 53

Nonimmediate talk, 70
Non-native English-speaking
parents, 253–254
Norm-referenced standardized
tests, 276–279
Norms, formulating, 8

O

Observation
language experience approach
to, 282–283
reading assessment through,
280–283
Optimal period, 102
Orff method, 266–267
Otitis media infections, 103, 118
Otoacoustic emissions test (OAE),
108
Overhearing, incidental learning
through, 59–60

P

Paraphrasing, 240
Parent(s)
advantaged vs. disadvantaged,
learning spoken
language and, 79–81
language experience book
participation by, 140, 195
listening by, 319
non-native English-speaking,
253–254
scaffolding use by, 131
vocabulary growth and, 131,
221
Parenting
celebrating the child, 323
developmental stages of
childhood, 317–318
focusing on child as an
individual, 316

friendships nurtured by, 320
listening to child with care and
respect, 319
overview of, 315
practical skills taught to child,
318–319
public speaking encouraged by,
320–321
refusal to accept low
expectations, 316–317
schoolwork and, 321–322
sense of responsibility
developed in child, 318
sibling relationships nurtured
by, 320
speaking for oneself
encouraged by, 320–321
speaking respectfully about the
child's teachers, 322
technology and, 319–320
"why me?" questions by child,
322
Paterson, D., 3–5, 7
Pattern guide, 301
Peabody Picture Vocabulary Test
(PPVT), 13, 70, 76, 131,
253
Pediatric Amplification Guideline
(American Academy of
Audiology), 50, 51
Pediatric Amplification Protocol
(American Academy of
Audiology), 51
Percentile ranks, on norm-
referenced standardized
tests, 276–277
Personal-worn FM technology,
55–56, 57, 58
Petro, Britt, 205–206
Phonemic awareness
pitch discrimination and, 265
vocabulary knowledge and,
220

Phonological awareness
  auditory-verbal therapy and, 92
  definition of, 44, 87
  description of, 103, 218–219, 266
  NRP designation of being
      important to beginning
      reading, 288
  pitch discrimination and,
      265–266
  reading acquisition and, 129
  vocabulary knowledge and, 220
Phonological information, 219
Phonological knowledge, 218
Phonological processing
      capabilities, 88–90
Pintner, R., 3–5, 7
Play, cognitive development and,
      113–114
Pollack, Doreen, 91
Poverty and learning spoken
      language
  advantaged vs. disadvantaged
      parents and, 79–81
  later academic achievement and,
      studies of, 75–79
Practical skills, 318–319
Predictability, during reading, 141
Pregnancy, reading aloud during,
      156
Prereaching, 115
Preschoolers, communication
      with, 244–245
Pretend activities, for teaching
      writing, 185
Principles of Auditory-Verbal
      Education, 360
Principles of Auditory-Verbal
      Therapy, 360
Print, teaching children about,
      158–160
Print knowledge, 159
Problem-solving negotiations,
      239–241

Proximodistal development, 114,
      115
Public speaking, 320–321

Q

Quotation share, 298, 301

R

Rancourt, David J. Jr., 328–330
Read-Aloud Handbook, The
      (Trelease), 167
Reading
  activities after, 294
  comprehension during, 29–34,
      137–138
  definitions of, 25–27
  dialogic, 132–133
  fluency in, 292–293
  interactive feedback used to
      develop, 286
  interactive theory of, 34–35
  language experience approach
      to, 140–150
  music perception and, 265–266
  National Reading Panel findings
      regarding areas of, 288
  in native language, in bilingual
      children, 254–256, 258
  postreading activities, 294, 297
  practical ideas for teaching,
      139–150
  practice with, 290
  predictability during, 141
  prereading phase of, 294
  reader's involvement in, 294
  reading aloud used to teach,
      139–140, 158–160, **159**
  rewards associated with, 190
  shared book. *See* Shared book
      reading
  spoken language affected by, 177

Reading *(continued)*
  study of, 35–40
    behaviorist psychology, 36
    cognitive psychology, 38–39
    critical theory and pedagogy,
      39–40
    linguistics and
      psycholinguistics, 36–38
    literary criticism, 39
    socialinguistics, 38
  theorizing about, 24–25
  thinking aspects of, 302–303
  word identification and, 27–29
  writing and, correlation
    between, 171
Reading achievement, 137
Reading aloud
  application questions after, 164
  benefits of, 139–140
  emotion questions after, 164
  examples of, 166–168
  follow-up questions after,
    163–165
  guidelines for, **165**
  implicit questions after, 164
  literal questions after, 163–164
  observing during, for reading
    assessment, 283
  parent–child bond development
    through, 166
  reading taught through,
    158–160, **159**
  reasons for, 157
  rhyme and rhythm learned
    through, 157
  technique for, with hearing-loss
    child, 139–140, 161–166
  with uncooperative child,
    165–166
  when to begin, 139, 156–157
Reading assessments
  description of, 279–280

  informal discussions with child
    about book, 285
  listening to child's language,
    281–282
  miscue analysis, 283–284
  observation, 280–283
  reading aloud observations for,
    283
  running records, 283–284
Reading instruction
  access to books, 291–292
  benefits of, 289
  classroom conditions for, 292
  practical ideas for, 139–150
  reading fluency, 292–293
  reading practice, 290
  suggestions for, 289–293
  thoughtful literacy, 293
  time management for, 291
Reading Recovery, 26, 280–281
"Reading Streak," 166–168
Receptive vocabulary, 18, 76
Reciprocal teaching, 224
Responsibility, sense of, 318
Retelling, 136
Rhyme and rhythm, in reading
  aloud, 157
Robbins, Amy McConkey, 268
Rosenblatt, Louise, 39
Rowling, J.K., 290
Running records, 283–284

S

Sagiv, Ari, 327–328
Scaffolding, 183, 204
Schema theory, 30, 39
Schemata, 30–34
School(s)
  educational sources other than,
    309–310
  mainstream classrooms, 310–312

optimal placement in, 306–309
Schoolbook language, 176
School-Home Early Language
     and Literacy Battery-
     Kindergarten (SHELL-K),
     76
Schoolwork, 321–322
Screening for early identification
     of hearing loss, 107–108
Scribbling, 179
Second language. *See also*
     Bilingualism; Multiple
     languages
  case example of, 257–258
  first language achievement
     effects on learning of,
     255
  in hearing-loss children,
     251–254, 258–259
  non-native English-speaking
     parents effect on
     learning of, 253–254
Segmental phonology, 69–70
Segmental restructuring, 219
Self-help skills, 115–116
Self-regulated comprehension, 33
Self-regulation, 104
Semantic map, 298, 301
Semantic mapping, 222–223
Semantic webbing, 222–223
Sense of responsibility, 318
Sensitivity, caregiver, 104–105
Sensorineural hearing loss (SNHL),
     108
Sentence construction, 7–8
Shared book reading
  learning from, 134
  listening during, 132, 134
  negotiating meaning during,
     135–136
  sharing constructions, 135–136
  story retelling, 129–134

Sibling relationships, 320
Sign language
  ASL, 71–73, 171, 338–339
  bilingual-bicultural approach to
     teaching of, 251
  as first language, in bilingual
     children, 254
  syntax and, 72
  window of opportunity and,
     72–73
Signal-to-noise ratio (S/N ratio),
     49–50, 56, 57, 59
Similes, 225
Smith, Frank, 26, 35, 37–38
Smoothing, 239
Social context, 116–117
Socialinguistics, 38
Sound-field technology. *See*
     Classroom Audio
     Distribution Systems
     (CADS)
Speaking for oneself, 320–321
Speech impairments, 117
Speech intelligibility, 49–50
Speech production, 69–70
Spelling, invented, 180, 182
Spoken language(s)
  ASL and, 71–73
  case studies of, 325–335
  connecting learning of, to
     learning to read, 7
  development of, 67–68. *See*
     also Learning, spoken
     language
  higher academic achievement
     and, 12–18
  at home, 136
  learning of
     description of, 158
     goals for, 151
     music learning and, 265–266
     poverty effects on, 75–81

Spoken language(s) *(continued)*
  multiple
    in hearing-loss children,
      251–254, 258–259
    non-native English-speaking
      parents effect on
      learning of, 253–254
  outcomes of, 325–335
  reading effects on, 177
Stanford Achievement Test, 7, 8–9,
  277
Story retelling, 129–134
Student learning
  scaffolding of, 204
  teacher's understanding of, 205
Studies
  of child development, 101–104
  of later academic achievement
    and, 75–79
  of reading. *See* Reading, study
    of
  review of selected, 3–12
Summarizing, 226
Sustained Silent Reading (SSR),
  291
Suzuki approach, for music
  teaching, 265, 270–272
Symbol-digit testing, 3–4, 5
Syndromes, co-occurring, 118
Synthesis level, in Bloom's
  taxonomy, 227

T

Teacher(s)
  speaking respectfully about, by
    parent, 322
  student learning and, 205
Teacher-to-student attunement,
  236
Team/team approach
  communication methods,
    244–246

description of, 235–236
Technology, parent's
  understanding of,
  319–320
Tenses, 195
Test of Early Reading Ability:
    Deaf or Hard of Hearing
    (TERA-D/HH), 277
Testing, fourth-grade slump
    caused by, 216, 218
Theorizing about reading, 24–25
Theory of mind (TOM), 110–111
Thoughtful literacy, 293
Top-down processing, 29–30, 34
Total Communication, 339
Traxler, C., 10
TuneUps, 268–270, 272

U

Uncooperative child, reading
    aloud to, 165–166
Understanding Reading (Smith),
    26
Unisensory program, 342
United States, early identification
    of hearing loss in,
    107–108
Universal Newborn Hearing
    Screening (UNHS), 107,
    108–109
University of Western Ontario
    Pediatric Audiological
    Monitoring Protocol 2011
    (UWO PedAMP), 51
Urbantschitsch, Victor, 340–341

V

Vocabulary
  learning of, 221
  listening, 219
  receptive, 18, 76

shared book reading study of, 129–132
Vocabulary growth
    associations used in, 151
    child's involvement in, 224
    description of, 220–225
    language building for, 224–225
    parents' role in, 221
    phonemic awareness for, 220
    segmental restructuring for, 219
    teacher's role in, 221
Vocabulary knowledge, 220
Vocabulary lists, 224
Vocabulary measure, 111

W

WAIS-III Digit Symbol-Coding, 4
Walking, complex behavior of, 115
Walter, Jean, 7–8
Werker, Janet, 45–46
Whetnal, E., 87
"Why me?" questions, 322
Win-lose negotiation, 239
Wireless connectivity, 53–54
Withdrawing, 239
Words
    high-frequency, 219
    identification of, 27–29, 288
    memorization of, 224
    memory storage of, 219
    neighborhoods of, 219
Wrightstone, J., 8, 12
Writing
    active participation in, 178
    areas of development, 180
    auditory-verbal approach, 173–178, 337–346

awkwardness of expression in, 176
in children with and without hearing loss, 198–201
development of, 176–178, 180, 182
drawing and, 179
first attempts at, by child, 179–180, **181**
focus on meaning during, 182
interactive, 172
learning to write
    authentic activities for, 183–185, **184**
    child's first attempts at writing, 179–180, **181**
    Language Experience Book, 180, 182–183
    practical ideas for, 179–185
    pretend activities for, 185
    summary of, 185–186
    teaching methods, 172
purposes of, 183
reading and, correlation between, 171
rewards associated with, 190
scribbling and, 179
studies of, 171–173
thinking aspects of, 302–303
Written communication, 183–185, **184**

Z

Zone of proximal development, 133, 192, 195
Zuckerman, Jeffrey, 334–335